Study Guide

Pharmacology

A Patient-Centered Nursing Process Approach

10th Edition

Study Guide prepared by
Mary B. Winton, PhD, RN, ACANP-BC
Assistant Professor
School of Nursing
Tarleton State University
Stephenville, Texas

Textbook prepared by
Linda E. McCuistion, PhD, MSN
NCLEX Live Review Presenter
Mandeville, Louisiana

Kathleen Vuljoin DiMaggio, RN, MSN
Professor Emerita
The University of Holy Cross
New Orleans, Louisiana

Mary B. Winton, PhD, RN, ACANP-BC
Assistant Professor
School of Nursing
Tarleton State University
Stephenville, Texas

Jennifer J. Yeager, PhD, RN, AGNP
Assistant Professor
Tarleton State University
Stephenville, Texas

ELSEVIER

Elsevier
3251 Riverport Lane
St. Louis, Missouri 63043

Notices

Knowledge and best practice in this field are constantly changing. As new research and experience broaden our
understanding, changes in research methods, professional practices, or medical treatment may become necessary.

Practitioners and researchers must always rely on their own experience and knowledge in evaluating
and using any information, methods, compounds, or experiments described herein. In using such information or methods they should be mindful of their own safety and the safety of others, including parties for
whom they have a professional responsibility.

With respect to any drug or pharmaceutical products identified, readers are advised to check the most
current information provided (i) on procedures featured or (ii) by the manufacturer of each product to be
administered, to verify the recommended dose or formula, the method and duration of administration, and
contraindications. It is the responsibility of practitioners, relying on their own experience and knowledge of
their patients, to make diagnoses, to determine dosages and the best treatment for each individual patient,
and to take all appropriate safety precautions.

To the fullest extent of the law, neither the Publisher nor the authors, contributors, or editors assume
any liability for any injury and/or damage to persons or property as a matter of products liability, negligence
or otherwise, or from any use or operation of any methods, products, instructions, or ideas contained in
the material herein.

Previous editions copyrighted 2018, 2015, 2012, 2009, 2006, 2003, 2000, 1997, 1993

Senior Content Development Specialist: Heather Bays
Content Strategist: Yvonne Alexopoulos
Publishing Services Manager: Deepthi Unni
Project Manager: Bharat Narang

Printed in the United States of America

Last digit is the print number: 9 8 7 6 5 4 3 2 1

Working together
to grow libraries in
developing countries

www.elsevier.com • www.bookaid.org

Reviewers

Travis Sonnet, PharmD
Adjunct Clinical Professor
WSU College of Pharmacy;
Inpatient Pharmacy Supervisor
Mann-Grandstaff VA Medical Center
Spokane, Washington

Kathleen Vuljoin DiMaggio, RN, MSN
Professor Emerita
The University of Holy Cross
New Orleans, Louisiana

Preface

This comprehensive *Study Guide* is designed to provide the learner with clinically based situation practice problems and questions. This book accompanies the text *Pharmacology: A Patient-Centered Nursing Process Approach*, Tenth Edition, and may also be used independently of the text.

Opportunities abound for the enhancement of critical thinking and decision-making abilities. Hundreds of study questions and answers are presented on nursing responsibilities in therapeutic pharmacology. Each chapter follows a format that includes NCLEX-style study questions (including multiple choice, matching, labeling, prioritizing, select all that apply, and completion exercises), and case studies.

This new edition provides more than 160 drug calculation problems and questions, many relating to actual patient care situations and enhanced with updated, real drug labels. The learner is also expected to recognize safe dosage parameters for the situation. The combination of the instructional material in the text and the multiplicity of a variety of practice problems in this *Study Guide* precludes the need for an additional drug dosage calculation book.

The tenth edition includes an updated step-by-step approach to using dimensional analysis on selected drug calculation problems, including critical care drugs. Multiple practice opportunities are provided in the areas of measurement, reading of drug labels, and calculation of oral and injectable dosages (including body surface area for pediatric and critical care drugs), and flow rates of intravenous fluids.

The nursing process is used throughout the patient situation–based questions and case studies. Chapters have questions that relate to assessment data, including laboratory data and side effects, planning and implementing care, patient/family teaching, cultural and nutritional considerations, and effectiveness of the drug therapy regimen.

Because of the ever-expanding number of drugs available, pharmacology can be an overwhelming subject. To help learners grasp essential content without becoming overwhelmed, chapters have been divided into multiple smaller sections. The result is a layout that is user-friendly.

Answers to all questions are presented in the Answer Key to make studying easier. The tenth edition provides rationales for every question, including the case studies.

The *Study Guide* is part of a comprehensive pharmacology package, including the textbook and Instructor and Student Resources available on the companion Evolve website. This package and each of its components were designed to promote critical thinking and learning. We are excited about this edition of the *Study Guide* because it offers the learner a variety of modalities for mastering the content.

Contents

1 The Nursing Process and Patient-Centered Care

STUDY QUESTIONS

Answer the following questions as true or false. If false, make the statement into a true statement.

1. A concept that influences patient care focuses on a disease-centered model of health care.

2. Concepts are related to patient's problems, the medications, or topic of care listed within the medical diagnosis.

3. The Nursing Alliance for Quality Care (NAQC) that supports quality patient-centered health care is partnered with the American Medical Association.

4. The Nursing Alliance for Quality Care (NAQC) believes that it is everyone's role to cultivate successful patient and family engagement.

5. The purpose of the nursing process is to diagnose and provide care.

Arrange the following actions of the nursing process in correct order.

6. a. Implementation
   b. Planning
   c. Evaluation
   d. Assessment
   e. Patient problem

Match the phrases in Column I to the step of the nursing process in Column II. The nursing process in Column II will be used more than once.

Column I

_____ 7. Decreased adherence

_____ 8. Current health history

_____ 9. Goal/outcome setting

_____ 10. Patient's environment

_____ 11. Action to accomplish goals

_____ 12. Drug allergies and reactions

_____ 13. Referral

_____ 14. Patient/significant other teaching

_____ 15. Use of teaching drug cards

_____ 16. Laboratory test results

_____ 17. Effectiveness of health teaching and drug therapy

Column II

a. Assessment
b. Patient problem
c. Planning
d. Implementation/intervention
e. Evaluation

Match the clinical manifestations in Column I with the data type in Column II. The data type in Column II will be used more than once.

Column I

_____ 18. Productive cough

_____ 19. Pain in left ear

_____ 20. Lab values

_____ 21. Nausea

_____ 22. Heart rate

_____ 23. Patient perception of drug's effectiveness

_____ 24. Reported allergies

Column II

a. Subjective

b. Objective

REVIEW QUESTIONS

Select the best response.

25. *Possible injury* would be included in which phase of the nursing process for a patient who is taking a sedative-hypnotic?
   a. Assessment
   b. Implementation
   c. Planning
   d. Patient problem

26. The patient has congestive heart failure and has been prescribed a diuretic. *Obtain patient's weight to be used for future comparison* is included in which phase of the nursing process?
   a. Assessment
   b. Evaluation
   c. Planning
   d. Patient problem

27. *The patient will receive adequate nutritional support through enteral feedings* is included in which phase of the nursing process?
   a. Assessment
   b. Implementation
   c. Planning
   d. Patient problem

28. *The patient will maintain a diastolic blood pressure between 60 to 80* is included in which phase of the nursing process?
   a. Assessment
   b. Evaluation
   c. Planning
   d. Patient problem

29. The patient has been diagnosed with angina and hypertension and has been started on a drug. *Instruct patient to avoid caffeine-containing beverages* is included in which phase of the nursing process?
   a. Evaluation
   b. Implementation
   c. Patient problem
   d. Planning

30. Revision of goals is included in which phase of the nursing process?
   a. Assessment
   b. Evaluation
   c. Implementation
   d. Planning

31. The patient has been prescribed a diuretic to treat hypertension. *Disturbed sleep* is included in which phase of the nursing process?
   a. Assessment
   b. Evaluation
   c. Implementation
   d. Patient problem

32. The pediatric patient has been started on antibiotics for strep throat. *Advise the child's parents to report adverse reactions such as nausea and vomiting to the health care provider* is included in which phase of the nursing process?
   a. Assessment
   b. Implementation
   c. Planning
   d. Potential Patient problem

33. The patient has been prescribed an opioid pain drug after hip surgery. *Psychological disturbance* is included in which phase of the nursing process?
    a. Implementation
    b. Evaluation
    c. Patient problem
    d. Planning

34. *Instruct patient not to discontinue drugs abruptly* is included in which part of the nursing process for a patient with epilepsy who is taking phenytoin?
    a. Assessment
    b. Evaluation
    c. Implementation
    d. Planning

CASE STUDY

Read the scenario and answer the following questions on a separate sheet of paper.

O.Y., 53 years old, has been diagnosed with diabetes and has been prescribed insulin. In speaking to the nurse, O.Y. says, "I don't think I can give myself shots. I can't stick myself with a needle."

1. Utilizing the nursing process, how will the nurse develop a teaching plan for O.Y.?

2. How will the nurse determine the effectiveness of the teaching plan?

2 Drug Development and Ethical Considerations

Match the description in Column I with the act or amendment in Column II.

Column I

a. Determines which drugs can be sold with or without a prescription
b. Attempts to control the abuse of depressants, stimulants, and hallucinogens
c. Tightened controls on drug safety and testing
d. Mandated physicians and pharmacists in keeping records of prescribed narcotics
e. Promotes the development of drugs used to treat rare illnesses
f. Tried to remedy the escalating problem of drug abuse
g. Empowered the FDA to monitor and regulate the manufacturing and marketing of drugs

Column II

_____ 1. Kefauver-Harris Amendment

_____ 2. Federal Food, Drug, and Cosmetic Act

_____ 3. The Orphan Drug Act

_____ 4. Durham-Humphrey Amendment

_____ 5. Harrison Narcotic Act

_____ 6. Drug Abuse Control Amendments

_____ 7. Comprehensive Drug Abuse Prevention and Control Act

Complete the following.

8. The _____ name, also known as the proprietary name, is usually a registered trademark.

9. Schedule _____ drugs are not approved for medical use.

10. The Health Insurance Portability and Accountability Act (HIPAA) allows patients more control over their

_____ _____.

11. The Food and Drug Administration Safety and Innovation Act (FDASIA) strengthens the _____ to

safeguard and advance public _____ by expediting development of _____,

_____, and _____ products.

12. Practicing nurses should be knowledgeable about the _____ _____ _____
to safely administer drugs.

Answer the following questions as true or false. If false, make the statement into a true statement.

_____ 13. Substance examples of Schedule II drugs include peyote, heroin, and *Cannabis*.

_____ 14. Examples of Schedule IV substances include the category of benzodiazepines.

_____ 15. All drugs become less effective over time.

_____ 16. A nurse advances the health care profession through research and scholarly inquiry.

_____ 17. A nurse will not be prosecuted for omitting a drug dose.

Select the best response.

18. Which ethical principle is being observed when a nurse explains to a research participant the risk versus the benefits of participating in the research?
    a. Justice
    b. Beneficence
    c. Autonomy
    d. Respect for persons

19. Before administering controlled drugs to a client, a nurse would perform which action?
    a. verify orders before drug administration
    b. not document all wasted drugs
    c. keep controlled drugs accessible for patient's convenience
    d. have a witness for wastage of only Scheduled III drugs

20. Which resource provides the basis for standards in drug strength and composition throughout the world?
    a. *United States Pharmacopeia/National Formulary*
    b. *American Hospital Formulary Service (AHFS) Drug Information*
    c. *MedlinePlus*
    d. *International Pharmacopeia*

21. Which primary purpose of federal legislation is related to drug standards?
    a. Provide consistency
    b. Establish cost controls
    c. Ensure safety
    d. Promote competition

22. The Kefauver-Harris Amendment was passed to improve safety by requiring which information to be included in the drug's literature?
    a. Recommended dose
    b. Pregnancy category
    c. Side effects and contraindications
    d. Adverse reactions and contraindications

23. The client presents to the emergency department with hallucinations. The client's friend states the client has been using lysergic acid diethylamide (LSD) and mescaline. To which schedule do these drugs belong?
    a. Schedule IV
    b. Schedule III
    c. Schedule II
    d. Schedule I

24. In which schedule would the nurse find codeine, an ingredient found in many cough syrup formulations?
    a. II
    b. III
    c. IV
    d. V

25. Where must controlled substances be stored in an institution/agency?
    a. In a double-wrapped and labeled container
    b. In the patient's drug bin
    c. Near the nurse's station
    d. In a locked, secured area

26. A client with advanced pancreatic cancer agrees to participate in a clinical research for a new chemotherapy regimen and asks the nurse which group will be assigned. The nurse answers, knowing that:
    a. he will receive information about the study through the mail.
    b. the nurse has the role in explaining the study to the patient.
    c. the patient must be alert and comprehend the information being provided.
    d. information should be vague because the patient does not need to know the study protocol.

27. The nurse must be alert for counterfeit prescription drugs. Which clues help identify counterfeit products? (*Select all that apply*).
    a. Different color
    b. Different dose
    c. Different taste
    d. Different labeling
    e. Different shape

CASE STUDY

Read the scenario and answer the following questions on a separate sheet of paper.

L.L. has received a prescription for a drug to treat hypertension and is preparing for discharge from the emergency department. L.L. says to the nurse, "I don't understand all of this paperwork that I have to sign. I sign this same form every time. What is HIPAA, and why should I even care?"

1. How will the nurse explain HIPAA to the patient as it pertains to the drugs prescribed?

2. What should the nurse tell the client about the boundaries on the use and release of the health records?

3 Pharmacokinetics and Pharmacodynamics

Complete the following.

1. The pharmacokinetic phase is composed of _____, _____, _____, and _____.

2. The $t_{1/2}$ or the _____ is when 50% of the drug concentration is eliminated.

3. _____ is the effect of drug action on cells.

4. Drug absorption is the movement of the drug into the _____ after _____.

5. Drugs that are _____ block responses.

6. Cell membranes contain _____ that enhance drug actions.

Match the terms in Column I with their descriptions in Column II.

Column I	Column II
_____ 7. Dissolution	a. Drug absorbed by diffusion
_____ 8. Hepatic first pass	b. Causes inactive drug action/response
_____ 9. Nonselective receptors	c. Drugs that affect various receptors
_____ 10. Passive absorption	d. Free active drug causing a pharmacologic response
_____ 11. Protein-bound drug	e. Proceeds directly from intestine to the liver
_____ 12. Unbound drug	f. Breakdown of a drug into smaller particles
_____ 13. Facilitated diffusion	g. Drug requiring a carrier for absorption

Match the terms in Column I with their descriptions in Column II.

Column I	Column II
_____ 14. Duration of action	a. Length of time a drug has a pharmacologic effect
_____ 15. Onset	b. The margin of safety of a drug
_____ 16. Peak action	c. Occurs when a drug has reached its highest plasma concentration
_____ 17. Therapeutic index	d. Time it takes a drug to reach minimum effective concentration

Select the best response.

18. Which drug form is most rapidly absorbed from the gastrointestinal (GI) tract?
   a. Capsule
   b. Sublingual
   c. Liquid
   d. Tablet

19. Disintegration of enteric-coated tablets occurs in the:
   a. colon.
   b. liver.
   c. small intestine.
   d. stomach.

20. Usually food _____ dissolution and absorption of drug.
    a. increases
    b. decreases
    c. has no effect on
    d. prevents

21. Which statement places the four processes of pharmacokinetics in the correct sequence?
    a. Absorption, metabolism, distribution, excretion
    b. Distribution, absorption, metabolism, excretion
    c. Distribution, metabolism, absorption, excretion
    d. Absorption, distribution, metabolism, excretion

22. Which type of drug passes rapidly through the gastrointestinal (GI) membrane?
    a. Lipid-soluble and ionized
    b. Lipid-soluble and nonionized
    c. Water-soluble and ionized
    d. Water-soluble and nonionized

23. Which factor(s) most commonly affect(s) a drug's absorption? (Select all that apply.)
    a. Body mass index
    b. Hypotension
    c. Pain
    d. Sleep
    e. Stress

24. Two days after starting diazepam for anxiety, the client is started on ampicillin with sulbactam for an infection. Which action will happen to the diazepam in the client's body?
    a. The diazepam remains highly protein bound.
    b. The diazepam is deactivated.
    c. Most of the diazepam is released, and it becomes more active.
    d. The diazepam is excreted in the urine unchanged.

25. Which body organ is the major site of drug metabolism?
    a. Kidney
    b. Liver
    c. Lung
    d. Skin

26. Which route of drug absorption has the greatest bioavailability?
    a. Intramuscular
    b. Intravenous
    c. Oral
    d. Subcutaneous

27. Which is the best description of a drug's serum half-life?
    a. The time required for half of a drug dose to be absorbed
    b. The time required after absorption for half of the drug to be eliminated
    c. The time required for a drug to be totally effective
    d. The time required for half of the drug dose to be completely distributed

28. A client is taking a drug that has a half-life of 24 to 30 hours. In preparing discharge teaching, which dosing schedule would the nurse anticipate will be prescribed for this drug?
    a. Daily
    b. Every other day
    c. Twice per day
    d. Three times per day

29. Which type of drug metabolite can be eliminated through the kidneys?
    a. Enteric-coated
    b. Lipid-soluble
    c. Protein-bound
    d. Water-soluble

30. An older adult client with a glomerular filtration rate (GFR) of less than 30 has been prescribed trimethoprim for a urinary tract infection. If the normal dose is 200 mg per day, which dosing would the nurse anticipate will occur with this client's dosing regimen?
    a. The dose will double.
    b. The dose will decrease by one-half.
    c. The dose will stay the same.
    d. The dose will increase to three times per day.

31. Which statement provides the best determinant of the biologic activity of a drug?
    a. The fit of the drug at the receptor site
    b. The misfit of the drug at the receptor site
    c. The inability of the drug to bind to a specific receptor
    d. The ability of the drug to be rapidly excreted

32. Which type of drug prevents or inhibits a cellular response?
    a. Agonist
    b. Antagonist
    c. Cholinergic
    d. Nonspecific drug

33. A drug effect on receptors located in different parts of the body may initiate a variety of responses depending on the anatomic site. Which type of drug responds in this manner?
    a. Ligand-gated
    b. Nonselective
    c. Nonspecific
    d. Placebo

34. Which term measures the margin of safety of a drug.
    a. Therapeutic range
    b. Therapeutic index
    c. Duration of action
    d. Biologic half-life

35. Which measurement checks for the highest plasma/serum concentration of the drug?
    a. Peak level
    b. Minimal effective concentration
    c. Half-life
    d. Trough level

36. Which data would be important for the nurse to check in a drug reference book or pamphlet before administering a drug? (Select all that apply.)
    a. Contraindications
    b. Half-life
    c. Maximum effective concentration
    d. Protein-binding effect
    e. Therapeutic range

37. Which types of physiologic effects are predictable or associated with the use of a specific drug?
    a. Severe adverse reactions
    b. Side effects
    c. Synergistic effects
    d. Toxic effects

38. Which term is illustrated when the nurse gives a large initial dose of a drug to rapidly achieve minimum effective concentration in the plasma?
    a. Therapeutic dose
    b. Toxic dose
    c. Loading dose
    d. Peak dose

39. A time-response curve evaluates parameters of a drug's action. Which parameter(s) is/are part of the time-response curve? (Select all that apply.)
    a. Duration of action
    b. Onset of action
    c. Peak action
    d. Therapeutic range
    e. Minimum effective concentration

40. Which intervention(s) regarding drug therapy would the nurse implement? (Select all that apply.)
    a. Assess for side effects, with a focus on undesirable side effects.
    b. Check reference books or drug inserts before administering the medication.
    c. Teach the patient to wait 1 week after the appearance of side effects to see if they disappear.
    d. Check the patient's serum therapeutic range of drugs that have a narrow therapeutic range.
    e. Evaluate peak and trough levels before administering drugs with a narrow therapeutic range.

CASE STUDY

Read the scenario and answer the following questions on a separate sheet of paper.

M.E. has been prescribed verapamil for angina. The nurse knows that this drug is part of the ligand-gated ion channel receptor family.

1. Explain the receptor theory and the four receptor families. What class of drug is verapamil, and how does it work?

2. What key teaching points will the nurse provide to M.E. regarding this drug?

4 Pharmacogenetics

Complete the following.

1. _____ is the study of how genomes affect an individual's drug response.

2. Persons with UGT1A1 gene variation will be unable to eliminate _____.

3. Clients with HLA-B*5701 allele can have fatal multi-organ hypersensitivity reactions with _____.

4. Life-threatening bleeds can occur with warfarin in clients with _____ and _____ genotypes.

Answer the following questions as true or false. If false, make it into a true statement.

5. Persons with genetic variation necessary to convert clopidogrel to the active metabolite are at risk for bleeding.

6. The CYP2D6 enzyme has little known variants slowing down drug metabolism.

7. Everyone within an ethnic group shares the same genetic variations.

8. Insurance companies are prohibited from requiring genetic testing to obtain health insurance.

REVIEW QUESTIONS

9. Which term is the study of how a person's genetics affect drug responses?
   a. Pharmacodynamics
   b. Pharmacotherapeutics
   c. Pharmacogenetics
   d. Ethnopharmacy

10. Which clients would benefit the most for the use of pharmacogenetics?
    a. A client with one disease process.
    b. A client who is not on any routine drugs.
    c. A client that is elderly.
    d. A client on multiple drugs.

11. Clients with which gene variation may not be able to eliminate irinotecan?
    a. UGT1A1 gene
    b. CYP2D6
    c. TPMT
    d. CYP2C19 enzyme

CASE STUDY

Read the scenario and answer the following questions on a separate sheet of paper.

R.J., an Asian who lives in a remote rural town, has fibromyalgia. R.J. was prescribed tramadol 50 mg by mouth every 6 hours as needed for pain. The dose was increased to 75 mg for unrelieved pain after 14 days of treatment. After another 14 days, the dose was increased to 100 mg. R.J. returns to the clinic for unrelieved pain after 2 months of treatment.

1. What is the nurse's first concern?

2. How should the nurse approach the client in treating the pain?

5 Complementary and Alternative Therapies

STUDY QUESTIONS

Match the description in Column I with the letter of the reference in Column II.

Column I

_____ 1. Therapeutic value of plants

_____ 2. Clarified marketing regulations for dietary supplements

_____ 3. Assures manufacturing quality controls

_____ 4. Reviews global literature on herbal studies by clinicians and researchers

_____ 5. Supports study of alternative therapies

Column II

a. Current Good Manufacturing Practices

b. Dietary Supplement Health and Education Act of 1994

c. National Center for Complementary and Integrative Health

d. Natural Standard Research Collaboration

e. Phytomedicine

Complete the following.

6. Pouring boiling water over _____ is called _____.

7. A(n) _____ is derived from soaking fresh or dried herbs in a solvent.

8. _____ of a plant added to a solvent and applied topically is called a(n) _____.

9. Tea made from boiling plants, such as bark, rhizomes, and roots, is called a(n)_____.

10. Aromatic _____ oils from plants are called _____ _____ _____.

Match the herb in Column I with the letter of its description in Column II. Some herbs may have more than one description.

Column I

_____11. Ginkgo biloba

_____12. Peppermint oil

_____13. Dong quai

_____14. Garlic

_____15. Cinnamon

_____16. Chamomile

_____17. Hawthorn

_____18. Echinacea

_____19. Ginger

_____20. St. John's wort

Column II

a. May be used to treat bronchitis and diabetes

b. May be used to treat kidney disease

c. Immune enhancer

d. May be helpful in intermittent claudication and Alzheimer disease

e. Relief from stiffness and pain of osteoarthritis and rheumatoid arthritis

f. May be used to induce sleep

g. May be effective treatment for tension headache

h. May interfere with anticoagulants

i. "Herbal Prozac"

j. May help lower cholesterol and prevent stomach cancer

Select the best response.

21. Which herb would the nurse recognize as one that provides relief of digestive and gastrointestinal distress?
    a. Chamomile
    b. Milk thistle
    c. *Echinacea*
    d. St. John's wort

22. The daughter of a parent with Alzheimer disease asks about a complementary therapy that can improve memory. The nurse provides information knowing that which substance has been used in clients with Alzheimer disease.
    a. *echinacea*
    b. ginger
    c. *Ginkgo biloba*
    d. peppermint

23. Health teaching for a client who was prescribed warfarin would include information on which herbal product(s)? *(Select all that apply.)*
    a. Bilberry
    b. Garlic
    c. Ginseng
    d. Licorice
    e. Turmeric

24. The nurse noticed a client has been taking ginseng. Which interventions would be appropriate by the nurse? *(Select all that apply.)*
    a. Discuss with the client the potential interactions of ginseng with anticoagulants.
    b. Tell the patient to stop taking the anticoagulant.
    c. Advise the client to continue taking the same brand of herbal therapy.
    d. Advise the client to report signs and symptoms of bleeding.
    e. Discuss with the client foods to avoid.

25. Which statement(s) by the client reflect(s) prudent use of herbs? *(Select all that apply.)*
    a. "Herbs are fine to use when breastfeeding."
    b. "Do not take a large quantity of any one herbal product."
    c. "Give the herb time to work for a persistent symptom before seeking care from a health care provider."
    d. "Do not give herbs to infants or young children."
    e. "Brands of herbal products are interchangeable."

26. The nurse is caring for a client who takes a variety of herbal products and is starting a prescription antidiabetic drug. The nurse teaches the client knowing that the effects of an antidiabetic drug are altered with which herbal products? *(Select all that apply.)*
    a. *Astragalus*
    b. *Echinacea*
    c. Ginseng
    d. Milk thistle
    e. Peppermint

27. Which drug(s) has/have negative interactions with St. John's wort? *(Select all that apply.)*
    a. Anticoagulants
    b. Anticonvulsants
    c. Antidepressants
    d. Birth control drugs
    e. Paralytic drugs

28. A client with a history of hypertension, atrial fibrillation, chronic obstructive pulmonary disease, and insomnia tells the nurse, "I really love the taste of licorice." What drug-herb interactions should the nurse inform the client can occur when given in combination with licorice? *(Select all that apply.)*
    a. Antihypertensive drug effects are decreased.
    b. Corticosteroid effects are increased.
    c. CNS depressant drug effects are decreased.
    d. Digoxin effects are increased.
    e. Rifampin effects are decreased.

CASE STUDY

Read the scenario and answer the following questions on a separate sheet of paper.

K.E., 21-year-old student presents to the student health clinic with a headache, accompanied by nausea and vomiting. K.E. has started missing classes and tells the nurse, "I really can't stand feeling terrible all the time" and has started trying "a bunch" of herbal remedies to attempt to get the symptoms under control. K.E. does not know the names of any of them.

1. Which drugs would the nurse suspect K.E is taking for these symptoms, and what is their presumed mechanism of action?

2. With which drugs do these herbals interact?

3. What health teaching will the nurse provide for K.E. regarding the use of herbal preparations?

6 Pediatric Considerations

Complete the following.

1. Infants have _____ protein sites than adults, resulting in _____ risk of toxicity.

2. The degree and rate of absorption of drugs in a pediatric patient are based on _____, _____, _____, and _____.

3. Gastric pH does not reach adult acidity until around _____ to _____ year(s) of age.

4. Distribution of a drug throughout the body is affected by _____, _____, _____, and effectiveness of various barriers to drug transport.

5. Until about the age of _____, the pediatric patient requires a(n) _____ dose of water-soluble drugs to achieve therapeutic levels.

Match the child's age group in Column I with a cognitive element to consider when administering drugs in Column II.

Column I

_____ 6. Infant

_____ 7. Toddler

_____ 8. Preschool

_____ 9. School-age

_____ 10. Adolescent

Column II

a. Allow some choice
b. Involve in administration process
c. Collaborate regarding plan of care
d. Provide simple explanation
e. Use minimum restraint necessary

REVIEW QUESTIONS

Select the best response.

11. The nurse is administering an oral drug with a low pH to a 2-week-old infant. Which action describes the impact of the infant's age on the absorption of this drug? (*Select all that apply.*)
    a. Absorption may be slower in this infant.
    b. Absorption may be quicker in this infant.
    c. This drug will be absorbed at the same rate as an older client.
    d. Oral drugs should not be administered to this age group.

12. The 18-month-old child has been prescribed an oral drug that is water-soluble. Based on the nurse's knowledge of drug distribution, how may the dosage need to be modified for the child to reach therapeutic level?
    a. Alternate route
    b. Decreased
    c. Increased
    d. No change

13. Since the blood-brain barrier in infants is immature, which drug outcome is more likely?
    a. Increased effect of drug
    b. More side effects from drug
    c. Quicker results of drug
    d. Higher toxicity risk

14. Which drug action does the nurse know about the rate of absorption for topical drugs to a 3-year-old child?
    a. The drug will absorb faster.
    b. The drug will absorb slower.
    c. There will be no difference.
    d. It depends on the sex of the child.

15. Which components are related to pharmacokinetics? (Select all that apply.)
    a. Absorption
    b. Distribution
    c. Excretion
    d. Metabolism
    e. Onset

16. A child has been admitted for nausea, vomiting, and diarrhea, and the health care provider has prescribed several drugs. Which concern(s) are appropriate for the nurse to have regarding drug administration? (Select all that apply.)
    a. Renal tubular function is decreased.
    b. Dehydration may lead to toxicity.
    c. The drugs should not be administered by the oral route.
    d. Rectal administration will promote quick absorption.
    e. Developmental levels must be considered.

17. The nurse is teaching a group of parents how to administer drugs to their children. Which element(s) of drug administration will be included in the teaching? (Select all that apply.)
    a. Allow the child to determine the time of drug administration.
    b. Lightly restrain the child as needed.
    c. Praise the child after successful administration.
    d. Never threaten the child into taking the drug.
    e. Never tell the child what to expect; just give the drug.
    f. Herbal preparations should not, in general, be given to children.

CASE STUDY

Read the scenario and answer the following questions on a separate sheet of paper.

A.M., 4 years old, fell from a tree branch and fractured her forearm. An intravenous (IV) site needs to be established and analgesia administered.

1. What strategies may the nurse implement to provide developmentally appropriate care for A.M.?

2. Discuss the utilization of topical anesthetics before inserting an IV.

3. How may the caregiver be involved in the child's care while the IV is established?

7 Older Adult Considerations

Complete the following.

1. Age-related factors among older adults influence drug _____, _____, _____, and excretion.

2. Drugs for older adults are prescribed at _____ dosages and _____ increase in dosage based on therapeutic _____.

3. Some of the characteristics in older adults that increase the risk for problems related to drugs include _____ and _____ changes associated with _____.

4. Pharmacodynamic responses to drugs are altered with aging as a result of changes in the number of _____ sites, which affects the _____ of certain drugs.

5. Identify at least five drugs that nurses should avoid administering to older adults with stage 4 or 5 chronic kidney disease.

Match the physiologic changes in Column I with the pharmacokinetic responses in Column II.

Column I	Column II
a. Altered by the decline in renal function	6. Absorption
b. Altered by a decline in muscle mass and an increase in fat	7. Distribution
c. Altered by decreased small-bowel surface area, decreased gastric emptying, and reduced gastric blood flow	8. Metabolism
d. Altered by the decline in hepatic circulation, liver atrophy, and a reduction in hepatic enzyme activity	9. Excretion

Identify the drug class for each group of drugs.

_____ 10. Lisinopril, benazepril, enalapril, quinapril

_____ 11. Acebutolol, atenolol, sotolol

_____ 12. Lithium, gabapentin, duloxetine, bupropion, venlafaxine, pregabalin

_____ 13. Irbesartan, losartan, valsartan

Answer the following questions as true or false. If false, rewrite the statement into a true statement.

_____ 14. Risk factors associated with polypharmacy do not include advanced age.

_____ 15. Risk factors associated with polypharmacy include being female.

_____ 16. Risk factors associated with polypharmacy include having more than one health care provider.

_____ 17. Risk factors associated with polypharmacy do not include the use of OTC drugs.

_____ 18. Beers criteria is a document that lists drugs that has negative interactions in older adults when they drink alcohol.

17

_____19.   Risk factors associated with polypharmacy include the use of vitamin and mineral supplements.

_____20.   Polypharmacy increases the risk of falls among older adults.

REVIEW QUESTIONS

Select the best response.

21. Which lab result is an indicator of normal glomerular filtration rate for an adult?
    a. Creatinine clearance: 100–125 mL/min
    b. Aspartate aminotransferase: 4–12 mL/min
    c. Troponin: 80–120 mL/min
    d. Urea: 1.2–4.5

22. The safest antihypertensive drugs for older adults have a low incidence of which side effect?
    a. Constipation
    b. Electrolyte imbalance
    c. Loss of appetite
    d. Vision disturbances

23. An older adult client recently started on diphenhydramine for runny nose, headache, sneezing, and scratchy eyes. List of drugs taken on a daily basis includes digoxin, fluoxetine, and a multivitamin on a daily basis.
    a. "I cannot work outside anymore because of the digoxin."
    b. "I think I need to find a different allergy drug to take."
    c. "I take fluoxetine because I have depression."
    d. "I should not take my wife's headache drug."

24. Which drug would have fewer adverse and toxic effects while maintaining its therapeutic effect?
    a. Half-life of 50 hours
    b. 90% protein bound
    c. Half-life of 4 hours
    d. Fat-soluble

25. Which lab value(s) will the nurse monitor in an older adult client to assess kidney function? (Select all that apply.)
    a. BUN
    b. Creatinine clearance
    c. CBC
    d. Lipase
    e. Triglycerides

26. An older adult client reports feeling dizzy every morning when getting out of bed. Which physiological effect does the nurse recognize the client is most likely experiencing?
    a. Bradycardia
    b. Intermittent claudication
    c. Hyperventilation
    d. Orthostatic hypotension

27. Which actions would the nurse recommend to a client who experiences dizziness when arising from bed?
    a. Change positions slowly.
    b. Move a chair close to the bed.
    c. Take deep breaths.
    d. Measure pulse before standing.

28. Following hospitalization, the older adult client receives a home visit from the nurse. The client asks if the drugs taken before hospitalization should continue. Which response would be appropriate by the nurse?
    a. "Yes, you should continue to take the drugs that you took before going to the hospital."
    b. "You should take one-half the dosage of each drug that you took prior to hospitalization."
    c. "You should take only the drugs that have been prescribed on discharge and not drugs that you took prior to hospitalization unless otherwise indicated."
    d. "You should continue to take those drugs that have been helpful to you."

29. The older adult client has difficulties opening the bottle of celecoxib. Which response is appropriate by the nurse?
    a. "Please ask your pharmacist to place your drug in a bottle with a non-childproof cap."
    b. "You can keep your drug in a glass cup in the medicine cabinet."
    c. "You could place your drug in an envelope."
    d. "A family member could help you with your daily drug regimen."

30. An older adult client is to take newly prescribed drugs at different times. Which suggestion by the nurse would be appropriate so that the client can adhere with the drug regimen?
    a. "Line up the bottles of medications on a table and take them in that order."
    b. "Obtain a weekly pill container with multiple time slots from the drugstore and fill the container the day or week before with the drugs."
    c. "Ask a neighbor to give the daily drugs."
    d. "Write down the drugs that you have taken each day."

31. In older adults, drug dosages are adjusted based on which factor(s)? (Select all that apply.)
    a. Amount of adipose tissue
    b. Height
    c. Nutritional status
    d. Laboratory results
    e. Response to drug

32. Before administering drugs to the older adult, which drug information(s) would the nurse know beforehand? *(Select all that apply.)*
    a. Whether the drug is highly protein bound
    b. Half-life of the drug
    c. Patient's last bowel movement
    d. Serum levels of drugs with a narrow therapeutic range
    e. Baseline vital signs

CASE STUDY

Read the scenario and answer the following questions on a separate sheet of paper.

M.Z., 80 years old, presents to the clinic for annual checkup. M.Z. has a medical history of diabetes, insomnia, and hypertension. Vital signs are temperature 99.2° F, heart rate 83 beats/minute, respiratory rate 16 breaths/minute, blood pressure 142/90 mm Hg, and blood glucose 96 mg/dL. While obtaining the health history, M.Z. complains of having trouble falling and staying asleep, and having to get up several times per night to go to the bathroom. Medications/supplements M.Z. is currently taking hydrochlorothiazide, triazolam, and chamomile tea. M.Z. states, "I try to remember to take my drugs, and sometimes I take an extra one, just in case I forgot one."

1. Which laboratory tests would the nurse anticipate for M.Z.?

2. Which suggestions would be appropriate for the nurse make to help with M.Z.'s sleeping difficulties?

3. What further teaching will the nurse provide about M.Z.'s drug regimen?

8 Drugs in Substance Use Disorder

Match the therapy in Column I to its description in Column II.

Column I

_____ 1. Cognitive behavioral therapy

_____ 2. Motivational enhancement therapy

_____ 3. Contingency management

Column II

a. Based on frequent behavior monitoring and removal of rewards for substance use

b. Recognize and stop negative patterns and enhance self-control

c. Develop motivation internally to commit to specific plan

Complete the following.

4. Misused drugs typically increase _____ and other _____ in the limbic system of the brain.

5. The _____ _____ is a structure within the brain that regulates the body's ability to feel pleasure.

6. The study of environmental influences on genetics is called _____.

7. Disulfiram _____ the enzyme involved in metabolizing alcohol.

8. Heroin addiction may be treated with _____.

9. Benzodiazepines are FDA approved to treat addiction to _____.

10. Opioids provide a sense of _____ and _____; methadone _____ these feelings.

11. _____ questionnaire can be used to screen for alcohol misuse.

12. Substance use disorder among nurses can be recognized by changes in _____, _____, _____, and _____.

Answer the following questions as true or false. If false, rewrite the statement into a true statement.

_____13. Electronic cigarettes are safer than tobacco products.

_____14. Dehydroepiandrosterone (DHEA) is found in many dietary supplements and is approved to slow aging.

_____15. Discrepancies in controlled-drug handling and records among health care professionals may indicate drug diversion.

Match the term in Column I with the definition in Column II.

Column I

_____ 16. Craving

_____ 17. Impaired control

_____ 18. Tolerance

_____ 19. Withdrawal syndrome

Column II

a. Diminished ability to control the use of a drug in terms of onset, level, or termination

b. A strong desire for the drug effects

c. A group of signs and symptoms of physiologic disturbance upon cessation or reduction of a drug

d. Requiring a significantly increased amount of a drug to achieve the desired effect

REVIEW QUESTIONS

Select the best response.

20. A client is seen in the emergency department for reportedly swallowing a small balloon full of cocaine. Which clinical manifestations would the nurse expect to see if the balloon ruptured?
   a. Dilated pupils and restlessness
   b. Hypotension and tachycardia
   c. Insomnia and fine tremors
   d. Respiratory depression and pinpoint pupils

21. Which drug can be given to aid a client with opioid withdrawal?
   a. Disulfiram
   b. Lorazepam
   c. Methadone
   d. Naloxone

22. The client has decided to quit smoking. Which key point(s) must the nurse include in the teaching plan? *(Select all that apply.)*
   a. Assess that the client is motivated to quit.
   b. Assist in setting a quit date of 1 month.
   c. Help the client identify what increases the desire to smoke.
   d. Advise the client to use chewing tobacco as a substitute.
   e. Provide the client with a list of smoking cessation aids.

23. Which percentage of nurses abuse drugs and demonstrate impaired practice attributable to that abuse?
   a. 1–2%
   b. 3–6%
   c. 7–10%
   d. 10–15%

24. "Bath salts" are classified as which type of drug?
   a. Amphetamine
   b. Benzodiazepine
   c. Hallucinogenic
   d. Synthetic cathinone

CASE STUDY

Read the scenario and answer the following questions on a separate sheet of paper.

C.L., 57 years old, presents to the emergency department (ED). C.L is unresponsive to verbal and painful stimuli and smells strongly of alcohol. Vital signs include temperature of 96.8° F, heart rate of 104 beats/minute, respiratory rate of 6 breaths/minute, blood pressure of 90/68 mm Hg, and oxygen saturation of 88% on room air.

1. What is the initial treatment for C.L.?

2. What are the potential complications for alcohol toxicity?

3. Describe the pharmacokinetics for disulfiram and the side effects if taken with any alcohol.

4. Identify the drug–drug interactions that can occur when taken concomitantly with disulfiram that would have similar reactions as if the person had been ingesting alcohol.

9 Safety and Quality

Identify the Quality and Safety Education for Nurses Institute (QSEN) competency for the following definition.

1. Minimizing risk to clients. _____

2. Respecting the client's rights. _____

3. Working collaboratively with inter-professional teams. _____

4. Improving client's delivery of care. _____

5. Using technology to improve care. _____

6. Delivering safe care based on current research. _____

Match the statement in Column I with the nursing implication for drug administration in Column II.

Column I

_____ 7. Right route

_____ 8. Right patient

_____ 9. Right time

_____ 10. Right documentation

_____ 11. Right assessment

_____ 12. Right drug

_____ 13. Right dose

_____ 14. Right education

_____ 15. Right to refuse

_____ 16. Right to evaluation

Column II

a. Measurement of a client's apical pulse
b. Amount of drug given as prescribed
c. Drug given intramuscularly (IM) as prescribed
d. Teaching a client about possible side effects of the drug
e. The client refuses to take drug
f. Verification of client identification (ID)
g. Nurse charts client's pain was decreased after drug administration
h. Client receives the prescribed drug
i. Nurse checks blood pressure following blood pressure drug administration
j. Drug given at the time prescribed

Match the situation in Column I with the instructions in Column II. Instructions in Column II will be used more than once.

Column I

_____ 17. Drugs poured by others

_____ 18. Client states the drug is different than usual

_____ 19. Bad-tasting drugs first, then pleasant-tasting drugs

_____ 20. Drugs in an unlabeled container

_____ 21. An opened multidose vial with date and time it was opened and initialed

_____ 22. Drugs left with visitors

Column II

a. Do not administer
b. Do administer

23. Provide the meaning of each abbreviation and determine if it is acceptable to use.
    a. ID
    b. MS
    c. q.o.d.
    d. gtt
    e. kg
    f. 1.0 mg
    g. mg
    h. qd
    i. KVO
    j. IVPB
    k. c̄
    l. ā
    m. bid

24. Provide the meaning of the following abbreviations on the drug type.

Abbreviation	Meaning
CR	
ER	
IM	
XR	
XT	

REVIEW QUESTIONS

Select the best response.

25. A client has been prescribed antibiotics that are scheduled for every 8 hours. Which statement by the client indicates the need for more teaching regarding the drug regimen?
    a. "I take this drug every 8 hours around the clock."
    b. "I have to take the drug even if I feel better."
    c. "I just take it divided into three doses while I'm awake."
    d. "I cannot take it more often even if I don't feel better."

26. The client has been prescribed a drug to be taken a.c. and h.s. Which instruction would the nurse give the client?
    a. "Take this drug every 6 hours."
    b. "Take this drug before meals and at bedtime."
    c. "Take this drug after meals and first thing in the morning."
    d. "Take this drug after meals and as needed."

27. Which statement describes the purpose of the "tall man" letters?
    a. To assist with drug reconciliation
    b. To aid in labeling drug allergies
    c. To promote safety between drugs with similar names
    d. To label differences in dosage strength of the same drug

28. The nurse is calculating an opioid dose for the client. The dose seems "large." Which action would the nurse take initially?
    a. Check the patient's name band and administer the drug.
    b. Call the health care provider.
    c. Recalculate the dose.
    d. Withhold the drug and document as not given.

29. The nurse working in a clinic will be administering flu shots from a multidose vial. Which information would the nurse include to label the bottle? (Select all that apply.)
    a. Nurse's initials
    b. Date vial opened
    c. Prescribing provider
    d. Time vial opened
    e. Expiration date

30. The older adult client tells the nurse, "I'm not taking that pill. I don't want it, and I won't take it!" Which action would the nurse take first?
    a. Document the client's refusal.
    b. Force the client to take the drug.
    c. Educate the client on the importance of the drug.
    d. Call the health care provider who prescribed the drug.

31. Which abbreviation(s) is/are not allowed by The Joint Commission? (*Select all that apply.*)
    a. IM
    b. U
    c. IU
    d. q.d.
    e. MS

32. A client tells the nurse the unused opioids were flushed down the toilet. Which response is best by the nurse?
    a. "Flushing unused drugs is okay."
    b. "Be sure to crush the drugs before flushing them."
    c. "Crush the drugs and throw them in the trash."
    d. "Throw them in the trash after mixing the drugs with unpalatable nonfood substance."

CASE STUDY

Read the scenario and answer the following questions on a separate sheet of paper.

A nurse is preparing to administer three of R.L.'s morning drugs. The nurse tells the client the drugs are for blood pressure, diabetes, and depression. When R.L. looked at the drugs, the client exclaims "these are not the pills I take."

1. What are the "six rights" in drug administration?

2. What methods can the nurse use to determine the "right patient" is receiving the drugs?

3. What is the nurse's best action when R.L. stated "these are not the pills I take?"

10 Drug Administration

Complete the following.

1. _____ and _____ drugs must be swallowed whole.

2. Handheld nebulizers deliver a very _____ _____ in a spray of drug.

3. When giving a client a drug via a handheld nebulizer, the client should be placed in _____ position.

4. A nasogastric tube should be flushed with _____ mL of water (or the prescribed amount) following drug administration.

5. Following insertion of a rectal suppository, the patient should remain in a side-lying position for at least _____ minutes.

Match the route in Column I with the correct length of needle in Column II.

Column I

_____ 6. Subcutaneous (subcut)

_____ 7. Intradermal (ID)

_____ 8. Intramuscular (IM)

Column II

a. ¼ to ½ inch in length
b. ⅝ to 1½ inch in length
c. ⅜ to ⅝ inch in length

Complete the following.

9. The injection site that is away from major nerves and is a preferred site for Z-track injections is the _____.

10. The preferred site for immunizations for infants and children who are not ambulating alone is the _____.

11. The site that is easily accessible but is suitable for only small-volume doses is the _____.

12. The preferred site for intramuscular injections in infants and children of any age is the _____.

13. Label the landmarks for ventrogluteal injection.

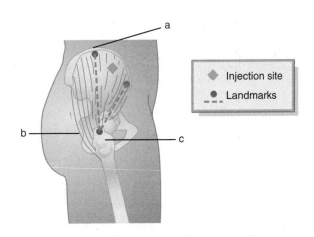

◆	Injection site
●	Landmarks

Select the best response.

14. A client is vomiting and has been prescribed an antiemetic. Which route does the nurse know is contraindicated for this client?
    a. Intradermal
    b. Intravenous
    c. Oral
    d. Rectal suppository

15. The 2-year-old child has been prescribed antibiotic eardrops. The nurse is providing education to the parents. Which instruction is correct in which to pull the auricle?
    a. Down and back
    b. Forward and back
    c. Forward and up
    d. Up and back

16. A client has been prescribed an intramuscular (IM) injection. The drug is thick and must be administered deep IM. Which does site would the nurse choose for the injection?
    a. Deltoid
    b. Dorsolateral
    c. Vastus lateralis
    d. Ventrogluteal

17. Which site is preferred for an immunization injection in an 8-week-old infant?
    a. Deltoid
    b. Dorsogluteal
    c. Vastus lateralis
    d. Ventrogluteal

18. A client is being discharged on new drugs. Which statement made by the client would indicate that more teaching is required?
    a. "I can take any over-the-counter drug or herbal preparation that I think would be helpful."
    b. "I need to make sure I keep appointments with my health care provider."
    c. "I need to report any side effects to my health care provider."
    d. "I will contact my pharmacy if I am going out of town to ensure that I have enough drug."

19. The client has been started on a new oral drug. Which information will the nurse include in the teaching? *(Select all that apply.)*
    a. Desired effect of the drug
    b. Dietary considerations
    c. Storage of all drugs in the refrigerator
    d. Research testing and development
    e. Written instructions on how to administer the drug

20. The client has been prescribed a steroid metered-dose inhaler (MDI) for asthma. Which statement by the client indicates understanding of how to use the MDI?
    a. "I can use it as often as I need it."
    b. "I need to rinse out my mouth after I use it."
    c. "I should put my mouth tightly over the end."
    d. "I can administer multiple puffs at one time."

CASE STUDY

Read the scenario and answer the following questions on a separate sheet of paper.

A.J., 20-year-old, is prescribed promethazine 12.5 mg intramuscular (IM) for intractable nausea. The nurse prepares to administer the drug.

1. Identify the size of the needle and syringe needed for IM injection.

2. What are the potential IM injection sites for this patient?

3. What method should the nurse use for this IM injection? Why?

11 Drug Calculations

INTRODUCTION

The Drug Calculations chapter in this Study Guide includes numerous drug labels to allow learners to become familiar with reading drug labels and calculating drug dosages from the information provided on the drug labels. Additionally, many practice problems in this Study Guide includes conversion factors with metric and household systems, drug reconstitutions for enteral and parenteral drugs, dosage calculations for enteral drugs, parenteral drugs, including insulin and intravenous flow rates. It is highly recommended to read and study Chapter 11 in the accompanying textbook prior to drug calculations in this Study Guide.

Drug calculation practice problems provide an opportunity to gain skill and competence in collecting and organizing the required data. Practice problems have examples of the administration of drugs via a variety of routes, including enteral (gastrointestinal) and parenteral (subcutaneous, intramuscular, and intravenous). Practice problems also include calculating dosages based on body weight and body surface area, intravenous heparin infusions, and critical care drugs.

When calculating dosages, select one of the three methods (basic formula, ratio and proportion/fractional equation, or dimensional analysis) presented in the accompanying textbook. After completing the required calculations, determine if the calculated answer is reasonable. In the event of a discrepancy, review both the thought process used in answering the problem and the actual mathematical calculation. It may be necessary to review the related section in Chapter 11 of the textbook. Practice problems provide reinforcement to gain expertise in the process of actually calculating drug dosages.

For methods other than dimensional analysis during calculations, round the numbers to the nearest *whole* number for drops; round to the nearest *tenth* for kilograms, pounds, milliliters, milligrams, and units; round to the nearest hundredths for body surface areas (m^2); and round to the nearest *minute* for time. Final answers for all drug calculations, round to the nearest *whole number* for milligrams, units, and drops. Round to the nearest *tenth* for kilograms, pounds, and milliliters. When doing dimensional analysis, conversion factors are already built into the equation and the final answer is the only number that is rounded. All calculations, except for the body surface area (BSA) using the West Nomogram, can be accomplished using dimensional analysis. Therefore, dimensional analysis is the recommended method for drug calculations.

The answers are in the back of the Study Guide. Some of the calculations will be illustrated in the Answer Key using dimensional analysis.

METRIC AND HOUSEHOLD SYSTEMS

Match the term in Column I with the appropriate abbreviation in Column II.

Column I

_____ 1. Gram

_____ 2. Milligram

_____ 3. Liter

_____ 4. Milliliter

_____ 5. Kilogram

_____ 6. Microgram

_____ 7. Meter

_____ 8. Fluid ounce

_____ 9. Quart

_____10. Pint

_____11. Pound

_____12. Cup

_____13. Tablespoon

_____14. Teaspoon

_____15. Drops

Column II

a. T or tbsp
b. g
c. mL
d. lb
e. fl oz
f. mg
g. L or l
h. gtt
i. kg
j. mcg
k. t or tsp
l. c
m. pt
n. qt
o. m

Complete the following.

16. The most frequently used conversions within the metric system are:

    A. 1 g = _____ mg

    B. 1 L = _____ mL

    C. 1 mg = _____ mcg

Convert the following unit of measurement.

17. 3 grams = _____ milligrams

18. 1.5 liters = _____ milliliters

19. 0.1 gram = _____ milligrams

20. 2500 milliliters = _____ liters

21. 250 milliliters = _____ liter

22. 500 milligrams = _____ gram

23. 2 quarts = _____ pints

24. 2 pints = _____ fluid ounces

25. 1½ quarts = _____ fluid ounces

26. 32 fluid ounces = _____ pints

27. 3000 micrograms = _____ milligrams

28. 3 teaspoons = _____ milliliters

29. 30 milliliters = _____ fluid ounce

30. 1 tablespoon = _____ teaspoon

31. 1 g = _____ mg

32. _____ g = 500 mg

33. 0.1 g = _____ mg

34. _____ L = 1000 mL, or _____ qt

35. 240 mL = _____ fl oz

36. 30 mL = _____ fl oz, or _____ T,

    or _____ t

37. 5 mL = _____ t

38. 3 T = _____ fl oz, or _____ t

39. 5 fl oz = _____ mL, or _____ T

DRUG CALCULATIONS FOR ENTERAL AND PARENTERAL DRUGS

For any drug calculations, use the basic formula, ratio and proportion/fractional equation, or dimensional analysis to calculate the following calculation problems. The recommended method is the dimensional analysis. Select the best response.

1. Before calculating drug dosages, all units of measurement must be converted to one system. Which system is the best method for the nurse to use?
   a. Any system the nurse prefers
   b. A system that fits with how the nurse will administer the drug
   c. A system that is easy to convert to
   d. The system on the drug label

2. Which methods are for administering drugs by parenteral routes? *(Select all that apply.)*
   a. Via a nasogastric tube
   b. Subcutaneous
   c. Intramuscular
   d. Intradermal
   e. Intravenous
   f. Any liquid drug via all routes

3. Which routes of administration can be used for insulin and heparin? *(Select all that apply.)*
   a. Oral
   b. Intramuscular
   c. Subcutaneous
   d. Intravenous
   e. Intradermal

4. Vials are glass containers with (self-sealing rubber tops/tapered glass necks). Vials are usually (discarded/reusable if properly stored). *(Circle correct answers.)*

5. Before drug reconstitution, the nurse should check the drug circular and/or drug label for instructions. After a drug has been reconstituted and additional doses are available, which information will the nurse write on the drug label? *(Select all that apply.)*
   a. Date to discard
   b. Initials
   c. The health care provider's order
   d. What it is reconstituted with

6. The nurse is preparing an intramuscular (IM) injection for an average adult. Which needle gauge and length could be used to administer the IM?
   a. 20, 21 gauge; ½, ⅝ inch in length
   b. 23, 25 gauge; ½, ⅝ inch in length
   c. 19, 20, 21 gauge; 1, 1½, 2 inches in length
   d. 25, 26 gauge; 1, 1½ inches in length

7. Which two parts of a syringe must remain sterile?
   a. Outside of syringe and plunger
   b. Tip of the syringe and plunger
   c. Both the tip and outside of the syringe
   d. Tip and outside of syringe and plunger

8. Subcutaneous injections can be administered at which degree angle(s)?
   a. 10-degree and 15-degree angles
   b. 45-degree, 60-degree, and 90-degree angles
   c. 45-degree angle only
   d. 90-degree angle only

9. The nurse calculates the drug dosage to be 0.25 milliliter. Which type of syringe should be selected?
   a. 3-mL syringe
   b. Insulin syringe
   c. Tuberculin syringe
   d. 10-mL syringe

10. To mix 3 milliliters of sterile saline solution in a vial containing a powdered drug, which size syringe should be selected?
    a. Tuberculin syringe
    b. Insulin syringe
    c. 3-mL syringe
    d. 5-mL syringe

11. Solutions in drug A and drug B are compatible. To combine 5 milliliters of drug A with 8 milliliters of drug B to be administered via syringe pump, the nurse would use which syringe size(s)?
    a. One 5-mL syringe and one 10-mL syringe
    b. Two 10-mL syringes
    c. One 20-mL syringe
    d. Two 5-mL syringes and one 10-mL syringe

Interpreting Drug Labels

Note: When converting a unit of measurement from one system to another, convert to the unit on the *drug label*.

Example:

Order: Penicillin V 0.5 g PO q8h

Available:

Convert _____ to _____ (unit of measurement to unit of measurement)

12. Provide the information requested on the following drug label.

A. What is the brand name of this drug? _____

B. What is the generic name of this drug? _____

C. What is the formulation of this drug? _____

D. What is the form of this drug? _____

13. Provide the information requested on the following drug label.

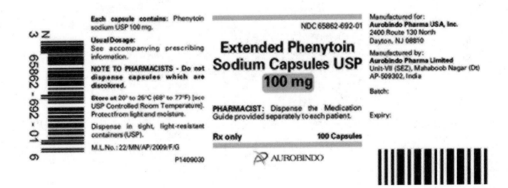

DO NOT USE IF INNER SEAL OVER BOTTLE OPENING IS BROKEN OR MISSING.

This package is not intended for household use.

Each tablet contains 5 mg of hydrocodone bitartrate and 300 mg of acetaminophen.

Usual adult dosage One or two tablets every four to six hours, as needed for pain. See package outsert for full prescribing information.

Protect from Light.

PHARMACIST: Dispense in a tight, light-resistant container with a child-resistant closure.

Store at 25°C (77°F); excursions permitted to 15°C to 30°C (59°F to 86°F) [see USP Controlled Room Temperature].

NDC 27808-114-02

Hydrocodone Bitartrate and Acetaminophen Tablets, USP CII

5 mg / 300 mg

Rx Only
500 Tablets

WARNING: Keep this and all medications out of the reach of children.

Manufactured by:
Tris PHARMA
Monmouth Junction, NJ 08852
www.trispharma.com

N S 27808-114-02 0

LOT
EXP

LB8440
Rev 00
03/16

A. What is the name of the drug? _____

B. What is the formulation of this drug? _____

C. Is this drug a controlled substance? _____

D. Circle on the label the marking that indicates it is a controlled substance.

E. What is the form of the drug? _____

F. How should the drug be stored? _____

G. What company manufactured the drug? _____

14. Provide the information requested on the following drug label.

Each capsule contains: Phenytoin sodium USP 100 mg.

Usual Dosage:
See accompanying prescribing information.

NOTE TO PHARMACISTS - Do not dispense capsules which are discolored.

Store at 20° to 26°C (68° to 77°F) [see USP Controlled Room Temperature]. Protect from light and moisture.

Dispense in tight, light-resistant containers (USP).

M.L.No.: 22/MN/AP/2009/F/G

P1409030

3 N
65862 - 692 - 01 6

NDC 65862-692-01

Extended Phenytoin Sodium Capsules USP
100 mg

PHARMACIST: Dispense the Medication Guide provided separately to each patient.

Rx only   100 Capsules

AUROBINDO

Manufactured for:
Aurobindo Pharma USA, Inc.
2400 Route 130 North
Dayton, NJ 08810

Manufactured by:
Aurobindo Pharma Limited
Unit-VII (SEZ), Mahaboob Nagar (Dt)
AP-509302, India

Batch:

Expiry:

A. What is the generic name of the drug? _____

B. Is the drug a controlled substance? _____

C. What is the form of the drug? _____

D. How much of the drug is in each capsule? _____

E. Circle the marking on the label that indicates whether a prescription is required.

F. How should the drug be stored? _____

15. Provide the information requested on the following drug label.

A. What is generic name of the drug? _____

B. What is the trade name? _____

C. Does this drug require a prescription? _____

D. What is the form of the drug? _____

E. What is the concentration of the drug? _____

F. What is the total volume in mL? _____

G. What is the usual dose for adults and children 12 years of age and over? _____

H. How many adult dosages are available? _____

16. Provide the information requested on the following drug label.

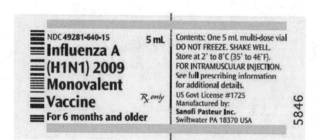

A. What is the name of the drug? _____

B. What is the form of the drug? _____

C. Is the vial a single dose vial or multi-dose vial? _____

D. How should the drug be stored? _____

E. How should this drug be administered? _____

17. Provide the information requested on the following drug label.

   A. What is the generic name? _____

   B. What is the trade name? _____

   C. How should it be stored? _____

18. Order: ritonavir 0.5 g PO bid
    Available:

   A. Is conversion needed to give this medication?
      a. No; it may be administered in grams.
      b. No; the pill may be broken if needed.
      c. Yes; it should be converted to grains.
      d. Yes; it should be converted to milligrams.
   B. How much of this medication should the nurse administer?
      a. ½ tablet
      b. 1 tablet
      c. 3 tablets
      d. 5 tablets

19. Order: diphenhydramine 25 mg PO q6h, PRN
    Available: diphenhydramine 12.5 mg/5 mL

A. Is conversion needed to give this drug?
   a. No; it can be administered in milligrams as ordered.
   b. No; you cannot mix mg and mL.
   c. Yes; it should be converted to grains.
   d. Yes; it should be converted to grams.
B. How many mL should the nurse give?
   a. 5 mL
   b. 10 mL
   c. 15 mL
   d. 20 mL

20. Order: clarithromycin 0.25 g PO bid
    Available:

A. Is conversion needed to give this medication?
   a. No; it may be administered in grams.
   b. No; you cannot mix mg and mL.
   c. Yes; it should be converted to grains.
   d. Yes; it should be converted to milligrams.
B. How many mL should be administered?
   a. 5 mL
   b. 10 mL
   c. 15 mL
   d. 20 mL

21. Order: hydroxyzine 25 mg PO q6h
    Available:

How many mL should be administered?
a. 5 mL
b. 7.5 mL
c. 10 mL
d. 12.5 mL

22. Order: ceftriaxone 500 mg IM
    Available:

A. How many mL should be administered?
   a. 1 mL
   b. 1.4 mL
   c. 2 mL
   d. 2.4 mL

B. What size syringe should be used? _____

23. Order: acarbose 50 mg PO tid
    Available:

How many tablets should be administered per dose?
a. 1 tablet
b. 2 tablets
c. 3 tablets
d. 4 tablets

24. Order: losartan potassium 100 mg daily
    Available:

A. What is the generic name? _____

B. What is the trade name? _____

C. How many tablets are in the container? _____

D. How many tablets should the patient receive per day?
    a. 1 tablet
    b. 2 tablets
    c. 3 tablets
    d. 4 tablets

25. Order: propranolol 15 mg PO q6h
    Available: propranolol 10-mg and 20-mg scored tablets

A. Which tablet strength should be administered? Why?
    a. 10-mg tablets
    b. 20-mg tablets

B. How many tablets should be administered?
    a. 1 tablet
    b. 1½ tablets
    c. 2 tablets
    d. 2½ tablets

38

26. Order: furosemide 80 mg PO daily
    Available:

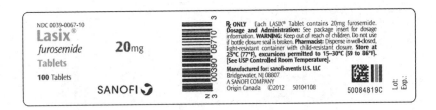

A. What is the generic name? _____

B. What is the trade name? _____

C. How should the medication be stored? _____

D. How many tablets should be administered?
   a. 2 tablets
   b. 3 tablets
   c. 4 tablets
   d. 5 tablets

27. Order: potassium ER 40 mEq PO daily
    Available:

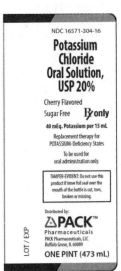

A. Which form should be used? Why?

B. Upon assessment, the nurse discovers the client has a nasogastric tube (NGT) and is unable to swallow. Which action is correct for the nurse to do?
   a. Give the drug as ordered.
   b. Give the oral liquid.
   c. Call the prescriber.
   d. Give the drug IV.

C. After calling the prescriber, the order was changed to 20 mEq via a nasogastric tube bid.

   a. Which form should be used? Why? _____

   b. How many milliliters should the nurse give per dose? _____

28. Order: verapamil 60 mg PO qid
Available:

   A. Which strength of verapamil should be selected?
      a. 120-mg tablet
      b. 80-mg tablet

   B. How many tablets should be administered?
      a. ½ tablet
      b. 1 tablet
      c. 1½ tablets
      d. 2 tablets

29. Order: trihexyphenidyl 4 mg/d PO in two divided doses q12h
Available:

   A. How many tablets per dose? _____

   B. How many tablets per 24 hours? _____

30. Order: oxacillin 400 mg IM q6h
    Available:

    A. How much diluent should be added for an intramuscular injection? _____

    B. How many milliliters should the patient receive?
        a. 0.5 mL
        b. 1.5 mL
        c. 2 mL
        d. 2.4 mL

31. Order: adalimumab 40 mg subcut every other week
    Available:

    A. What is the route of administration?_____

    B. What is the dosage strength? _____

    C. How many milliliters should the patient receive? _____

    D. What size syringe(s) should be used? *(Select all that apply.)*
        a. Tuberculin
        b. Insulin
        c. 1-mL syringe
        d. 3-mL syringe

32. Order: trazodone 150 mg PO daily
    Available: trazodone in 50-mg tablets and 100-mg tablets

    A. How many tablets should be administered if the 50-mg tablet is used?
        a. 1 tablet
        b. 2 tablets
        c. 3 tablets
        d. 4 tablets

    B. How many tablets should be administered if the 100-mg tablet is used?
        a. ½ tablet
        b. 1 tablet
        c. 1½ tablets
        d. 2 tablets

33. Order: warfarin 7.5 mg PO daily
    Available:

A. Which dosage strength should be selected?
   a. Warfarin 2.5 mg
   b. Warfarin 5 mg

B. How many tablet(s) should be administered? *(Consider all the possible combinations).*

34. Order: lithium carbonate 300 mg PO tid
    Available: lithium carbonate in 150- and 300-mg capsules and 300-mg tablets. The patient's lithium level is 1.8 mEq/L (normal value is 0.5–1.5 mEq/L).

    What is the best action by the nurse?
    a. Give 150 mg (half the dose).
    b. Give 300-mg tablet and not the capsule.
    c. Advise the patient not to take the dose for a week.
    d. Withhold the drug and contact the health care provider.

35. Order: carvedilol 6.25 mg PO bid
    Available:

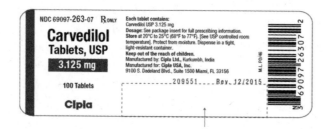

A. How many tablets should be administered per dose?
   a. 1 tablet
   b. 2 tablets
   c. 3 tablets
   d. Call the pharmacy to bring 6.25 tabs

B. How many tablets should the patient receive in 24 hours?
   a. 4 tablets
   b. 6 tablets
   c. 8 tablets
   d. 10 tablets

36. Order: azithromycin 500 mg PO on day 1, then 250 mg PO daily for next 4 days
Available:

A. Circle the route on the label.

B. How many milliliters should be administered the first day?
   a. 2.5 mL
   b. 6.5 mL
   c. 12.5 mL
   d. 25 mL

C. How many milliliters should be administered per day for the next 4 days?
   a. 5 mL/day
   b. 6.25 mL/day
   c. 10 mL/day
   d. 12.5 mL/day

37. Order: trihexyphenidyl elixir 1 mg PO tid
Available: trihexyphenidyl 2 mg/5 mL

What amount should be administered per dose?
   a. 2 mL
   b. 2.5 mL
   c. 3 mL
   d. 5 mL

38. Order: trimethobenzamide 200 mg IM STAT
Available: trimethobenzamide ampule, 100 mg/1 mL

How many milliliters should be administered?
   a. 0.5 mL
   b. 0.8 mL
   c. 1 mL
   d. 2 mL

39. Order: chlorpromazine 20 mg deep IM tid
    Available:

How many milliliters should be administered?
a. 0.3 mL
b. 0.5 mL
c. 0.8 mL
d. 1 mL

40. A client is scheduled to take digoxin 0.25 mg. The hospital is currently out of stock of digoxin 0.25 mg and has only 0.125-mg doses on hand. The client is concerned when the pills were received because they are a different color and a different amount from those she takes daily. When the client questions the tablets, what is the nurse's best response?
a. "Please don't worry; it is because we use generic drugs."
b. "Please don't worry; I calculated this carefully and it is your regular dose."
c. "We don't have the 0.25-mg tablets available, so I brought you two pills of 0.125 mg to equal your 0.25 mg dose."
d. "You are right, this is the wrong dosage. I will be right back with the correct one."

41. Order: carbidopa 12.5mg/levodopa 125 mg PO bid
    Available:

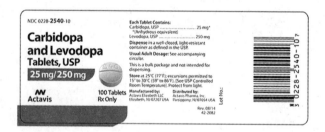

How many tablets should be administered per dose?
a. ½ tablet should be given.
b. 1 tablet should be given.
c. 1½ tablets should be given.
d. Do not administer the medication, and call the pharmacy for the correct dose.

42. Order: lactulose 25 g PO q6h
Available:

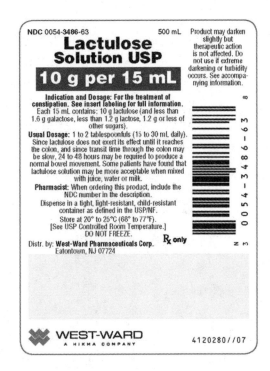

How many milliliters should the patient receive per dose?
a. 10 mL
b. 16.7 mL
c. 25 mL
d. 37.5 mL

43. Order: hydromorphone 2 mg subcut q4h PRN for pain
Available:

A. Are the drugs on the label interchangeable?

B. How many mL would you give of the correct drug?
a. 0.5 mL
b. 1 mL
c. 1.5 mL
d. 2 mL

44. Order: cyanocobalamin 1000 mcg IM daily for 5 days
    Available: cyanocobalamin 10,000 mcg/10 mL

    How many milliliters should be administered?
    a. 0.4 mL
    b. 0.6 mL
    c. 0.8 mL
    d. 1 mL

45. Order: heparin 3000 units subcut q6h
    Available:

    How many milliliters should be administered?
    a. 0.2 mL
    b. 0.4 mL
    c. 0.6 mL
    d. 0.8 mL

46. Order: insulin regular 15 units subcut before breakfast
    Available:

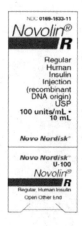

    Shade in the dosage on the syringe.

47. Order: topiramate 50 mg per day PO administered in 2 divided doses
Available:

A. What is the trade name? _____

B. What is the generic name? _____

C. What is the form? _____

D. How many capsules per dose? _____

DRUG CALCULATIONS USING BODY WEIGHT

48. Order: penicillin V potassium 200,000 units PO q6h
Child weighs 46 pounds.
Recommended child's drug dosage: 25,000–90,000 units/kg/day in 3–6 divided doses.
Available: (NOTE: The dosage per 5 mL is in mg and units.)

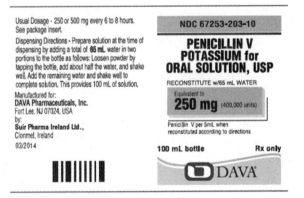

A. Is the prescribed dose in a safe range?
   a. No
   b. Yes

B. How many milliliters should the child receive for each dose?
   a. 1 mL
   b. 1.5 mL
   c. 2 mL
   d. 2.5 mL

49. Order: cefuroxime axetil 200 mg PO q12h
    Child's age: 8 years; weight: 75 pounds
    Recommended child's drug dosage (3 months–12 years): 10–15 mg/kg/day
    Available:

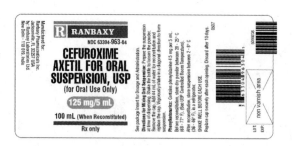

   A. Is the prescribed dose appropriate?
      a. No
      b. Yes

   B. If the 200-mg dose is given, how many milliliters should the child receive per dose?
      a. 2 mL
      b. 4 mL
      c. 6 mL
      d. 8 mL

50. Order: amoxicillin 75 mg PO q8h
    Child weighs 5 kg.
    Recommended child's drug dosage: 80–90 mg/kg/day in divided doses

   A. Is the prescribed dose appropriate?
      a. No
      b. Yes

   B. According to the order, how many milligrams would the child receive per day (24 hours)?
      a. 225 mg
      b. 400 mg
      c. 450 mg
      d. 600 mg

51. Order: acetaminophen 250 mg PO q6h PRN
    Available: 160 mg/5 mL

   How many milliliters should be administered?
      a. 3.2 mL
      b. 6 mL
      c. 7.8 mL
      d. 10 mL
      e. 12 mL

52. Order: ceftriaxone 50 mg/kg IM daily
Child weighs 8 kg.
Available:

A. How much diluent is needed? _____

B. What is the final concentration? _____

C. How many milliliters should the child receive per dose?
    a. 0.5 mL
    b. 1.1 mL
    c. 1.5 mL
    d. 2 mL
    e. 2.4 mL

53. Order: erythromycin suspension 160 mg PO q6h
Child weighs 25 kg.
Recommended child's drug dosage: 30–50 mg/kg/day in divided doses q6h
Available:

A. Is the prescribed dosage within dose parameters?
    a. Yes, the dosage is safe.
    b. No, the dosage is too low.
    c. No, the dosage is too high.

B. How many milliliters should the child receive for the ordered dosage?
    a. 0.25 mL
    b. 2 mL
    c. 3 mL
    d. 4 mL

54. Order: cefaclor 75 mg PO q8h
    Child weighs 22 pounds.
    Recommended child's drug dosage: 20–40 mg/kg/day in 3 divided doses.
    Available:

A. Calculate the minimum and maximum recommended dosage range per dose. _____

B. Is the ordered dosage appropriate? _____

C. How many milliliters per dose should be given?
   a. 2 mL
   b. 3 mL
   c. 4 mL
   d. 5 mL
   e. 6 mL

55. Order: amoxicillin/clavulanate potassium 150 mg (amoxicillin component) PO q8h
    Child weighs 26 pounds.
    Recommended child's drug dosage: 45 mg/kg/day in 3 divided doses.
    Available:

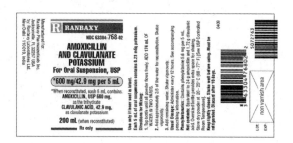

A. How many kilograms does the child weigh?
   a. 10 kg
   b. 12 kg
   c. 14 kg
   d. 15 kg

B. Is the prescribed dosage within dose parameters?
   a. Yes, the dosage is safe.
   b. No, the dosage is too low.
   c. No, the dosage is too high.

C. How many milliliters of the ordered dosage should the child receive per dose?
   a. 1.3 mL
   b. 1.5 mL
   c. 2 mL
   d. 3.5 mL

56. Order: acetaminophen 135 mg PO q6h PRN for fever
Child weighs 25 pounds.
Recommended dosage range is 10–15 mg/kg/dose q4–6h PRN.

A. What is the child's weight in kilograms? _____

B. What are the minimum and maximum safe dosage ranges? _____

C. Is the ordered dose safe? _____

57. A 3-year-old is ordered ticarcillin/clavulanic acid 50 mg/kg (ticarcillin component) IV q6h. The child weighs 23 pounds. How many milligrams will the child receive per dose? _____

58. A child with meningitis is ordered ceftriaxone 100 mg/kg/day IV divided q12h. The child weighs 65 pounds.

A. How many milligrams will the child receive per day? _____

B. How many milligrams will the child receive per dose? _____

Use the West nomogram as indicated in the following drug calculations.

59. Refer to the West nomogram and determine the BSA for the following children of normal height and weight.

A. Child weighs 5 pounds. _____

B. Child weighs 25 pounds. _____

C. Child weighs 53 pounds. _____

60. Refer to the West nomogram to determine the following BSAs.

A. A child who is 43 inches tall and weighs 54 pounds _____

B. A child who is 39 inches tall and weighs 60 pounds _____

C. A child who is 56 centimeters tall and weighs 15 kilograms _____

61. Calculate the following BSA using the square root method for inches and pounds.

A. A child weighs 25 pounds and is 32 inches tall. _____

B. A child weighs 58 pounds and is 48 inches tall. _____

C. A child is 40 inches tall and weighs 34 pounds. _____

62. Calculate the following BSAs using the square root method for centimeters and kilograms.

A. A child weighs 8 kilograms and is 28.2 centimeters long. _____

B. A child weighs 28.1 kilograms and is 133.4 centimeters tall. _____

C. A child is 85.5 centimeters tall and weighs 25 kilograms. _____

63. Order: lomustine 100 mg/m^2
Child's weight is 80 pounds; height is 40 inches tall.

A. Calculate the BSA using the West nomogram. _____

B. Calculate the BSA using the square root method and using the child's height and weight in inches and pounds.

_____

C. Using the calculated answer from B, determine the milligrams the child should receive per dose.

_____

64. Drug X 50 mg/m^2 is ordered for a child who weighs 70 pounds and is 54 inches tall.

A. What is the BSA using the square root method? _____

B. How many milligrams should the child receive? _____

65. Drug X 35 mg/m^2 is ordered for a child who weighs 43 pounds and is 52 inches tall.

A. What is the BSA using the square root method? _____

B. What is the dosage? _____

66. Drug X 134 mg/m^2 is ordered for a child who is 100 pounds and is 54 inches tall.

A. What is the BSA using the square root method? _____

B. What is the dosage? _____

67. Carmustine 225 mg/m^2 IV as a single dose every 4 weeks is ordered for a child who weighs 71 pounds and is 60 inches tall.

A. What is the BSA using the square root method? _____

B. How many milligrams should the child receive? _____

68. Methotrexate 3.3 mg/m^2 IV daily every 4 weeks is ordered for an adolescent who is 104 pounds and is 64 inches tall.

A. What is the BSA using the square root method? _____

B. How many milligrams should the adolescent receive? _____

69. Order: cyclophosphamide 350 mg/m^2
     Child's weight: 36.9 kg; height: 59 centimeters

     A. What is the child's BSA using the square root method? _____

     B. How many milligrams should the child receive? _____

70. Order: imatinib 340 mg/m^2/day PO divided into two doses
     Child weighs 47.5 kilograms and is 160 centimeters tall.

     A. What is the BSA using the square root method? _____

     B. How many milligrams should the child receive per dose? _____

DRUG CALCULATIONS FOR DRUGS REQUIRING RECONSTITUTION

71. Order: oxacillin sodium 300 mg IM q6h
     Available:

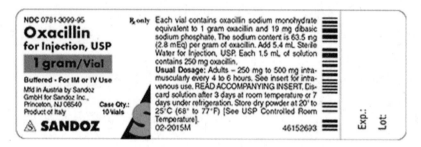

     A. The nurse must add _____ mL of sterile water to yield _____ mg/_____mL of drug solution.

     B. How many milliliters should be administered?
        a. 0.5 mL
        b. 1 mL
        c. 1.8 mL
        d. 2 mL

72. Order: nafcillin 500 mg IM q4h
     Available:

     A. The nurse must add _____ mL of diluent to yield _____ mg/mL of drug solution.

     B. How many milliliters should be administered?
        a. 1 mL
        b. 2 mL
        c. 3 mL
        d. 4 mL

73. Order: cefotetan disodium 500 mg IM q12h
    Available: (NOTE: Mix 2 mL of diluent. Once reconstituted, each mL of solution contains cefotetan 400 mg.)

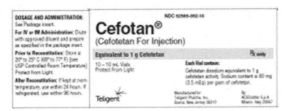

How many milliliters should be administered per dose?
a. 1 mL
b. 1.3 mL
c. 2 mL
d. 2.3 mL

74. Order: ampicillin sodium 350 mg IM q6h
    Available:

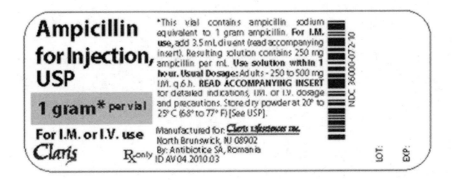

How many milliliters should be administered per dose?
a. 0.8 mL
b. 1 mL
c. 1.4 mL
d. 2 mL

75. Order: tobramycin 3 mg/kg IM in three divided doses
    Patient's weight: 184 pounds
    Available:

How many milliliters should be administered per dose?
a. 1.5 mL
b. 2.8 mL
c. 4.2 mL
d. 6.3 mL

76. The health care provider orders heparin infusion. The nurse will calculate the dosage for infusion in which of the following units of measurement?
    a. mL/h
    b. gtt/min
    c. units/h
    d. units/kg/h

77. The best method for calculating critical care drugs is:
    a. ratio and proportion method because they contain multiple steps.
    b. fractional equation method because conversion factors are not needed.
    c. basic formula method because it is the easiest.
    d. dimensional analysis because all the units of measurement and conversion factors are included in one equation.

78. When an electronic infusion device is used to deliver intravenous fluids or drugs, the nurse will calculate the flow rate in which of the following units of measurement?
    a. gtt/min
    b. units/h
    c. gtt/mL
    d. mL/h

79. When infusing intravenous fluids by gravity, the nurse will calculate the flow rate in which of the following units of measurement?
    a. gtt/min
    b. gtt/mL
    c. units/h
    d. mL/h

Match the common fluid abbreviation in Column I to the appropriate IV solution bags in Column II.

Column I

_____ 80. D$_5$ 1/2NS

_____ 81. LR or RL

_____ 82. D$_5$W

_____ 83. D$_5$NS

Column II

a.

LOT   EXP

◉   ◉   2B2324
NDC 0338-0117-04
DIN 00061085   **1**

2

Lactated Ringer's Injection USP

3

4

1000 mL
EACH 100 mL CONTAINS 600 mg SODIUM CHLORIDE USP
310 mg SODIUM LACTATE 30 mg POTASSIUM CHLORIDE USP
20 mg CALCIUM CHLORIDE USP pH 6.5 (6.0 TO 7.5) mEq/L
SODIUM 130 POTASSIUM 4 CALCIUM 2.7 CHLORIDE 109
LACTATE 28 OSMOLARITY 273 mOsmol/L (CALC) STERILE
NONPYROGENIC SINGLE DOSE CONTAINER **NOT FOR USE IN THE
TREATMENT OF LACTIC ACIDOSIS** ADDITIVES MAY BE
INCOMPATIBLE CONSULT WITH PHARMACIST IF AVAILABLE WHEN
INTRODUCING ADDITIVES USE ASEPTIC TECHNIQUE MIX
THOROUGHLY DO NOT STORE DOSAGE INTRAVENOUSLY AS
DIRECTED BY A PHYSICIAN SEE DIRECTIONS CAUTIONS
SQUEEZE AND INSPECT INNER BAG WHICH MAINTAINS PRODUCT
STERILITY DISCARD IF LEAKS ARE FOUND MUST NOT BE USED IN
SERIES CONNECTIONS DO NOT ADMINISTER SIMULTANEOUSLY
WITH BLOOD DO NOT USE UNLESS SOLUTION IS CLEAR FEDERAL
(USA) LAW PROHIBITS DISPENSING WITHOUT PRESCRIPTION
STORE UNIT IN MOISTURE BARRIER OVERWRAP AT ROOM
TEMPERATURE (25°C/77°F) UNTIL READY TO USE AVOID
EXCESSIVE HEAT SEE INSERT

5

6

7

Baxter
BAXTER HEALTHCARE CORPORATION
DEERFIELD IL 60015 USA
MADE IN USA
DISTRIBUTED IN CANADA BY
BAXTER CORPORATION
TORONTO ONTARIO CANADA
Viaflex® CONTAINER
PL 146® PLASTIC
FOR PRODUCT INFORMATION
CALL 1-800-933-0303

8

◉   ◉   **9**

b.

LOT   EXP

◉   ◉   2B0064
NDC 0338-0017-04   **1**

2

5% Dextrose Injection USP

3

4

1000 mL
EACH 100 mL CONTAINS 5 g DEXTROSE HYDROUS USP
pH 4.0 (3.2 TO 6.5) OSMOLARITY 252 mOsmol/L (CALC)
STERILE NONPYROGENIC SINGLE DOSE CONTAINER ADDITIVES
MAY BE INCOMPATIBLE CONSULT WITH PHARMACIST IF AVAILABLE
WHEN INTRODUCING ADDITIVES USE ASEPTIC TECHNIQUE MIX
THOROUGHLY DO NOT STORE DOSAGE INTRAVENOUSLY AS
DIRECTED BY A PHYSICIAN SEE DIRECTIONS CAUTIONS SQUEEZE
AND INSPECT INNER BAG WHICH MAINTAINS PRODUCT STERILITY
DISCARD IF LEAKS ARE FOUND MUST NOT BE USED IN SERIES
CONNECTIONS DO NOT ADMINISTER SIMULTANEOUSLY WITH BLOOD
DO NOT USE UNLESS SOLUTION IS CLEAR FEDERAL (USA) LAW
PROHIBITS DISPENSING WITHOUT PRESCRIPTION STORE UNIT IN
MOISTURE BARRIER OVERWRAP AT ROOM TEMPERATURE
(25°C/77°F) UNTIL READY TO USE AVOID EXCESSIVE HEAT SEE
INSERT

5

6

7

Baxter
BAXTER HEALTHCARE CORPORATION Viaflex® CONTAINER
DEERFIELD IL 60015 USA   PL 146® PLASTIC
MADE IN USA   FOR PRODUCT INFORMATION
CALL 1-800-933-0303

8

◉   ◉   **9**

c.

LOT   EXP

◉   ◉   2B1073
NDC 0338-0085-03   **–1**

–2

5% Dextrose and 0.45% Sodium Chloride Injection USP

–3

500 mL
EACH 100 mL CONTAINS 5 g DEXTROSE HYDROUS USP 450 mg SODIUM
CHLORIDE USP pH 4.0 (3.2 TO 6.5) mEq/L SODIUM 77 CHLORIDE 77
HYPERTONIC OSMOLARITY 406 mOsmol/L (CALC) STERILE
NONPYROGENIC SINGLE DOSE CONTAINER ADDITIVES MAY BE INCOMPATIBLE
CONSULT WITH PHARMACIST IF AVAILABLE WHEN INTRODUCING ADDITIVES USE
ASEPTIC TECHNIQUE MIX THOROUGHLY DO NOT STORE DOSAGE
INTRAVENOUSLY AS DIRECTED BY A PHYSICIAN SEE DIRECTIONS CAUTIONS
SQUEEZE AND INSPECT INNER BAG WHICH MAINTAINS PRODUCT STERILITY
DISCARD IF LEAKS ARE FOUND MUST NOT BE USED IN SERIES CONNECTIONS
DO NOT USE UNLESS SOLUTION IS CLEAR FEDERAL (USA) LAW PROHIBITS
DISPENSING WITHOUT PRESCRIPTION STORE UNIT IN MOISTURE BARRIER
OVERWRAP AT ROOM TEMPERATURE (25°C/77°F) UNTIL READY TO USE
AVOID EXCESSIVE HEAT SEE INSERT

–4

Baxter
BAXTER HEALTHCARE CORPORATION Viaflex® CONTAINER
DEERFIELD IL 60015 USA   PL 146® PLASTIC
MADE IN USA   FOR PRODUCT INFORMATION
CALL 1-800-933-0303

d.

LOT   EXP

◉   ◉   2B1064
NDC 0338-0089-04   **1**

2

5% Dextrose and 0.9% Sodium Chloride Injection USP

3

4

1000 mL
EACH 100 mL CONTAINS 5 g DEXTROSE HYDROUS USP
900 mg SODIUM CHLORIDE USP pH 4.0 (3.2 TO 6.5)
mEq/L SODIUM 154 CHLORIDE 154 HYPERTONIC
OSMOLARITY 560 mOsmol/L (CALC) STERILE NONPYROGENIC
SINGLE DOSE CONTAINER ADDITIVES MAY BE INCOMPATIBLE
CONSULT WITH PHARMACIST IF AVAILABLE WHEN INTRODUCING
ADDITIVES USE ASEPTIC TECHNIQUE MIX THOROUGHLY DO NOT
STORE DOSAGE INTRAVENOUSLY AS DIRECTED BY A PHYSICIAN
SEE DIRECTIONS CAUTIONS SQUEEZE AND INSPECT INNER BAG
WHICH MAINTAINS PRODUCT STERILITY DISCARD IF LEAKS ARE
FOUND MUST NOT BE USED IN SERIES CONNECTIONS DO NOT
USE UNLESS SOLUTION IS CLEAR FEDERAL (USA) LAW PROHIBITS
DISPENSING WITHOUT PRESCRIPTION STORE UNIT IN MOISTURE
BARRIER OVERWRAP AT ROOM TEMPERATURE (25°C/77°F) UNTIL
READY TO USE AVOID EXCESSIVE HEAT SEE INSERT

5

6

7

Baxter
BAXTER HEALTHCARE CORPORATION Viaflex® CONTAINER
DEERFIELD IL 60015 USA   PL 146® PLASTIC
MADE IN USA   FOR PRODUCT INFORMATION
CALL 1-800-933-0303

8

◉   ◉   **9**

Complete the following.

84. Macrodrip infusion sets deliver _____ gtt/mL; microdrip infusion sets deliver _____ gtt/mL.

85. KVO means _____. The preferred size of IV bag for KVO is (1000 mL/500 mL/250 mL). *(Circle correct answer.)*

86. The Buretrol is a (calibrated cylinder with tubing/small IV bag of solution with short tubing). *(Circle correct answer.)*

87. The pump infusion regulator that delivers mL/h is a (volumetric/nonvolumetric) IV regulator. *(Circle correct answer.)*

88. Patient-controlled analgesia is a method used to administer drugs intravenously. The purpose is to provide _____

   _____.

89. Order: 1 liter or 1000 mL of D_5W to infuse over 6 hours
   Available: Macrodrip set: 10 gtt/mL

   The IV flow rate should be _____ gtt/min.

90. Order: 1000 mL of $D_5\frac{1}{2}NS$ with 1 ampule of multiple vitamins to infuse over 8 hours
   Available: Macrodrip set: 15 gtt/mL

   Calculate the IV flow rate in gtt/min. _____

91. Order: ceftriaxone 2 g in 100 mL of 0.9% NaCl (normal saline solution) over 30 minutes
   Available: Macrodrip set: 15 gtt/mL

   Calculate the IV flow rate in gtt/min. _____

92. Order: The following IV fluids to infuse over 24 hours are ordered. They include 1 L of D_5W, 1 L of $D_5\frac{1}{2}NS$, and 500 mL of 5% D/LR.
   Available:

   A. One liter is equal to _____ milliliters.

   B. Total number of milliliters of IV solutions to infuse in 24 hours is _____ milliliters.

   C. What is the flow rate? _____

93. A liter of IV fluid was started at 7:00 am and was to infuse for 8 hours. The IV set delivers 10 gtt/mL. At 12:00 pm, only 500 mL were infused.

   A. How much IV fluid is left?
      a. 100 mL
      b. 200 mL
      c. 300 mL
      d. 400 mL
      e. 500 mL

   B. Recalculate the flow rate for the remaining IV fluids in gtt/min. _____

94. Order: cimetidine 200 mg IV q6h
     Set and solution: Buretrol with drop factor 60 gtt/mL; primary IV fluid of 500 mL of 0.9% NaCl
     Instruction: Dilute cimetidine 200 mg in 50 mL of normal saline and infuse in 15 minutes.

     A. How much cimetidine will be infused per mL?
        a. 2 mg
        b. 3 mg
        c. 4 mg
        d. 5 mg

     B. Calculate the flow rate in gtt/min.
        a. 50 gtt/min
        b. 100 gtt/min
        c. 150 gtt/min
        d. 200 gtt/min

95. Order: cefazolin 1000 mg IV q8h
     Available:

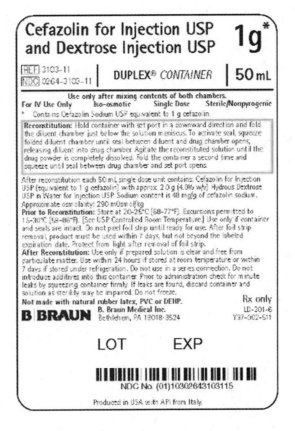

     IV tubing with drop factor, 15 gtt/mL
     Calculate IV flow rate in gtt/min to be infused over 1 hour.
     a. 6.5 gtt/min
     b. 7 gtt/min
     c. 12.5 gtt/min
     d. 13 gtt/min

96. Order: nafcillin 1000 mg IV q4h
Available:

A. How many mL of diluent should be added? _____

B. What is the drug's concentration? _____
   IV tubing available: Secondary set with drop factor 15 gtt/mL
   Instruction: Dilute nafcillin 1000 mg in 100 mL of D$_5$W and infuse in 40 minutes.

C. Calculate the flow rate.
   a. 22 gtt/min
   b. 38 gtt/min
   c. 53 gtt/min
   d. 69 gtt/min

97. Order: fluconazole 400 mg IV daily
Available:

IV tubing available: Secondary set with drop factor 15 gtt/mL

Instruction: Infuse over 2 hours.

What is the flow rate? _____

Chapter **11** **Drug Calculations**

98. Order: imipenem; cilastatin 500 mg IV q8h
    Available: imipenem; cilastatin 500 mg in 100-mL solution

NDC 63323-322-25   342025

IMIPENEM AND CILASTATIN
FOR INJECTION, USP (I.V.)

500 mg/ 500 mg* per vial   Not to be divided

* Each vial contains imipenem 500 mg (Anhydrous Equivalent) and Cilastatin Sodium equivalent to 500 mg of Cilastatin.
Inactive ingredient: sodium bicarbonate 20 mg added to each vial as a buffer. The sodium content is approximately 37.5 mg (1.6 mEq).
After suspension, vial contents must be transferred to 100 mL of infusion solution prior to intravenous infusion.

CAUTION: SINGLE DOSE VIAL / FOR I.V. USE ONLY / NOT FOR DIRECT INFUSION

Rx only   1 PACKAGE (25 Single Dose Vials)   FRESENIUS KABI

Instruction: Infuse over 30 minutes.

Calculate the gtt/min with an infusion set, 20 gtt/mL. _____

99. Order: sulfamethoxazole/trimethoprim 10 mcg/kg/d (trimethoprim component), IV divided in 2 doses. Client weighs 135 pounds.
    Available: sulfamethoxazole/trimethoprim 400 mg/80 mg per 5 mL

    Instruction: Further dilute in 250 mL of D_5W and infuse over 2 hours.

    A. What is the total dosage in micrograms for the day? _____

    B. How many micrograms for each dose?_____

    C. What is the flow rate?_____

    D. The hospital is experiencing a power failure after 20 minutes of infusion. Recalculate the flow rate in gtt/min with IV tubing, 20 gtt/mL to be infused over 1 hour and 40 minutes.

100. Order: metronidazole 500 mg IV q6h
     Available:

100 mL   NDC 0409-7811-27

METRONIDazole
Injection, USP
500 mg/100 mL (5 mg/mL)

EACH mL CONTAINS METRONIDAZOLE 5 mg; SODIUM
CHLORIDE 7.9 mg; DIBASIC SODIUM PHOSPHATE,
ANHYDROUS 0.48 mg; CITRIC ACID, ANHYDROUS
0.23 mg. SODIUM 14 mEq/100 mL. 314 mOsmol/LITER
(CALC.). pH 5.8 (4.5 to 7.0).
ADDITIVES SHOULD NOT BE MADE TO THIS SOLUTION.
DO NOT REFRIGERATE
SINGLE-DOSE CONTAINER. FOR I.V. USE. USUAL DOSAGE:
SEE INSERT. STERILE, NONPYROGENIC. PROTECT FROM
LIGHT. USE ONLY IF SOLUTION IS CLEAR AND CONTAINER
IS UNDAMAGED. MUST NOT BE USED IN
SERIES CONNECTIONS.

Rx ONLY   3 V
IM-2347   CONTAINS DEHP
MANUFACTURED BY HOSPIRA, INC., LAKE FOREST, IL 60045 USA
N+ AND NOVAPLUS ARE REGISTERED TRADEMARKS
OF NOVATION, LLC.

Instruction: Infuse in 30 minutes.

What is the flow rate?_____

101. Order: amikacin sulfate 7.5 mg/kg q12h
     Adult weight: 64 kg
     Available:

   A. How many mL would equal amikacin 400 mg? _____

       Instruction: Dilute amikacin 400 mg in 100 mL of D$_5$W and infuse in 30 min.

   B. What is the flow rate?_____

102. Order: minocycline 100 mg IV q12h
     Available: Add 5 mL of sterile water.

   Instruction: Further dilute minocycline 100 mg in 500 mL of D$_5$W and infuse in 6 hours.

   What is the flow rate? _____

103. Order: cefepime hydrochloride 1 g IV q12h
     Available:

Instruction: Drop factor, 60 gtt/mL. Infuse over 30 minutes.

What is the flow rate?_____

104. Order: ampicillin sodium/sulbactam sodium 1.5 g IV q6h
     Available: (NOTE: ADD-Vantage vials do not need further dilution.)

NDC 0409-2689-01   R$_x$ only

Ampicillin and Sulbactam for Injection, USP

1.5 grams

Sterile   For I.V. use only

Single Dose   ADD-Vantage® Vial

equivalent to
1 g of ampicillin plus
0.5 g of sulbactam   Hospira

Set and solution: IV tubing with drop factor of 15 gtt/mL

Instruction: Infuse ampicillin sodium/sulbactam sodium 1.5 g solution in 100 mL of D$_5$W over 30 minutes.

What is the flow rate? _____

105. Order: heparin 30,000 units/d continuous infusion
Available:

250 mL SINGLE-DOSE CONTAINER   NDC 0409-7794-52
RX ONLY

HEPARIN

12,500 USP Units/250 mL
(50 USP Units/mL)

**HEPARIN SODIUM IN
5% DEXTROSE INJECTION**

WARNING: CONTAINS SULFITES — 50
EACH 100 mL CONTAINS
HEPARIN SODIUM 5,000 USP
UNITS (PORCINE INTESTINAL
MUCOSA); DEXTROSE,   100
HYDROUS 5 g; CITRIC ACID,
ANHYDROUS 51 mg; SODIUM
CITRATE, DIHYDRATE
334 mg; SODIUM METABISULFITE
20 mg; ELECTROLYTES: SODIUM 150
38 mEq/L; CITRATE 42 mEq/L.
STERILE. USUAL DOSAGE: SEE
INSERT. ADDITIVES SHOULD
NOT BE MADE TO THIS
SOLUTION. LATEX-FREE. SINGLE
DOSE CONTAINER. DISCARD
UNUSED PORTION. FOR   200
INTRAVENOUS USE ONLY.

OTHER

IM-3490
HOSPIRA, INC., LAKE FOREST, IL 60045 USA   Hospira

A. How many units/h is the client receiving? _____

B. What is the flow rate? _____

106. Order: heparin bolus 80 units/kg, then maintenance infusion of 18 units/kg/h
Client's weight: 180 pounds
Available:

HEPARIN SODIUM
25,000 USP units per 250 mL
(100 USP units per mL)
in 5% Dextrose Injection

NDC 0264-9587-20

250 mL EXCEL® CONTAINER

Each 100 mL contains: Heparin
Sodium USP (porcine intestinal mucosa)
10,000 USP Heparin units; Hydrous
Dextrose USP 5 g; Dibasic Sodium
Phosphate•7H₂O USP 0.41 g; Citric
Acid Anhydrous USP 0.093 g; Sodium
Metabisulfite NF (antioxidant) <0.07 g;
Water for Injection USP qs
Electrolytes (mEq/liter): Sodium 38;
Phosphate (HPO₄⁼) 30; Citrate 15

WARNING: CONTAINS SULFITES.
Do not admix with other drugs.
Sterile. Single dose container.
For intravenous use only.
Recommended Storage: Room temperature
(25°C). Avoid excessive heat. Protect from
freezing. See Package Insert. Do not remove
overwrap until ready for use.
Not made with natural rubber latex, PVC or DEHP.
REF P5872   Rx only   OTHER

25,000 USP units per 250 mL
(100 USP units per mL)

50
100
150

BARCODE

BARCODE
200

B. Braun Medical Inc.
Bethlehem, PA 18018-3524 USA
B|BRAUN   API from Spain

A. What is the client's weight in kg? _____

B. How many units for the bolus? _____

C. Calculate the maintenance infusion flow rate. _____

107. A client was prescribed heparin sodium 18 units/kg/h; titrate according to the weight-based heparin protocol. The client's weight is 123 pounds. Heparin 25,000 units/250 mL (100 unit/mL) is available.

A. Calculate the flow rate in mL/h _____

B. aPTT is 40, and the protocol states to rebolus with 40 units/kg and increase the infusion rate by 2 units/kg/h.

How many more units did the client receive? _____ What is the new flow rate? _____

108. A client was prescribed heparin sodium 18 units/kg/h; titrate according to the weight-based heparin protocol for a patient with pulmonary embolus. The client's weight is 63 kilograms. Heparin 25,000 units/250 mL (100 units/mL) is available.

A. Calculate the flow rate in mL/h _____

B. aPTT is 45, and the protocol states to rebolus with 40 units/kg and increase infusion by 2 units/kg.

How many more units did the patient receive? _____ What is the new flow rate? _____

109. A client was prescribed heparin sodium 18 units/kg/h; titrate according to the weight-based heparin protocol. The client's weight is 70 kilograms. Heparin 12,500/250 mL (50 unit/mL) is available.

A. Calculate the flow rate in mL/h _____

B. aPTT is >90, and the protocol states to hold the infusion for 1 hour and decrease rate by 3 units/kg/h.

What is the new flow rate? _____

110. Order: diltiazem 0.25 mg/kg bolus over 2 minutes, then 15 minutes later, rebolus with 0.35 mg/kg IV, then start maintenance infusion at 10 mg/h.
Weight: 65 kg
Available:
For bolus:

For maintenance infusion:

A. What is the total bolus in milligrams? _____

B. What is the flow rate for the maintenance infusion? _____

111. Order: dobutamine 2 mcg/kg/min as a continuous infusion. Titrate according to client's hemodynamic response.
Weight: 63 kg
Available:

What is the flow rate? _____

112. Order: dobutamine 5 mcg/kg/min as a continuous infusion. Titrate according to patient's hemodynamic response.
Weight: 78 kg
Available:

A. What is the flow rate? _____

B. Nurse is to increase the dobutamine infusion by 2 mcg/kg/min. What is the new flow rate? _____

113. Order: amiodarone 0.5 mg/min
Available:

What is the flow rate? _____

114. Client is receiving nitroglycerin 0.25 mg/min for unstable angina.
Available:

LIFT HERE

250 mL
NITROGLYCERIN
200 mcg/mL
(50 mg total per container)
in 5% Dextrose Injection

℞ only   LATEX

Printed in USA
Hospira, Inc., Lake Forest, IL 60045 USA   Hospira

What is the flow rate? _____

115. Client is receiving nitroglycerin 55 mcg/min.
Available:

What is the flow rate? _____

116. Order: dobutamine 5 mcg/kg/min

Client's weight: 152 lb

Available: dobutamine 500 mg in 250 mL D_5W

What is the flow rate? _____

117. Order: dobutamine 10 mcg/kg/min

    Client's weight: 95 kg

    Available: dobutamine 1000 mg in 250 mL D$_5$W

    What is the flow rate? _____

118. Order: dopamine 5 mcg/kg/min

    Patient weights 130 lb

    Available: dopamine 800 mg in 500 mL of D$_5$W

    What is the flow rate? _____

119. Order: dopamine 300 mcg/min

    Available: dopamine 400 mg in 250 mL of D$_5$W

    What is the flow rate? _____

120. Order: heparin at 800 units/h

    Available: heparin 25,000 units in 250 mL of D$_5$W

    What is the flow rate? _____

121. Order: lidocaine 2 g in 250 mL of D$_5$W at 30 mL/h
    A. How many mg/min is the client receiving? _____
    B. What is the flow rate? _____

122. Order: nitroprusside 100 mg/250 mL D$_5$W at 29 mL/hour for hypertension

    The patient weighs 143 lb.
    A. How many mcg/kg/min of nitroprusside is the client receiving? _____
    B. What is the flow rate? _____

12 Fluid Volume and Electrolytes

Match the electrolyte in Column I with its normal value in Column II.

Column I

_____ 1. Magnesium

_____ 2. Calcium

_____ 3. Sodium

_____ 4. Potassium

_____ 5. Chloride

_____ 6. Phosphorus

Column II

a. 96–106 mEq/L
b. 135–145 mEq/L
c. 2.4–4.4 mEq/L
d. 1.5–2.5 mEq/L
e. 3.5–5 mEq/L
f. 8.6–10.2 mg/dL

Match the description in Column I with its term in Column II.

Column I

_____ 7. Similar to plasma concentration

_____ 8. Based on milliosmoles per kilogram of water

_____ 9. Solutions containing fewer particles and more water

_____ 10. Solutions having a higher solute/particle concentration

Column II

a. Osmolality
b. Isoosmolar
c. Hypoosmolar
d. Hyperosmolar

REVIEW QUESTIONS

11. The nurse has taught a client how to take oral potassium supplement. Which statement by the client indicates that more education is required?
    a. "I can take this with a few sips of water."
    b. "It may upset my stomach."
    c. "I should drink at least six ounces of water or juice when I take it."
    d. "I must not chew up the tablet."

12. A client has been diagnosed with hypokalemia and will be admitted to the hospital for potassium replacement intravenously (IV). Which action is appropriate by the nurse when preparing to give this drug?
    a. Prepare the syringe to give IV push.
    b. Push the potassium into the IV bag and do not mix before administration.
    c. Push the potassium into the IV bag and shake vigorously.
    d. Obtain an IV pump and pump tubing.

13. The nurse notices that the client's intravenous (IV) site has become erythematous and edematous while IV potassium was infusing. Which action is most appropriate by the nurse?
    a. Flush the IV site with normal saline and continue the infusion.
    b. Flush the IV site with heparin.
    c. Stop the IV and check for blood return.
    d. Discontinue the IV and restart in another site.

14. A client has been receiving intravenous potassium. The nurse notices the client is now tachycardic. What other symptom(s) might the nurse expect to see if the client is becoming hyperkalemic? *(Select all that apply.)*
    a. Abdominal distention
    b. Nausea
    c. Numbness in extremities
    d. Polyuria
    e. Hypoglycemia

15. A client is found to be hyperkalemic. Which medication will the nurse anticipate administering?
    a. Magnesium mixed in 250 mL of normal saline
    b. 0.9% saline (NS) bolus of 500 mL
    c. A fluid challenge of 250 mL of 10% dextrose in water ($D_{10}W$).
    d. Sodium bicarbonate

16. A client has been started on a enteral potassium supplement. Which teaching should be included for this patient? (*Select all that apply.*)
    a. List the signs and symptoms of both hypokalemia and hyperkalemia.
    b. Regular testing of serum potassium levels is required.
    c. The patient should increase his intake of potassium-rich foods.
    d. The drug must be taken on a full stomach or with a glass of water.
    e. The patient should sit up for 30 minutes after taking the drug.

17. Which value indicates normal range for serum osmolality?
    a. 175–195 mOsm/kg
    b. 275–295 mOsm/kg
    c. 330–350 mOsm/kg
    d. 475–495 mOsm/kg

18. Which term is used to describe the body fluid when the serum osmolality is 285 mOsm/kg?
    a. Hypoosmolar
    b. Hyperosmolar
    c. Isoosmolar
    d. Neoosmolar

19. A client with severe head trauma is receiving 3% saline. It has an osmolality of 900 mOsm/kg. This is considered to be which type of solution?
    a. Hypotonic
    b. Hypertonic
    c. Isotonic
    d. Neotonic

20. By which route is the majority of potassium excreted?
    a. Feces
    b. Kidneys
    c. Liver
    d. Lungs

21. A client has pancreatitis. The nurse knows the client is at risk for which electrolyte abnormality? (*Select all that apply.*)
    a. Hypocalcemia
    b. Hypernatremia
    c. Hypomagnesemia
    d. Hyperkalemia

22. The nurse is teaching the client about calcium absorption and includes the health teaching that vitamin D is needed for calcium absorption. Which area the body does vitamin D help in calcium absorption?
    a. Large intestine
    b. Small intestine
    c. Kidneys
    d. Liver

23. Calcium is distributed bound and unbound to proteins in which proportions?
    a. 25%:75%
    b. 50%:50%
    c. 75%:25%
    d. 90%:10%

24. A client is prescribed 2 liters of intravenous (IV) fluids: 1000 milliliters (mL) of 5% dextrose in water (D_5W) followed by 1000 mL of 5% dextrose in 0.45% sodium chloride ($D_5\frac{1}{2}$ NS). Which term classifies these fluids?
    a. Colloids
    b. Crystalloids
    c. Lipids
    d. Parenteral nutrition

25. A client is in the hospital overnight after having surgery and the nurse has received an order to start 5% dextrose in 0.45% sodium chloride ($D_5\frac{1}{2}$ NS) intravenously. $D_5\frac{1}{2}$ NS is considered which type of fluid?
    a. Hypotonic
    b. Hypertonic
    c. Isotonic
    d. Normotonic

26. A client is receiving high-molecular-weight dextran after an explosion has burned over 50% of the body. Which action describes the purpose of dextran?
    a. Temporarily restore circulating volume
    b. Serve as a line to infuse blood into
    c. Piggyback fluid for antibiotics
    d. Whole blood substitute

27. Which body fluid has a similar electrolyte composition to lactated Ringer solution?
    a. Plasma
    b. Skin
    c. Tears
    d. White blood cells

28. A client is taking potassium chloride and hydrochlorothiazide. The client's serum potassium level is 2.4 mEq/L. Which clinical manifestations would the nurse expect to see in this client? *(Select all that apply.)*
    a. Bradycardia
    b. Headache
    c. Muscle weakness
    d. Nausea
    e. Anorexia

29. Magnesium deficiencies are frequently associated with which other electrolyte imbalance?
    a. Hypocalcemia
    b. Hyperkalemia
    c. Hyponatremia
    d. Hyperphosphatemia

30. A client with a serum potassium level of 3.2 mEq/L asks why potassium supplement was prescribed. Which response by the nurse is most appropriate?
    a. "Your potassium level is 3.2 mEq/L which is low and should be corrected."
    b. "You will only be on the drug for a few days, so don't worry."
    c. "You obviously aren't taking enough in your diet, so you have to take this."
    d. "Have you been constipated lately? Constipation will cause a low potassium level."

31. A client with lab results of Na$^+$ 150 mEq/L, K$^+$ 4.2 mEq/L, Cl$^-$ 100 mEq/L, Ca^{++} 9.8 mEq/L, Mg$^+$+ 1.8 mg/dL, PO$_4^-$ 3.1 mEq/L has which electrolyte abnormality?
    a. Hypocalcemia
    b. Hyperkalemia
    c. Hypernatremia
    d. Hypomagnesemia

32. A client with a serum potassium level of 6.1 mEq/L will exhibit which clinical manifestation(s)? *(Select all that apply.)*
    a. Abdominal cramps
    b. Muscle weakness
    c. Oliguria
    d. Paresthesias of the face
    e. Tachycardia and later bradycardia

33. Which drugs are used to treat hyperkalemia? *(Select all that apply.)*
    a. Digoxin and furosemide
    b. Glucagon and magnesium
    c. Glucose and insulin
    d. Sodium polystyrene sulfonate and sorbitol
    e. Sodium bicarbonate and calcium gluconate

34. A client has had diarrhea for several days and has a serum calcium level of 7.2 mg/dL. Which clinical manifestations will the nurse expect to see in this client? *(Select all that apply.)*
    a. Hyperactive deep tendon reflexes
    b. Irritability
    c. Numbness of the fingers
    d. Pathologic fractures
    e. Tetany

CASE STUDY

Read the scenario and answer the following questions on a separate sheet of paper.

D.M., 28 years old, has been stabbed multiple times in the chest and abdomen. Vital signs on arrival include blood pressure 84/62 mm Hg, heart rate 118 beats/minute, respiratory rate 30 breaths/minute, pulse oximetry 94% on room air, and temperature 96.4° F.

1. What is the priority assessment for this client?

2. What types of fluids would the nurse anticipate to be ordered?

3. Explain the advantage of using whole blood versus packed red blood cells.

13 Vitamin and Mineral Replacement

Match the appropriate word or phrase in Column I with the letter of the fat- or water-soluble vitamins in Column II. The vitamin listed in Column II will be used more than once.

Column I

_____ 1.   Vitamin A

_____ 2.   Vitamin B complex

_____ 3.   Vitamin C

_____ 4.   Vitamin D

_____ 5.   Vitamin E

_____ 6.   Vitamin K

_____ 7.   Toxic in excessive amounts

_____ 8.   Metabolized slowly

_____ 9.   Minimal protein binding

_____ 10. Readily excreted in urine

_____ 11. Slowly excreted in urine

Column II

a.   Fat-soluble vitamins
b.   Water-soluble vitamins

Match the appropriate vitamin in Column I with the letter of the common food sources in Column II.

Column I

_____ 12. Vitamin A

_____ 13. Vitamin B_{12}

_____ 14. Vitamin C

_____ 15. Vitamin D

_____ 16. Vitamin E

Column II

a.   Salmon, egg yolk, milk
b.   Wheat germ, egg yolk, avocado
c.   Fish, liver, egg yolk
d.   Green and yellow vegetables
e.   Tomatoes, pepper, citrus fruits

Label the *ChooseMyPlate* diagram with the appropriate food groups.

17.

a. _____

b. _____

c. _____

d. _____

e. _____

REVIEW QUESTIONS

Select the best response.

18. Regulation of calcium and phosphorous metabolism and calcium absorption from the intestine is a major role of which vitamin?
    a. A
    b. B_{12}
    c. C
    d. D

19. A client who just gave birth wants to know why the baby needs vitamin K. Which response is appropriate by the nurse?
    a. "It will help the baby's digestive tract work better."
    b. "Vitamin K helps a baby maintain its temperature."
    c. "Vitamin K helps the blood to clot."
    d. "This will help prevent infections for the first month."

20. Protection of red blood cells from hemolysis is a role of which vitamin?
    a. A
    b. D
    c. E
    d. K

21. During a well-woman exam, a young female client is interested in becoming pregnant and asks the nurse what supplements she should take. Which response is best for the nurse to provide?
    a. "Folic acid supplements are recommended in women who may become pregnant to prevent neural tube defects."
    b. "Vitamin A 8000 units should be taken to promote bone growth."
    c. "Megadoses of iron are important for blood formation."
    d. "Vitamin C 1600 mg should be taken to prevent colds, which are more common in pregnancy."

22. The client has been involved in a motorcycle collision and has lost 1500 mL of blood from a pelvic fracture. Which mineral is essential for regeneration of hemoglobin?
    a. Chromium
    b. Copper
    c. Iron
    d. Selenium

23. The client has a history of heavy alcohol abuse. The client presents to the emergency department confused, combative, and complaining of double vision. The family states the client has become very forgetful recently. The nurse will anticipate that the prescriber will order which substance for this client?
    a. Vitamin C
    b. Vitamin B_1
    c. Dextrose
    d. Vitamin B_6

24. Which vitamin or mineral is responsible for collagen synthesis?
    a. Vitamin C
    b. Vitamin D
    c. Iron
    d. Zinc

25. The client takes an antacid for reflux and an iron supplement for anemia. Which information will the nurse include in client education regarding these drugs?
    a. "The drugs help each other do its job."
    b. "Iron and antacids must be taken on alternate days."
    c. "Antacids will decrease iron absorption."
    d. "Iron will decrease the effectiveness of the antacids."

26. A client is advised to drink a liquid iron preparation through a straw because it may cause which side effect?
    a. Bleeding gums
    b. Esophageal varices
    c. Corroded tooth enamel
    d. Tooth discoloration

27. Which client might be at most risk for vitamin A deficiency?
    a. A 36-year-old pregnant client
    b. An 18-year-old client with celiac disease
    c. A 74-year-old client with a urinary tract infection
    d. A 33-year-old client with sickle cell anemia

28. Vitamin A is stored in the liver, kidneys, and fat. By which route is it excreted?
    a. Rapidly through the bile and feces
    b. Slowly through the urine and feces
    c. Rapidly through the bile only
    d. Slowly through the feces only

29. A 24-year-old client has been prescribed large doses of vitamin A as treatment for acne. Which advise will the nurse provide to this client? *(Select all that apply.)*
    a. Contact the health care provider concerning drug dosing.
    b. Report peeling skin, anorexia, or nausea and vomiting to the health care provider.
    c. Do not exceed the recommended dosage without consulting the health care provider.
    d. Avoid alcohol consumption.
    e. Megadoses of vitamin A are necessary for several months to alleviate acne.

30. The client has a history of tuberculosis and is on isoniazid therapy. The client presents to the clinic with complaints of numbness and weakness in to the hands and feet. Which vitamin supplement might be considered for his condition?
    a. Niacin
    b. Pyridoxine
    c. Riboflavin
    d. Thiamine

31. The client with sustained burns to 40% of his body and is receiving long-term parenteral nutrition would be at risk for which mineral deficiency?
    a. Copper
    b. Iron
    c. Selenium
    d. Zinc

32. Chromium is thought to be helpful in control of which condition?
    a. Alzheimer disease
    b. Common cold
    c. Type 2 diabetes
    d. Raynaud phenomenon

33. Which food is high in copper?
    a. Broccoli
    b. Grapefruit
    c. Lamb
    d. Shellfish

34. The client presents to the emergency department with an overdose of the oral anticoagulant warfarin. The nurse will anticipate administration of which vitamin for this client?
    a. B_2
    b. C
    c. E
    d. K

CASE STUDY

Read the scenario and answer the following questions on a separate sheet of paper.

A client with a history of atrial fibrillation and on the anticoagulant warfarin is seen in the clinic for routine blood work to monitor the international normalized ratio (INR). While obtaining client's drug history, it was discovered that the client has been taking various vitamins, including vitamins E, C, and A. The client also has been on a "health conscious" diet, consuming large amounts of fresh fruits and vegetables and fresh fish.

1. Describe the mechanisms of action for vitamins A, C, and E and the potential complications of hyper-vitaminosis.

2. Discuss the drug–drug and drug–food interactions that can occur with warfarin.

3. What education should the nurse provide?

14 Nutritional Support

STUDY QUESTIONS

Complete the following.

1. Adequate nutritional support is needed for the body's _____ _____.

2. A critically ill person requires _____ more than the normal energy requirement.

3. In addition to nutritional support, _____ and _____ balance must be considered.

4. A _____ _____ _____ should be used when considering enteral nutrition.

5. The gastrostomy tube, also known as a _____ tube, is placed _____, _____,

    or _____.

Answer the following questions as true or false. If the statement is false, reword the sentence to make it true.

_____ 6. Early enteral nutrition restores intestinal motility and maintains GI function.

_____ 7. Nutritional support is considered if the patient has had little or no nutrition for more than 5 days.

_____ 8. Parenteral and enteral nutrition are synonymous and are delivered through the same route.

_____ 9. Nasoduodenal, nasojejunal, and jejunostomy enteral nutrition deliver food below the pyloric sphincter.

Label the following.

10. Label the routes for enteral feedings.

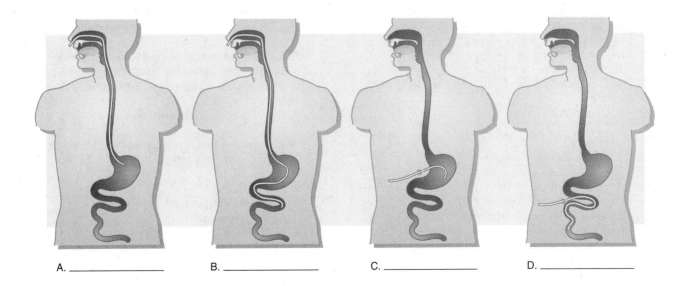

A. _____   B. _____   C. _____   D. _____

Match the terms in Column I with the descriptions in Column II.

Column I

_____ 11. Bolus

_____ 12. Intermittent

_____ 13. Continuous

_____ 14. Cyclic

Column II

a. Feeding given every 3–6 hours for 30–60 minutes by gravity infusion
b. Feeding given continuously into the small intestine
c. Feeding infused over 8–16 hours per day
d. 250–400 mL given at one time; used for ambulatory patients

REVIEW QUESTIONS

Select the best response.

15. The older adult client has a history of hypertension, arthritis, and diabetes. Which category of formula for enteral feeding would the nurse anticipate?
    a. Specialty
    b. Polymeric
    c. Immune modulating
    d. Modular

16. The client with a functional gastrointestinal (GI) system is at risk for aspiration because of difficulty swallowing. Which supplemental nutrition does the nurse anticipate will be ordered?
    a. Enteral via nasogastric tube
    b. Parenteral via peripheral IV
    c. Parenteral via central IV
    d. Enteral via jejunostomy tube

17. Which enteral feeding is administered over 30–60 minutes by pump infusion?
    a. Bolus
    b. Continuous
    c. Gravity
    d. Intermittent

18. The client who sustained full-thickness burns to the face 2 months ago is now undergoing skin grafting and wound repair and requires nutritional support. The nurse understands that the best way to administer nutrition to this patient is through which route?
    a. Continuous.
    b. Cyclic.
    c. Gravity.
    d. total parenteral nutrition (TPN).

19. A client with ulcerative colitis exacerbation has been prescribed total parenteral nutrition (TPN) for 8 weeks. Which site will the nurse select to administer TPN?
    a. Accessory vein
    b. Brachiocephalic vein
    c. Radial vein
    d. Subclavian vein

20. Which percentage of carbohydrates is provided by total parenteral nutrition (TPN)?
    a. < 10%
    b. 10–20%
    c. 25–50%
    d. 60–70%

21. The client sustained a severe head injury and is on continuous enteral tube feedings. These feedings are commonly administered over which time frame?
    a. over 30–60 minutes.
    b. over 24 hours.
    c. over 15 minutes.
    d. over 8–16 hours.

22. Which side effect is commonly associated with enteral nutrition? *(Select all that apply.)*
    a. Constipation
    b. Diarrhea
    c. Urinary retention
    d. Yeast infection

23. The nurse withdraws 170 mL of gastric residual in a client receiving enteral nutrition by means of continual feeding. Which action is most appropriate by the nurse?
    a. Discontinue enteral nutrition and change to TPN.
    b. Immediately notify the health care provider.
    c. Stop the feeding for 30–60 minutes and recheck.
    d. Switch to a formula with more fiber.

24. Which reasons would enteral feedings be used before total parenteral nutrition (TPN)? *(Select all that apply.)*
    a. Less costly
    b. Less risk of aspiration
    c. Lower risk of infection
    d. Maintenance of GI integrity
    e. Promotes better wound healing

25. Which complication(s) is/are associated with the use of total parenteral nutrition (TPN)? *(Select all that apply.)*
   a. Air embolism
   b. Aspiration
   c. Hyperglycemia
   d. Pneumothorax

CASE STUDY

Read the scenario and answer the following questions on a separate sheet of paper.

M.B., 35 years old, sustained severe trauma from a roll-over motor vehicle collision. M.B. has been on total parenteral nutrition (TPN) for several weeks and is being transitioned to enteral feeding through a nasogastric tube before a gastrostomy tube is placed.

1. What steps must be performed to transition a patient from TPN to enteral nutrition?

2. What precautions will the nurse take to prevent aspiration?

15 Adrenergic Agonists and Antagonists

Match the term in Column I with the letter of the description in Column II.

Column I

_____ 1. Alpha$_1$ blocker

_____ 2. Beta blocker

_____ 3. Selectivity

_____ 4. Sympathomimetic

_____ 5. Sympatholytic

Column II

a. Blocks action of sympathetic nervous system
b. Has a greater affinity for certain receptors
c. Causes vasodilation
d. Causes decreased heart rate
e. Similar in action to stimulation of the sympathetic nervous system

Complete the following.

6. Adrenergic receptors are located on the _____ cells of smooth muscles.

7. Bladder relaxation and urinary sphincter constriction resulting in urinary retention may occur with high doses of _____ agonists.

8. Sympathomimetics (do/do not) pass into the breast milk. *(Circle correct answer.)*

9. Adrenergic blockers are also called _____.

10. The antidote for infiltration intravenously (IV) of alpha- and beta-adrenergic drugs such as norepinephrine and dopamine is _____.

11. A beta-adrenergic blocker that can be given for migraine or hypertension is _____.

12. Mood changes such as depression and suicidal tendencies are possible when taking which type of adrenergic blocker? _____

13. Carvedilol, penbutolol, and pindolol are examples of selective/nonselective beta blockers. *(Circle correct answer.)*

14. Nonselective beta blockers, such as propranolol, are contraindicated in patients with _____ and _____.

15. What is most likely to occur if a patient is taking an adrenergic agonist with an adrenergic blocker? _____

Match the letter of the adrenergic response in Column I to the associated receptor in Column II (Receptors in Column II may be used more than once, and response may affect more than one receptor type.)

Column I

_____ 16. Increases gastrointestinal relaxation

_____ 17. Increases force of heart contraction

_____ 18. Dilates pupils

_____ 19. Decreases salivary secretions

_____ 20. Inhibits release of norepinephrine

_____ 21. Dilates bronchioles

_____ 22. Increases heart rate

_____ 23. Promotes uterine relaxation

_____ 24. Dilates blood vessels

Column II

a. Alpha$_1$
b. Alpha$_2$
c. Beta$_1$
d. Beta$_2$

REVIEW QUESTIONS

Select the best response.

25. A client with asthma asks the nurse how albuterol inhaler will work to help breathe better. Which response by the nurse best explains the action of the drug?
   a. "Albuterol will increase your heart rate so you will feel like you are able to breathe better."
   b. "Albuterol causes the airways to open up more in the lungs, improving function."
   c. "Albuterol will cause an increase in urinary output to remove extra fluid from the lungs."
   d. "Albuterol causes bronchial smooth muscle contraction that forces air into the lungs."

26. A client presents to the clinic with a swollen face and tongue, difficulty breathing, and audible wheezes after eating a peanut butter sandwich for lunch. Which action would the nurse first take?
   a. Ensure a patent airway.
   b. Obtain an electrocardiogram (ECG).
   c. Administer 1 mg of 1:1000 epinephrine subcutaneously.
   d. Start an intravenous (IV) normal saline.

27. A client calls the home health agency to tell the nurse about shaking and trembling after using the albuterol inhaler. Which question would the nurse first ask the client?
   a. "Are you having any other symptoms?"
   b. "How long ago did this start?"
   c. "When was the last time you used your inhaler?"
   d. "How many puffs on the inhaler did you take?"

28. Which drug(s) is/are classified as beta blockers? (*Select all that apply.*)
   a. Albuterol
   b. Atenolol
   c. Propranolol
   d. Amphetamine
   e. Acebutolol

29. The nurse discovers an intravenous (IV) site has infiltrated on a client receiving intravenous (IV) dopamine. The nurse prepares to administer which drug as an antidote.
   a. dobutamine
   b. epinephrine
   c. phentolamine
   d. reserpine

30. When completing the client health history, the nurse finds a history of narrow-angle glaucoma. When performing the drug reconciliation, which drug would concern the nurse? (*Select all that apply.*)
   a. Pseudoephedrine
   b. Midodrine
   c. Albuterol
   d. Carvedilol

31. Some over-the-counter (OTC) drugs for cold symptoms contain substances that have sympathetic properties. These drugs are contraindicated in clients with which disease process?
   a. Allergic rhinitis
   b. Hypertension
   c. Orthostatic hypotension
   d. Chronic bronchitis

32. Which adrenergic drug used in emergency settings does not decrease renal function?
    a. Norepinephrine
    b. Dopamine
    c. Phenylephrine
    d. Dobutamine

33. Beta$_1$ receptors are located in which area of the body? (*Select all that apply.*)
    a. Gastrointestinal tract
    b. Lungs
    c. Kidneys
    d. Brain
    e. Heart

34. A client tells the nurse during the admitting history that alternative and complementary therapies are used to help manage medical conditions. Which drug would raise a concern in a client taking St. John's wort?
    a. Reserpine
    b. Albuterol
    c. Propranolol
    d. Pseudoephedrine

35. A nurse received an order for timolol 100 mg b.i.d. Which action is most appropriate by the nurse?
    a. Give the client the drug after proper identification.
    b. Hold the drug, and contact the health care provider regarding the dosage.
    c. Give the drug now, and request a new order during patient rounds.
    d. Assess the client's vital signs, and give the drug.

36. Catecholamine can be best defined by which statement?
    a. A substance that can produce a sympathomimetic response
    b. Another name for a beta blocker
    c. A type of decongestant
    d. A receptor site in the lungs

CASE STUDY

Read the scenario, and answer the following questions on a separate sheet of paper.

R.G. is a 34-year-old client who sustained a bee sting and had an allergic reaction. R.G. has been prescribed an epinephrine auto-injector.

1. What are the mechanisms of action and indications for the epinephrine auto-injector?

2. How should the drug be stored?

3. Describe how the client should administer the drug.

16 Cholinergic Agonists and Antagonists

STUDY QUESTIONS

Match the term in Column I with the mechanism of action in Column II.

Column I

_____ 1.   Acetylcholine (ACh)

_____ 2.   Anticholinergic

_____ 3.   Anticholinesterase

_____ 4.   Cholinergic agonists

_____ 5.   Cholinesterase

_____ 6.   Muscarinic receptor

_____ 7.   Nicotinic receptor

_____ 8.   Direct-acting parasympathomimetic

Column II

a.   Stimulates smooth muscle and slows heart rate
b.   Impacts skeletal muscles
c.   Stimulates muscarinic and nicotinic receptors
d.   Stimulate the parasympathetic system
e.   Blocks the action of acetylcholine
f.   Mimics cholinergic actions
g.   Blocks the breakdown of acetylcholine
h.   Causes the breakdown of acetylcholine

Labeling

9.   Identify cholinergic effects to the different organs affected by the parasympathetic nervous system.

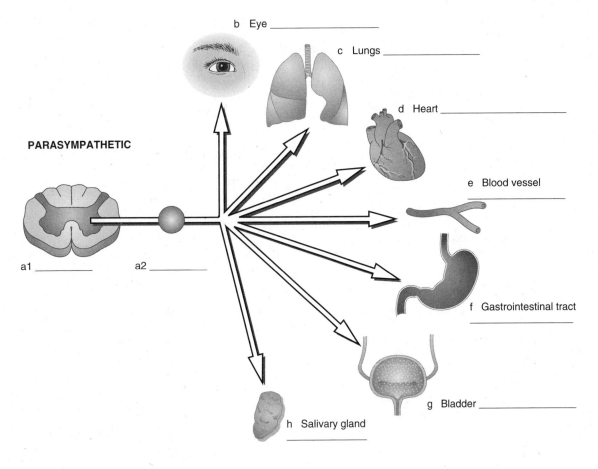

b Eye _____

c Lungs _____

d Heart _____

e Blood vessel _____

PARASYMPATHETIC

a1 _____   a2 _____

f Gastrointestinal tract _____

g Bladder _____

h Salivary gland _____

Select the best response.

10. Which drug would the nurse anticipate administering to a client who ingested an organophosphate poison?
    a. Bethanechol
    b. Edrophonium chloride
    c. Metoclopramide
    d. Pralidoxime chloride

11. The pediatric client has urinary retention. Which cholinergic drug does the nurse anticipate will be prescribed to increase urination?
    a. Bethanechol
    b. Edrophonium chloride
    c. Metoclopramide
    d. Neostigmine bromide

12. Anticholinergic eyedrops are used for which purpose?
    a. Constrict the pupils
    b. Dilate the pupils
    c. Decrease the intraocular pressure
    d. Detect astigmatism

13. A client with narrow-angle glaucoma is prescribed an anticholinergic drug. Which action would be a priority by the nurse?
    a. Administer the medication as ordered after verifying the patient's identity.
    b. Give only one-half of the prescribed dose.
    c. Hold the dose and contact the health care provider.
    d. Wait until after the patient has taken glaucoma medication and then give the drug.

14. Which type of medication is bethanechol?
    a. Anticholinergic
    b. Cholinergic agonist
    c. Cholinesterase inhibitor
    d. Sympatholytic

15. Which statement describes the mechanism of action for bethanechol?
    a. Inhibits muscarinic receptors
    b. Inhibits nicotinic receptors
    c. Stimulates muscarinic receptors
    d. Stimulates nicotinic receptors

16. The client who was prescribed bethanechol asks the nurse how it works. Which response would be most appropriate by the nurse?
    a. "This drug decreases bladder tone."
    b. "This drug inhibits bladder contraction."
    c. "This drug promotes contraction of the bladder."
    d. "This drug stimulates urine production."

17. Which outcome to the body would occur from receiving large doses of cholinergic drugs? *(Select all that apply.)*
    a. Decreased blood pressure
    b. Decreased salivation
    c. Increased bronchial secretions
    d. Mydriasis
    e. Urinary retention

18. The client has been prescribed bethanechol and is experiencing decreased urinary output. Which action would be a priority by the nurse?
    a. Catheterize the client to drain the bladder and measure output.
    b. Encourage the client to increase fluid intake to increase urinary output.
    c. Encourage the client to relax when urinating.
    d. Notify the health care provider with current intake and output values.

19. The client has been taking bethanechol and is experiencing flushing, sweating, nausea, and abdominal cramps. Which action would be best for the nurse to take?
    a. Document the client's manifestations.
    b. Give the client a laxative.
    c. Increase the client's fluid intake.
    d. Obtain an order to administer atropine.

20. Which drug treats myasthenia gravis by increasing muscle strength?
    a. Bethanechol
    b. Edrophonium chloride
    c. Neostigmine bromide
    d. Pilocarpine

21. The nurse is taking care of five clients in the emergency department. Which client(s) would be candidate(s) to receive atropine? *(Select all that apply.)*
    a. A client having surgery for appendicitis
    b. A client with a heart rate of 38 beats/minute and dizziness
    c. A client with paralytic ileus
    d. A client with urinary retention
    e. A client with gastric ulcers

22. The nurse would question an order for atropine for which client?
    a. A client with a peptic ulcer
    b. A client with parkinsonism
    c. A client with cirrhosis
    d. A client with narrow-angle glaucoma

23. The client with new diagnosis of peptic ulcers was prescribed propantheline. Which substance would the nurse teach that is a priority point for nutrition?
   a. Calcium
   b. Fat
   c. Fiber
   d. Protein

24. Which teaching point(s) will the nurse include for a client taking hyoscyamine for irritable bowel syndrome? *(Select all that apply.)*
   a. Ensure adequate fluid intake.
   b. Do not drive until you are aware of how this drug will affect your vision.
   c. Sucking on hard candy may help with dry mouth.
   d. Increased sweating is a common side effect.
   e. Report a rapid heart rate to your health care provider.

25. Anticholinergic drugs are contraindicated in clients with which disease processes? *(Select all that apply.)*
   a. Coronary artery disease
   b. Diabetes mellitus
   c. Gastrointestinal obstruction
   d. Supraventricular tachycardia

26. A specific group of anticholinergics may be prescribed in the early treatment of which neuromuscular disorder?
   a. Multiple sclerosis
   b. Muscular dystrophy
   c. Myasthenia gravis
   d. Parkinsonism

27. The older adult client is taking benztropine for symptoms associated with parkinsonism. The nurse will instruct the client to report which clinical manifestation(s) to the health care provider? *(Select all that apply.)*
   a. Diarrhea
   b. Dizziness
   c. Hallucinations
   d. Hyperthermia
   e. Palpitations

CASE STUDY

Read the scenario and answer the following questions on a separate sheet of paper.

H.H., 65 years old, has just received a prescription for tolterodine tartrate for treatment of urinary incontinence.

1. What is the mechanism of action of this drug?

2. What are some of the major side effects?

3. What are some contraindications for tolterodine tartrate?

4. Discuss key teaching points for the nurse to provide when educating H.H.

17 Stimulants

STUDY QUESTIONS

Complete the following.

1. The central nervous system involves the _____ and the _____ _____.

2. Attention-deficit/hyperactivity disorder can be caused by a _____ of neurotransmitters.

3. Amphetamines stimulate the release of neurotransmitters _____ and _____, and can lead to cardiovascular problems.

4. Anorexiants have a/an _____ effect on the brain to _____ _____.

5. Central nervous system stimulants, also referred to as _____, stimulate respiration.

REVIEW QUESTIONS

Select the best response.

6. Which medical condition(s) is/are central nervous system (CNS) stimulants approved to treat? *(Select all that apply.)*
   a. Attention-deficit/hyperactivity disorder (ADHD)
   b. Anorexia
   c. Narcolepsy
   d. Obesity
   e. Posttraumatic stress disorder (PTSD)

7. An adult client has been prescribed methylphenidate for the treatment of narcolepsy. The client presents to the clinic with hand tremors and feelings of nervousness. Which priority teaching consideration(s) should be included for this client? *(Select all that apply.)*
   a. Avoid operating hazardous equipment.
   b. Caffeine should be avoided.
   c. Nervousness and tremors may occur.
   d. Take the medication before meals.
   e. Report any weight gain.

8. Which drug group acts on the brainstem and medulla to stimulate respiration?
   a. Amphetamine
   b. Analeptic
   c. Anorexiant
   d. Triptan

9. An adolescent client is being treated with methylphenidate for attention-deficit/hyperactivity disorder (ADHD). What common effects should the client and family be informed might occur? *(Select all that apply.)*
   a. Euphoria
   b. Headache
   c. Hypertension
   d. Irritability
   e. Hypotension
   f. Vomiting

10. To maintain the half-life of immediate-release methylphenidate, how often should this drug be taken?
    a. Daily
    b. 2 to 3 times a day
    c. 4 times a day
    d. Every other day

11. The client has been prescribed phentermine hydrochloride for obesity. The client also has Parkinson disease and takes selegiline. Which nursing action would the nurse do before the client starts the new drug?
    a. Contact the client's primary health care provider to verify the prescription.
    b. Have baseline lab work drawn to assess liver function.
    c. Tell the client to immediately stop taking the selegiline.
    d. Tell the client to increase fluid intake with the next meal.

12. An overweight client has a history of migraines, depression, and hypertension and has been started on phentermine-topiramate. For which condition is phentermine-topiramate used?
   a. Attention-deficit/hyperactivity disorder (ADHD)
   b. Asthma
   c. Narcolepsy
   d. Short-term weight management

13. The pediatric client has been started on methylphenidate for attention-deficit/hyperactivity disorder (ADHD). Which information should the nurse include in the health teaching?
   a. Constipation is a common side effect.
   b. Counseling should be combined with drug.
   c. This drug will only be used for a few weeks.
   d. Weight gain is to be expected.

14. Which statement(s) is/are true of methylphenidate? (Select all that apply.)
   a. If taken with monoamine oxidase inhibitors (MAOIs), it may increase a hypertensive crisis.
   b. The effects of anticoagulants may increase.
   c. Hyperglycemia may occur.
   d. Insulin will be more effective.
   e. There may be increased effects if taken with caffeinated beverages.

15. An 18-year-old client is brought to the emergency department by the roommates. Blood pressure is 220/136 mm Hg, heart rate 142 beats/minute, and respiratory rate 20 breaths/minute. the client is responsive only to deep pain. Client's roommates report the client was trying to lose weight and has been taking "these pills obtained over the Internet." Which medical condition would the nurse consider as the most likely cause for this client's symptoms?
   a. Cardiac arrest
   b. Food poisoning
   c. Hemorrhagic stroke
   d. Pregnancy-induced hypertension

16. Central nervous system (CNS) stimulants are absolutely contraindicated for clients with a history of which condition(s)? (Select all that apply.)
   a. Coronary artery disease
   b. Diabetes
   c. Hypothyroidism
   d. Hypertension
   e. Glaucoma

17. A neonate born at 28 weeks' gestation is scheduled to receive caffeine citrate 20 mg/kg intravenously shortly after birth. The neonate's mother asks, "Why are you giving my baby stuff that is in coffee?" Which statement made by the nurse is most appropriate?
   a. "Caffeine can help your baby breathe better."
   b. "It will help your baby gain weight faster."
   c. "The baby's temperature will be warmer with caffeine."
   d. "This isn't the same substance that is in coffee."

CASE STUDY

Read the scenario, and answer the following questions on a separate sheet of paper.

A new nurse started at a school where more than 75 students take methylphenidate for attention-deficit/hyperactivity disorder (ADHD). The majority of the students come in between 11:30 AM and 12:30 PM for their medication.

1. What are the pharmacokinetics and pharmacodynamics for methylphenidate?

2. What are the nursing implications for giving these drugs at school regarding timing, monitoring, and health teaching for the students, families, and teachers?

18 Depressants

Identify the induction time for the following anesthetics—slow or rapid:

1. Halothane _____

2. Enflurane _____

3. Methoxyflurane _____

4. Midazolam _____

5. Propofol _____

6. Nitrous oxide _____

Complete the following.

7. The broad classification of CNS depressants includes the following seven groups: _____, _____, _____, _____, _____, _____, and _____.

8. The two phases of sleep are _____ and _____.

9. The mildest form of CNS depression is _____.

10. Anesthesia (may/may not) be achieved with high doses of sedative-hypnotics. *(Circle correct answer.)*

11. Procaine hydrochloride is used in local anesthesia as a short/moderate/long-acting anesthetic *(Circle correct answer.)*

12. General anesthesia depresses the _____ system, alleviates _____, and causes a loss of _____.

13. Surgery is performed during the _____ stage of anesthesia. The other three stages are _____, _____, and _____.

14. Bupivacaine and tetracaine are drugs commonly used for _____ anesthesia.

15. A major potential adverse effect of spinal anesthesia is _____.

16. A type of spinal anesthesia used for patients in labor is a(n) _____.

17. Muscle relaxants (are/are not) part of balanced anesthesia. *(Circle correct answer.)*

18. Drugs used to induce sleep in those who have difficulty getting to sleep are _____-acting barbiturates.

19. One example of a nonbenzodiazepine drug for the treatment of insomnia is _____. *(Answers may vary.)*.

20. The drug of choice for the management of benzodiazepine overdose is _____.

21. Local anesthetics are divided into two groups: _____ and _____.

Match the common side effect of sedative-hypnotics in Column I with the letter of the description in Column II .

Column I		Column II
_____ 22.	Hangover	a. Need to increase dosage to get desired effect
_____ 23.	REM rebound	b. Suppression of respiratory center in the medulla
_____ 24.	Dependence	c. Skin rashes
_____ 25.	Tolerance	d. Residual drowsiness
_____ 26.	Respiratory depression	e. Results in withdrawal symptoms
_____ 27.	Hypersensitivity	f. Vivid dreams and nightmares

REVIEW QUESTIONS

Select the best response.

28. Which class of drug is the most commonly pre-scribed drug to assist patients with sleep disorders?
    a. Analeptic
    b. Anesthetic
    c. Sedative-hypnotic
    d. Triptan

29. Which drugs may be prescribed to control seizures?
    a. Intermediate-acting barbiturates
    b. Long-acting barbiturates
    c. Short-acting barbiturates
    d. Ultra–short-acting barbiturates

30. A client returns to the unit after having surgery with spinal anesthesia. Which action(s) would be best for the nurse to take to decrease the possibility of spinal headache? *(Select all that apply.)*
    a. Administer morphine 1 to 2 mg intravenously (IV).
    b. Ambulate the client as soon as she regains sensation.
    c. Encourage the client to stay flat in bed.
    d. Increase fluid intake.
    e. Position the patient in high-Fowler's position.

31. The client who will be receiving spinal anesthesia for surgery is positioned with the back arched. The client asks "Why do I have to sit a certain way? Why can't I just be comfortable?" Which statement would be best for the nurse to provide to the client?
    a. "It is easier for the anesthesiologist if you sit this way."
    b. "Because of your age, you have to sit straight up."
    c. "The anesthesia is injected in a specific area so it distributes evenly."
    d. "You can sit however you like."

32. The client is postoperative day 3 from major ortho-pedic surgery and is unable to sleep. If nonpharma-cologic measures have not been effective, what drug does the nurse anticipate may be ordered?
    a. Flumazenil
    b. Phenobarbital
    c. Triazolam
    d. Zolpidem

33. Which type(s) of anesthesia is/are administered us-ing lidocaine? *(Select all that apply.)*
    a. General
    b. Inhaled
    c. Intravenous
    d. Local
    e. Spinal

34. The client works 12-hour night shifts one week and 12-hour day shifts the next week. the client tells the nurse that "some kind of sleeping pill from the drugstore" is used to help with sleep. What does the nurse suspect is the most likely main ingredient in the over-the-counter sleep drug?
    a. Antihistamines
    b. Barbiturates
    c. Benzodiazepines
    d. Opioid agonists

35. The 71-year-old client presents to the health care provider with complaints of inability to go to sleep and inability to stay asleep. Which question(s) will the nurse ask to further evaluate the complaint? *(Select all that apply.)*
   a. "What are your bedtime routine?"
   b. "How many caffeinated beverages do you drink per day?"
   c. "Do you take naps?"
   d. "Do you sleep with the windows open?"
   e. "Are you taking diuretics?"

CASE STUDY

Read the scenario and answer the following questions on a separate sheet of paper.

F.B., 42-years-old, is scheduled for a laparoscopic chole-cystectomy. F.B. has had a bad experience with anesthesia before and is very anxious.

1. What drugs might be prescribed before F.B.'s surgery for anxiety?

2. Explain the principles of balanced anesthesia.

19 Antiseizure Drugs

STUDY QUESTIONS

Match the seizure type in Column I with its definition in Column II.

_____ 1. Absence seizure

_____ 2. Partial seizure

_____ 3. Generalized seizure

_____ 4. Myoclonic seizure

_____ 5. Simple seizure

a. Involves one hemisphere of the brain with no loss of consciousness

b. Can be focal or massive with jerky movements lasting 10 seconds or less

c. No loss of consciousness and can have a motor, sensory, autonomic, or psychic form

d. Loss of consciousness usually lasts less than 10 seconds; also called petit mal seizures

e. A seizure that involves both hemispheres of the brain with loss of consciousness

Complete the following.

6. To diagnose epilepsy, results of a(n) _____ are useful.

7. Seventy-five percent of all epilepsy is primary or _____.

8. The International Classification of Seizures describes the two categories of seizures as _____ and _____.

9. Antiseizure drugs suppress abnormal electrical impulses, thus _____ the seizure, but they (do/do not) eliminate the cause. *(Circle correct answer.)*

10. Antiseizure drugs (are/are not) used for all types of seizures. *(Circle correct answer.)*

11. The first anticonvulsant used to treat seizures was _____, discovered in 1938, and today is the most commonly used drug for seizures.

12. It is strongly recommended that the patient check with the health care provider before taking _____ products.

13. Administration of phenytoin via the (oral/intramuscular/intravenous) route is not recommended because of its erratic absorption rate. *(Circle correct answer.)*

REVIEW QUESTIONS

Select the best response.

14. The client with a history of bipolar disorder recently experienced tonic-clonic seizures. Which drug would the nurse expect to be prescribed for this client? *(Select all that apply.)*
    a. Carbamazepine
    b. Diazepam
    c. Ethosuximide
    d. Acetazolamide

15. The client has a seizure disorder and has just discovered that she is pregnant. At her first prenatal visit, she tells the nurse, "I quit taking all of my drugs because I don't want anything to be wrong with my baby." What is the nurse's best response?
    a. "You can't do that. You have to take your medications."
    b. "What drugs have been prescribed for you?"
    c. "How long have you had seizures?"
    d. "When was your last seizure?"

16. Which anticonvulsant(s) is/are appropriate for status epilepticus? *(Select all that apply.)*
    a. Fosphenytoin
    b. Carbamazepine
    c. Phenobarbital
    d. Diazepam
    e. Topiramate

17. The client has just been diagnosed with epilepsy and will be starting phenytoin. The client's spouse asks how this drug works in the body. What is the nurse's best response?
    a. "It inhibits the enzyme that destroys one of the neurotransmitters."
    b. "It helps stop the entry of sodium into the cell."
    c. "It has not been determined exactly how it prevents seizures."
    d. "It increases the amount of calcium that enters the cell."

18. The client has just been diagnosed with a seizure disorder and has been started on valproic acid. What statement(s) by the client indicate(s) to the nurse more instruction regarding the drug is needed? *(Select all that apply.)*
    a. "I just have to remember to take it once a day."
    b. "I do not have to worry about labs."
    c. "I need to take it at the same times every day."
    d. "This drug will cure my seizures."

19. The nurse has received an order to administer an initial dose of intravenous (IV) phenytoin to a client with new-onset seizures. What will the nurse check before administering the first dose? *(Select all that apply.)*
    a. Hourly urine output
    b. Blood glucose levels
    c. Cardiac rhythm
    d. Blood pressure measurements

20. The client receiving intravenous (IV) phenytoin for grand mal seizures complains of burning at the IV site. What is the nurse's best action?
    a. Call the health care provider immediately to change the drug to oral.
    b. Continue the infusion and reassure the patient.
    c. Flush the line with 10 mL of normal saline and continue the infusion.
    d. Discontinue the IV and restart the IV infusion at a different site.

21. A client was started on an antiseizure drug for a seizure disorder of unknown cause and asks how long the drug will need to be taken. Which response is appropriate by the nurse?
    a. "You will need to take an anticonvulsant of some type for your lifetime."
    b. "This drug should be taken until you haven't had a seizure for a month."
    c. "Seizures are unpredictable and so is the duration of the treatment."
    d. "You will only need to take it for a short period of time because antiseizures will cure the seizure disorder."

22. Which result is within the therapeutic range for phenytoin?
    a. 8 mcg/mL of bound phenytoin
    b. 18 mcg/mL of bound phenytoin
    c. 28 mcg/mL of unbound phenytoin
    d. 38 mcg/mL of unbound phenytoin

23. Which information would the nurse document after witnessing a client having seizure?? *(Select all that apply.)*
    a. Types of movements
    b. Duration of movements
    c. Ability to stop movements
    d. Progression of movements
    e. Preceding events

24. The nurse is preparing discharge teaching for a client who has been started on phenytoin for a seizure disorder. Which information about the side effects of this drug will the nurse provide to the client and family member?
    a. "There may be a green discoloration of the patient's urine."
    b. "It is best to use a hard-bristle toothbrush for dental care."
    c. "Nosebleeds and sore throats should be reported to the health care provider."
    d. "The patient should get up slowly to prevent fainting."

25. Which effect would the nurse expect to see if the client is experiencing a common side effect of phenytoin?
    a. Gingival hyperplasia
    b. Excessive thirst
    c. Weight gain
    d. Muscle tremors

26. A client presents to the emergency department in status epilepticus. Which drug would the nurse anticipate being ordered first?
    a. Diazepam
    b. Midazolam
    c. Propofol
    d. Phenobarbital

27. Which statement(s) is/are true about seizures and antiseizure uses in pregnancy? *(Select all that apply.)*
    a. Seizures may increase up to 33% in women with history of seizures.
    b. Many antiseizure drugs have teratogenic properties.
    c. Antiseizure drug use increases the loss of folic acid.
    d. Antiseizure drugs increase the effects of vitamin K.
    e. Valproic acid causes malformation in 40% to 80% of fetuses.

28. Which antiseizure drug may also be used as prophylaxis for migraine headaches?
    a. Diazepam
    b. Phenytoin
    c. Valproic acid
    d. Clorazepate

CASE STUDY

Read the scenario and answer the following questions on a separate sheet of paper.

A.R., a 30-year-old elementary school teacher, missed several appointments with the primary care provider for management of tonic-clonic seizures. A.R. states, "I just can't take the carbamazepine. I can't function with it." Primary care provider prescribes oxcarbazepine, instead.

1. What will the nurse discuss with the patient regarding oxcarbazepine?

2. What information should the nurse provide about antiseizure drugs and pregnancy?

20 Drugs for Parkinson's and Alzheimer Disease

Match the description in Column I with the letter of the reference in Column II.

Column I

_____ 1. Acetylcholinesterase (AChE) inhibitor

_____ 2. Dopamine agonist

_____ 3. Dystonic movement

_____ 4. Bradykinesia

_____ 5. Pseudo parkinsonism

Column II

a. Stimulates dopamine receptors
b. Drug-induced parkinsonism
c. Allows more acetylcholine in the neuron receptors
d. Involuntary abnormal movements
e. Slowed movements

Complete the following.

6. The two neurotransmitters within the neurons of the striatum of the brain that have opposing effects are _____ and _____.

7. Which of the neurotransmitters is deficient in Parkinson disease? _____

8. A drug used in a combination therapy to treat Parkinson disease by replacing the neurotransmitter is _____.

9. The substance that inhibits the enzyme dopa decarboxylase and allows more levodopa to reach the brain is _____.

10. An example of an acetylcholinesterase inhibitor is _____.

11. Acetylcholinesterase inhibitors _____ transmission at the cholinergic synapses.

12. The drug _____ prolongs action of levodopa and can decrease "on-off" fluctuations in patients with parkinsonism.

13. The drugs that are a combination of dopaminergic and a catechol-*O*-methyltransferase (COMT) inhibitor that provides the greatest dosing flexibility include _____, _____, and _____.

14. An example of a Food and Drug Administration (FDA)–approved anticholinergic drug used for Parkinson disease is _____.

Select the best response.

15. A client taking carbidopa-levodopa tablets for parkinsonism is complaining of dizziness, diarrhea, anxiety, and nasal stuffiness. Which complaints would the nurse recognize as a possible side effect of carbidopa-levodopa?
    a. Dizziness
    b. Diarrhea
    c. Anxiety
    d. Nasal stuffiness

16. The nurse is teaching a client with parkinsonism about extended-release carbidopa-levodopa. Which statement(s) by the client indicate(s) the need for further teaching? *(Select all that apply.)*
    a. "This drug may make my movements smoother."
    b. "My skin may turn yellow if I miss too many doses."
    c. "If I have trouble swallowing, I can crush my drug and mix it with applesauce."
    d. "I must take this medicine on an empty stomach."
    e. "I need to check my blood sugar regularly while taking this drug."

17. The nurse is helping a family prepare for a grocery shopping trip for a client who has been prescribed selegiline for Parkinson disease. Which food(s) should be avoided? *(Select all that apply.)*
    a. Aged cheeses
    b. Chocolate
    c. Peanut butter
    d. Wheat bread
    e. Yogurt

18. A client with Alzheimer disease is taking rivastigmine and has also been started on a drug for depression. Which order will the nurse question before administering the new drug?
    a. Atypical antidepressant
    b. Monoamine oxidase inhibitor (MAOI) antidepressant
    c. Selective serotonin reuptake inhibitor (SSRI) antidepressant
    d. Tricyclic antidepressant

19. A client with parkinsonism currently takes carbidopa-levodopa, and the client's health care provider adds entacapone to the drug regimen. Which change in the dosing of carbidopa-levodopa would the nurse expect to occur?
    a. There should be no change in the drug dosage.
    b. Both carbidopa and levodopa dosages should be decreased.
    c. Only the levodopa dosage should decrease.
    d. Only the carbidopa dosage should decrease.

20. Anticholinergics are contraindicated for which client?
    a. A client with glaucoma
    b. A client with shingles
    c. A client with urinary frequency
    d. A client with diabetes
    e. A client with angina

21. A client with a history of Parkinson disease is brought into the emergency department after the family reports the client is talking to "rabbits coming out of the walls" at home. Which drug does the nurse suspect may have caused this symptom? *(Select all that apply.)*
    a. Bromocriptine mesylate
    b. Selegiline hydrochloride
    c. Pramipexole dihydrochloride
    d. Tolcapone

22. A client's wandering and hostility levels have increased per family reports. Which dosing information would concern the nurse in this client who is taking memantine 10 mg/day?
    a. The dose is too high a daily dose to maintain mental status.
    b. The client has taken an overdose of the drug.
    c. The client is not taking enough of the drug.
    d. A combination of memantine and amantadine may be needed.

23. Which statement by the client indicates an understanding of how to relieve some of the side effects associated with the use of benztropine mesylate?
    a. "I can suck on hard candy or chew sugarless gum to prevent dry mouth."
    b. "I need to take my drug every 6 hours so I don't get constipated."
    c. "I should decrease the doses of all of my other drugs so I don't get dizzy."
    d. "I should urinate after meals so I do not retain urine."

CASE STUDY

Read the scenario and answer the following questions on a separate sheet of paper.

J.T. is a 75-year-old who has been diagnosed with Alzheimer disease. J.T. will be living with the daughter and granddaughter. J.T.'s health care provider has prescribed rivastigmine 3 mg bid.

1. Explain the progressive decline of Alzheimer disease.

2. How does rivastigmine work?

3. What are some of the safety measures the daughter and granddaughter can utilize to help J.T. stay safe in the new home?

21 Drugs for Neuromuscular Disorders and Muscle Spasms

Match the classifications of multiple sclerosis (MS) in Column I with the definition in Column II.

Column I

_____ 1.   Relapsing remitting MS

_____ 2.   Primary progressive MS

_____ 3.   Secondary progressive MS

_____ 4.   Progressive relapsing MS

Column II

a.   May have relapses, remissions, and plateaus
b.   Relapse with full recovery and residual deficit
c.   Clear acute relapses with or without full recovery
d.   Will have slowly worsening symptoms with no relapses or remissions

Complete the following.

5.   Muscle spasms can result from _____ injuries and spasticity from chronic _____ _____.

6.   Muscle relaxants suppress the _____ reflex and are prescribed for muscle spasms that do not respond

     to _____ drugs or other forms of therapy.

7.   Baclofen, dantrolene, and tizanidine are some drugs to _____ pain and _____ mobility
     for hyperexcitable, spastic muscles.

SHORT ANSWER QUESTIONS

Identify the affected neuromuscular site(s) for each of the autoimmune neuromuscular disorders and the drugs to treat the disorders.

8.   Myasthenia gravis

9.   Multiple sclerosis

Select the best response.

10. The nurse is assessing a client who is receiving treatment for myasthenia gravis with pyridostigmine. Which clinical manifestations would be noted if the drug is working?
    a. Increased salivation
    b. Maintenance of muscle strength
    c. Miosis
    d. Tachycardia

11. The client is receiving treatment for myasthenia gravis with an acetylcholinesterase (AChE) inhibitor. The nurse observes that the client is diaphoretic, drooling, and eyes are tearing. What will concern The nurse would be most concerned about the client exhibiting these clinical manifestations in which medical condition?
    a. Client is having an anaphylactic reaction.
    b. Client is having a cholinergic crisis.
    c. Client is in the early stages of myasthenic crisis.
    d. Client is having a vascular spasm.

12. Which emergency drug will be administered to a client exhibiting signs of cholinergic crisis?
    a. Atropine
    b. Diazepam
    c. Neostigmine
    d. Pyridostigmine

13. The client presents to the health care provider with complaints of double vision, headache, and muscle weakness. The client states that these symptoms come and go every few weeks, but these "spells" seem to be getting closer together. Which diagnostic test is likely to be ordered if multiple sclerosis is considered?
    a. Angiography
    b. Computerized tomography (CT) scan
    c. Magnetic resonance imaging (MRI)
    d. Myelogram

14. The client has been receiving pyridostigmine. Which drug when ordered by the health care provider should the nurse question before administering to the client?
    a. Histamine$_2$ blocker
    b. Propranolol
    c. Cephalosporin
    d. Tetracycline

15. The client has been prescribed azathioprine and interferon-β for remissions and exacerbations of multiple sclerosis. The client inquires, "How will this help me feel better?" Which response is appropriate by the nurse?
    a. "These drugs will help form new neurons and axons."
    b. "They will improve muscle strength."
    c. "They will reduce spasticity and improve muscular movement."
    d. "They will stop the progression of the disease."

16. The client has multiple sclerosis and is experiencing muscle spasms. Centrally acting muscle relaxants improve spasms by which mechanism?
    a. They affect *mu* receptors to decrease pain.
    b. They decrease pain and increase range of motion.
    c. They decrease inflammation of the peripheral nerves.
    d. They speed conduction to improve flexibility.

17. The client has been involved in a motor vehicle collision and has been prescribed methocarbamol for muscle spasms of the neck and back. Which side effect(s) should the nurse discuss with the client before discharge? *(Select all that apply.)*
    a. Urine discoloration
    b. Diarrhea
    c. Drowsiness
    d. Increased appetite

18. Which drug order should the nurse question before administration?
    a. Dantrolene sodium for muscle spasms
    b. Diazepam for narrow-angle glaucoma
    c. Acetylcholine receptor (AChR) antibody for diagnostic testing for myasthenia gravis
    d. Chlorzoxazone for muscle trauma

CASE STUDY

Read the scenario and answer the following questions on a separate sheet of paper.

G.D., 24-years-old, was involved in a high-speed rollover motor vehicle accident and has a spinal cord injury. G.D. has muscle spasms and some spasticity to the lower extremities bilaterally. G.D. has intermittently been prescribed carisoprodol and will be started on baclofen.

1. Why do muscle spasms occur in patients with spinal cord injuries?

2. What is the mechanism of carisoprodol? How does baclofen work?

3. What are the side effects of each drug?

Antipsychotics and Anxiolytics

STUDY QUESTIONS

Match the term in Column I to the corresponding statement in Column II.

Column I

_____ 1. Acute dystonia

_____ 2. Akathisia

_____ 3. Anxiolytics

_____ 4. Neuroleptic

_____ 5. Psychosis

_____ 6. Schizophrenia

_____ 7. Tardive dyskinesia

_____ 8. Extrapyramidal symptoms

Column II

a. Losing contact with reality
b. Protrusion and rolling of the tongue, sucking and smacking movements of the lips, chewing motion
c. Muscle tremors, rigidity, shuffling gait
d. Restlessness, inability to sit still, foot-tapping
e. Spasms of tongue, face, neck, and back
f. Used to treat anxiety and insomnia
g. Drug that modifies psychotic behavior
h. Chronic psychotic disorder

Complete the following.

9. Antipsychotic drugs were developed to improve the _____ _____, _____, and _____ of patients with psychotic symptoms resulting from an imbalance of _____, a neurotransmitter.

10. Typical antipsychotics are subdivided into phenothiazines and nonphenothiazines. Nonphenothiazines are divided into four classes: _____, _____, _____, and _____.

11. The most common side effect of all antipsychotics is _____.

12. Antipsychotics may lead to dermatologic side effects early in drug therapy that include _____ and _____.

13. Phenothiazines (increase/decrease) the seizure threshold; adjustment of anticonvulsants may be required. *(Circle correct answer.)*

14. Anxiolytics (are/are not) usually given for secondary anxiety. *(Circle correct answer.)*

15. Long-term use of anxiolytics is not recommended because _____ may develop within weeks or months.

16. The action of anxiolytics resembles that of _____, not antipsychotics.

Match the following drugs in Column I with their drug classification in Column II. Drug classifications in Column II may be used more than once.

Column I

_____ 17. Clozapine

_____ 18. Chlorpromazine

_____ 19. Fluphenazine

_____ 20. Molindone hydrochloride

_____ 21. Haloperidol

_____ 22. Risperidone

Column II

a. Phenothiazine
b. Nonphenothiazine
c. Atypical antipsychotic

REVIEW QUESTIONS

Select the best response.

23. Neuroleptic drugs are useful in the management of which type of medical condition?
    a. Anxiety disorders
    b. Depressive disorders
    c. Psychotic disorders
    d. Psychosomatic disorders

24. A client who was started on antipsychotic drugs asks the nurse when the drug will take effect. Which response is best by the nurse?
    a. "It may take up to one week to start to feel the full effects."
    b. "Responses vary, but it may be about 6 weeks."
    c. "You will only feel better when you start psychotherapy, too."
    d. "You should start to feel better within 30-60 minutes."

25. The client has been started on chlorpromazine hydrochloride for treatment of intractable hiccups. Which information will the nurse include in client education about this class of drug?
    a. "A therapeutic response to this drug will be immediate."
    b. "Change positions slowly from sitting to standing to prevent orthostatic hypotension."
    c. "It is all right to have alcohol when taking this drug."
    d. "This drug may be stopped abruptly as soon as your pain stops."

26. Typical antipsychotics may cause extrapyramidal symptoms (EPS) or pseudoparkinsonism. Which symptom is considered an extrapyramidal symptom?
    a. Downward eye movement
    b. Intentional tremors
    c. Loss of hearing
    d. Shuffling gait

27. Which drug would the nurse expect to give to decrease extrapyramidal symptoms (EPS)?
    a. Benztropine
    b. Bethanechol
    c. Buspirone hydrochloride
    d. Doxepin

28. Phenothiazines are grouped into three categories based on their side effects. In which group is fluphenazine?
    a. Aliphatic
    b. Piperazine
    c. Piperidine
    d. Thioxanthene

29. The client has been prescribed fluphenazine for treatment of schizophrenia. Which information should the nurse include in the client teaching for this drug? *(Select all that apply.)*
    a. "Blood pressure changes are not an indication of an adverse reaction."
    b. "It is all right to take all herbal drugs when taking fluphenazine."
    c. "Notify your health care provider if you have dizziness, headache, or nausea."
    d. "This medication must be taken every day."
    e. "You should not drink alcohol when taking this drug."

30. An 80-year-old client with diminished renal and hepatic function is prescribed fluphenazine 5 mg every 8 hours for a newly diagnosed schizophrenia. Which statement is correct about the amount of the drug prescribed?
    a. Nothing. The client is an adult, and this is in the normal adult range.
    b. The client's dose should be 10% less than the young and middle - adult dose.
    c. The client's dose should be 25% to 50% less than the usual young and middle-adult dose.
    d. This drug is contraindicated in clients who are greater than 70 years old.

31. A client presents to the emergency department with an overdose of chlorpromazine hydrochloride. Which action is a priority for the nurse to take?
    a. Administer activated charcoal.
    b. Administer anticholinergic drugs.
    c. Establish an intravenous (IV) site.
    d. Maintain the airway.

32. A highly agitated and combative client presents to the emergency department. The health care provider has ordered haloperidol 5 mg intramuscularly (IM). Which statement is correct about this medication when giving it as an antipsychotic?
    a. It has a sedative effect on agitated, combative patients.
    b. It is the drug of choice for older patients with liver disease.
    c. It will not cause extrapyramidal syndrome (EPS).
    d. It can safely be used in patients with narrow-angle glaucoma.

33. Which drug class consists of atypical antipsychotics?
    a. Butyrophenones
    b. Phenothiazines
    c. Serotonin/dopamine antagonists
    d. Thioxanthenes

34. The atypical antipsychotics have a weak affinity for the dopamine subtype 2 (D_2) receptors. Consequently, which outcome to the occurrence of extrapyramidal syndrome (EPS) is correct?
    a. An absence of EPS
    b. An increase in EPS
    c. Fewer EPS
    d. No effect on EPS

35. Atypical antipsychotics have a stronger affinity for which type of dopamine subtype receptors that block serotonin receptors?
    a. D_1
    b. D_2
    c. D_3
    d. D_4

36. A young adult client with bipolar disorder has just been prescribed risperidone. Which side effect should the nurse include in the health teaching about this drug?
    a. Hepatotoxicity
    b. Hyperglycemia
    c. Hearing loss
    d. Urinary frequency

37. The drug alprazolam belongs to which anxiolytic drug group?
    a. Antihistamines
    b. Benzodiazepines
    c. Buspirones
    d. Phenothiazines

38. In which patient(s) is/are fluphenazine contraindicated? (Select all that apply.)
    a. A client with narrow-angle glaucoma
    b. A client in a coma
    c. A client with subcortical brain damage
    d. A client with continued blood dyscrasias despite lowering dose
    e. A client with neuromuscular pain

39. Lorazepam is an anxiolytic drug; however, it may be prescribed for other purposes. For which other condition(s) might it be prescribed? (Select all that apply.)
    a. Alcohol withdrawal
    b. Anxiety associated with depression
    c. Muscle spasms
    d. Preoperative induction
    e. Status epilepticus

CASE STUDY

Read the scenario, and answer the following questions on a separate sheet of paper.

H.K., a young college student, is brought to the emergency department. H.K.'s friends say H.K. had been trying to "cram for finals." They have been unable to awaken H.K. after sleeping for 18 hours. An empty bottle of clonazepam and a bottle of vodka were found at the bedside. Vital signs are temperature 99° F, heart rate 64 beats/minute, respiratory rate 8 breaths/minute, blood pressure 82/40 mm Hg, O_2 saturation 78% on room air. H.K. is only responsive to deep pain.

1. What class of drug is clonazepam?

2. What is its mechanism of action?

3. What are the side effects associated with this category of drug?

4. With the above history, what is concerning to the nurse, and what are the priority actions?

23 Antidepressants and Mood Stabilizers

Answer the following questions as true or false. If false, make it into a true statement.

1. _____ Herbal supplements, such as St. John's wort, do not interact with selective serotonin reuptake inhibitors.

2. _____ Tyramine-rich foods include aged cheese, yogurt, and soy sauce.

3. _____ Monoamine oxidase inhibitors (MAOIs) are considered first-line therapy for depression.

4. _____ Amitriptyline is considered a serotonin norepinephrine reuptake inhibitor (SNRI).

5. _____ Causes of depression include decreased circulating neurotransmitter levels or the occurrence of major stressors such as the recent death of a family member.

Complete the following.

6. Clinical response of tricyclic antidepressants (TCAs) occurs after _____ of drug therapy.

7. TCAs _____ mood, _____ interest in daily living, and _____ insomnia.

8. Herbal supplements that can be used to treat mild depression include _____.

9. Atypical antidepressants or _____ _____ affect one or two of the three neurotransmitters: _____, _____, and _____.

10. Any drugs that _____ the _____ can cause a hypertensive crisis when taken with an MAOI.

11. _____ was the first drug used to treat _____ _____ disorder.

12. Lithium's therapeutic index has a _____ range from _____.

13. Nonsteroidal antiinflammatory drugs (NSAIDs) can _____ lithium level whereas _____ and _____ diuretics can _____ lithium levels.

14. SNRIs are used for major depression, _____, and _____.

15. Many antidepressants interact with _____ _____ that can lead to _____.

Match the drugs in Column I with the neurotransmitters affected in Column II. The neurotransmitters in Column II may be used more than once.

Column I

_____ 16. Amitriptyline

_____ 17. Fluoxetine

_____ 18. Venlafaxine

_____ 19. Doxepin

_____ 20. Citalopram

_____ 21. Duloxetine

_____ 22. Selegiline

Column II

a. Dopamine
b. Norepinephrine
c. Serotonin

Match the drugs in Column I with their drug classification in Column II. The drug classifications in Column II may be used more than once.

Column I

_____ 23. Trazodone

_____ 24. Maprotiline

_____ 25. Citalopram

_____ 26. Amitriptyline

_____ 27. Tranylcypromine

_____ 28. Paroxetine

Column II

a. Atypical antidepressants
b. Selective serotonin reuptake inhibitors (SSRIs)
c. Monoamine oxidase inhibitors (MAOIs)
d. Tricyclic antidepressants (TCAs)

REVIEW QUESTIONS

Select the best response.

29. Which drug would the nurse expect to administer to a young client with enuresis?
    a. Citalopram
    b. Fluvoxamine
    c. Imipramine
    d. Sertraline

30. The client has been taking phenelzine for several months for depression, which has not improved. Which dose is the maximum daily dose for this drug?
    a. 15 mg/day
    b. 45 mg/day
    c. 60 mg/day
    d. 90 mg/day

31. The client has been prescribed amitriptyline as an adjunct to therapy for depression. Which information will the nurse include in the health teaching regarding this drug?
    a. "Check your heart rate daily. It may become very slow."
    b. "Stand up slowly because your blood pressure can drop suddenly."
    c. "You should start to feel less depressed within 12 hours."
    d. "Take your drug in the morning because it will make you alert."

32. Which food(s) or beverage(s) is/are contraindicated in a client that is prescribed isocarboxazid? *(Select all that apply.)*
    a. Bananas
    b. Chocolate
    c. Chicken
    d. Milk
    e. Wine

33. A client who has been taking fluoxetine and "some herb" for depression is complaining of a severe headache. The client is diaphoretic and restless. Which herb does the nurse suspect the client has been taking?
    a. Ephedra
    b. Ginseng
    c. Garlic
    d. St. John's wort

34. Which effect is an advantage of taking selective serotonin reuptake inhibitors (SSRIs) over tricyclic antidepressants (TCAs)?
    a. Fewer sexual side effects
    b. Increased appetite
    c. Less sedation
    d. Less tachycardia

35. Which nursing intervention is most important for a client taking lithium?
    a. Advising the client that the drug can be stopped when not in a manic phase
    b. Emphasizing the importance of client-adjusted dosage
    c. Monitoring for excessive thirst, weight gain, and increased urination
    d. Teaching the client to limit fluid intake to prevent weight gain

36. The client is currently taking lithium for bipolar disorder, manic phase. Which laboratory value would the nurse monitor?
    a. BUN
    b. Blood glucose
    c. INR
    d. Platelet count

37. The client has been taking lithium 1800 mg/day in three divided doses for 10 days. The client remains agitated and hyperactive, with a lithium level of 0.7 mEq/L. Which client condition would the nurse suspect is occurring?
    a. The patient is experiencing lithium toxicity.
    b. The patient's lithium level is subtherapeutic.
    c. The patient's lithium level is therapeutic.
    d. The patient is allergic to lithium.

38. The nurse is teaching the client about lithium. Which statement by the client indicates a need for more education?
    a. "I can stop my drug if I have not been manic for 2 weeks."
    b. "I should avoid caffeine products that may aggravate the manic phase."
    c. "I should take my drug with food."
    d. "It is important that I wear or carry ID indicating that I am taking lithium."

39. The client has been prescribed venlafaxine for generalized anxiety disorder. Which statement by the client indicates the need for further health teaching?
    a. "I need to take my drug even if I am not feeling anxious."
    b. "I need to wear sunscreen when I am outdoors."
    c. "If I have any issues with my sexual performance, I can ask my health care provider."
    d. "It is OK if I keep taking my herbal drugs for my depression and anxiety."

40. The client with a history of bipolar disorder and is taking lithium is considering pregnancy. Which teratogenic effects can occur when taking lithium while pregnant? *(Select all that apply.)*
    a. Congenital anomaly
    b. Excessive weight gain
    c. Hyperemesis gravidarum
    d. Heart defects
    e. Multiple gestation

CASE STUDY

Read the scenario and answer the following questions on a separate sheet of paper.

F.K., 53-years-old female, has recently relocated to start a new job after the current position of 20 years was eliminated. F.K. was prescribed fluoxetine 20 mg at bedtime for complaints of insomnia, sadness, tearfulness, and inability to concentrate. F.K. tells the nurse, "I can't believe I lost my job and have to start over. I feel like such a failure." She is postmenopausal and has a history of hypertension and migraines.

1. Discuss SSRIs and their mechanism of action.

2. What questions should the nurse ask in the initial interview?

3. What discharge health education regarding fluoxetine should the nurse provide?

24 Antiinflammatories

Match the term in Column I with the definition in Column II.

Column I

_____ 1. Acetylsalicylic acid (ASA)

_____ 2. Indomethacin

_____ 3. Ketorolac

_____ 4. Fenamate

_____ 5. Oxicam

_____ 6. Immunomodulator

_____ 7. Colchicine

_____ 8. Allopurinol

_____ 9. Celecoxib

Column II

a. Disrupts the inflammatory process and delays disease progression

b. Indicated for long-term arthritic conditions

c. One of the first nonsteroidal antiinflammatory drugs (NSAIDs) introduced

d. Oldest antiinflammatory drug

e. The first injectable NSAID

f. The first drug used to treat gout

g. Drug of choice for patients with chronic tophaceous gout

h. Potent class of NSAID used for acute and chronic arthritic conditions

i. Cyclooxygenase inhibitor

Complete the following.

10. Inflammation is a response to tissue _____ and _____.

11. The five cardinal signs of inflammation are _____, _____, _____,

_____, and _____.

12. Leukocyte infiltration of the inflamed tissue occurs during the _____ phase of inflammation.

13. The half-life of each NSAID (does/does not) differ greatly. *(Circle correct answer.)*

14. When using NSAIDs for inflammation, the dosage is generally _____ than that for pain relief.

15. Corticosteroids are indicated to control _____ flareups.

Select the best response.

16. Which body response occurs during the vascular phase of inflammation?
    a. Leukocyte and protein infiltration into inflamed tissue
    b. Vasoconstriction with leukocyte infiltration into inflamed tissue
    c. Vasoconstriction and fluid influx into the interstitial space
    d. Vasodilation with increased capillary permeability

17. A client who is taking nonsteroidal antiinflammatory drugs (NSAIDs) for arthritis complains of persistent heartburn. What further question(s) should the nurse ask the client about the heartburn? *(Select all that apply.)*
    a. "Do you take your drug with food?"
    b. "Have you been drinking an increased amount of water?"
    c. "Have you noticed a change in the color of your bowel movements?"
    d. "What dosage of the NSAID are you taking?"
    e. "Where is the heartburn located?"

18. When preparing discharge teaching for a client who has been prescribed ibuprofen for arthritis, Which statement would the nurse provide to the client on the mechanism of action?
    a. "Ibuprofen is a COX-2 inhibitor, so it blocks prostaglandin synthesis."
    b. "Ibuprofen inhibits prostaglandin synthesis."
    c. "Ibuprofen binds with opiate receptor sites."
    d. "Ibuprofen promotes vasodilation to increase blood flow."

19. A client with a complicated medical history including hypertension, atrial fibrillation, and arthritis calls the health care provider's office to speak with a nurse about "all of these bruises I have all of a sudden." Which potential drug interaction should concern the nurse with these symptoms?
    a. Aspirin and warfarin
    b. Sulfasalazine and acetaminophen
    c. Tolmetin and propranolol
    d. Meloxicam and amlodipine

20. A 4-year-old child was brought to the emergency room for continued fever despite taking aspirin. Which statement is correct about a 4-year-old receiving aspirin?
    a. Aspirin has the potential to cause gastrointestinal (GI) bleeding in children.
    b. Aspirin has the potential to cause ringing in the ears in children.
    c. Aspirin has the potential to cause hyperglycemia in children.
    d. Aspirin has the potential to cause Reye syndrome in children.

21. A client with a history of asthma has been prescribed sulfasalazine, a salicylate derivative, for arthritis. Which effects can salicylic acid and salicylate derivatives cause that would concern the nurse?
    a. Tachycardia
    b. Increased secretions
    c. Bronchospasm
    d. Fluid retention

22. Which statement is correct about the positive aspect of ibuprofen in relation to other nonsteroidal antiinflammatory drugs (NSAIDs)?
    a. It tends to cause less gastrointestinal (GI) irritation.
    b. It may be taken between meals.
    c. It has a long half-life of 20–30 hours.
    d. It has no drug-drug interactions.

23. A client has been prescribed ibuprofen 400 mg three times a day (tid) for arthritis. Which statement by the client would indicate a need for further education?
    a. "This drug may cause gastrointestinal (GI) upset."
    b. "Now I won't have to drink so much water."
    c. "I know this drug might cause some diarrhea."
    d. "I will need to stop taking this drug if I get pregnant."

24. What advantage does piroxicam have over other nonsteroidal antiinflammatory drugs (NSAIDs)?
    a. Piroxicam does not cause any GI irritation
    b. Piroxicam has fewer drug-drug interactions
    c. Piroxicam has a long half-life
    d. Piroxicam has a rapid onset

25. By which action does colchicine relieve the symptoms of gout?
    a. Colchicine inhibits the migration of leukocytes to the inflamed area.
    b. Colchicine blocks reabsorption of uric acid.
    c. Colchicine blocks prostaglandin release.
    d. Colchicine inhibits uric acid synthesis.

26. Which mechanism of action is primary for probenecid in the treatment of gout?
    a. Probenecid is used for the retention of urate crystals in the body
    b. Probenecid is used for the inhibition of the reabsorption of uric acid
    c. Probenecid is used for the promotion of uric acid removal in the ureters
    d. Probenecid is used for the increasing the release of uric acid

27. Which describes the mechanism of action for etanercept for the treatment of severe rheumatoid arthritis?
    a. Etanercept neutralizes tumor necrosis factor (TNF), thereby altering the inflammatory response.
    b. Etanercept inhibits IL-1 from binding to interleukin receptor sites in cartilage and bone.
    c. Etanercept blocks COX-2 receptors, which are needed for biosynthesis of prostaglandins.
    d. Etanercept promotes uric acid reabsorption.

28. When discontinuing steroid therapy, which time frame would the dosage be tapered?
    a. No tapering is necessary
    b. 1–4 days
    c. 5–10 days
    d. More than 10 days

29. A client has started taking corticosteroids for an arthritic condition. Which information should the nurse include in a health teaching plan? *(Select all that apply.)*
    a. Corticosteroids are used to control arthritic flare-ups in severe cases.
    b. Corticosteroids have a short half-life.
    c. Corticosteroids are usually administered once a day.
    d. Corticosteroids are tapered over the course of 5–10 days.
    e. Corticosteroids may not be taken with prostaglandin inhibitors.

30. Which information should the nurse include when teaching about antigout drug? *(Select all that apply.)*
    a. Include large doses of vitamin C supplements.
    b. Increase fluid intake.
    c. Avoid alcoholic beverages.
    d. Avoid foods high in purine.
    e. Take the drug with food.
    f. Avoid direct sunlight.

31. A client who has been prescribed infliximab for severe rheumatoid arthritis has developed temperature of 101.9° F, chills, nausea, vomiting, and dizziness. Which advise would the nurse provide for the client to do?
    a. The nurse does not need to advise anything. These are common side effects of infliximab.
    b. Instruct the client take a cool bath.
    c. The client should wait 24 hours and, if symptoms continue, call the clinic back.
    d. The client should contact the health care provider for further evaluation.

CASE STUDY

Read the scenario, and answer the following questions on a separate sheet of paper.

F.E., 54-years-old, comes to the clinic for treatment of an inflammatory condition. F.E. reports taking 975 mg of aspirin combined with 65 mg of caffeine every 4 hours for the past week for joint pain without relief. F.E. now reports bloody stools. Vital signs include blood pressure 90/62 mm Hg, heart rate 118 beats/min, respiratory rate 24 breaths/min, temperature 100.0° F, and pulse oximetry 98% on room air. Other assessment includes pale and cool skin.

1. What is the therapeutic dosage range for aspirin? What is the maximum dose?

2. What are the common side effects of aspirin?

3. What are the signs and symptoms of aspirin overdose?

4. Discuss the possible causes for the client's abnormal vital signs.

25 Analgesics

Complete the following.

1. The _____ theory proposes tissue injury activates _____ and causes the release of chemical mediators.

2. Opioids such as morphine activate the same receptors as _____ to reduce pain.

3. Nonsteroidal antiinflammatory drugs (NSAIDs) control pain at the _____ level by blocking pain-sensitizing chemicals and interfering with the production of _____.

4. As a result of unrelieved pain, a client may develop glucose intolerance and _____ respiratory rate, heart rate, blood pressure, and stress response.

Match the term in Column I to its definition in Column II.

Column I

_____ 5. Pain threshold

_____ 6. Pain tolerance

_____ 7. Neuropathic pain

_____ 8. Endorphins

_____ 9. Analgesics

_____ 10. Nociceptors

Column II

a. Neurohormones that naturally suppress pain conduction
b. Class of drugs that relieve pain
c. Level of stimulus needed to create a painful sensation
d. Sensory receptors for pain
e. Pain due to disease or injury of the peripheral nervous system (PNS) or central nervous system (CNS)
f. Amount of pain a person can endure without interfering with normal functioning

Complete the following.

11. Opioids act primarily on the _____ and nonopioid analgesics act on the _____ at the pain receptor sites.

12. In addition to suppressing pain impulses, opioids also suppress _____ and _____.

13. In addition to pain relief, many opioids have _____ and _____ effects.

14. Opioids are contraindicated for use in clients with _____ and _____.

15. The client taking meperidine reports blurred vision. The nurse knows this is a(n) _____ and would report this finding to the _____.

16. Pentazocine, an opioid agonist-antagonist, is classified as a Schedule _____ drug.

Match the term in Column I to its definition in Column II.

Column I

_____17. Acute pain

_____18. Cancer pain

_____19. Somatic pain

_____20. Visceral pain

_____21. Chronic pain

_____22. Superficial pain

_____23. Vascular pain

Column II

a. Originates from smooth muscle and organs
b. Occurs from pressure on nerves and organs
c. Occurs suddenly and is usually less than 3 months in duration
d. Contributes to headaches or migraines
e. Originates in skeletal muscle, ligaments, and joints
f. Persists for more than 3 months and is difficult to treat
g. Originates on surface areas such as skin and mucous membranes

REVIEW QUESTIONS

Select the best response.

24. Which drug effect is considered a major side effect of meperidine?
a. Decreased blood pressure
b. Decreased pulse rate
c. Increased respiration
d. Increased urine output

25. Which assessment finding is an indication of opioid overdose?
a. Dilated pupils
b. Increased urinary output
c. Pinpoint pupils
d. Diarrhea

26. Which nursing assessment would be least important when monitoring a client who is receiving hydromorphone?
a. Bowel sounds
b. Fluid intake
c. Pain scale
d. Vital signs

27. Which information will the nurse include in a teaching plan for a client who is being discharged home after knee surgery with a prescription for an opioid? *(Select all that apply.)*
a. Dietary restrictions while taking hydrocodone
b. Instructions not to exceed recommended dosage
c. Instructions not to use alcohol or central nervous system depressants while taking hydrocodone
d. Instructions on how to prevent constipation
e. Side effects to report

28. Which factor is most relevant to the relief of chronic pain?
a. Administration of drugs at client's request
b. Use of opioid analgesics
c. Use of injectable drugs
d. Use of drugs with long duration of action

29. The client is brought to the emergency department with a reported overdose of morphine. Which drug will the nurse anticipate be prescribed?
a. Butorphanol
b. Naloxone
c. Flumazenil
d. Pentazocine

30. Mixed opioid agonist-antagonists were developed in hopes of decreasing which problem?
a. Chronic pain
b. Opioid abuse
c. Renal failure
d. Respiratory depression

31. The client abruptly stopped taking an opioid after taking it 8 weeks for a mild back injury sustained at work. Which time frame would the nurse anticipate withdrawal symptoms attributable to physical dependence to begin?
a. 6–12 hours
b. 24–48 hours
c. 48–72 hours
d. 72–96 hours

32. Which time frame is correct on the duration of pain relief for controlled-release morphine?
a. 1–2 hours
b. 4–5 hours
c. 8–12 hours
d. 24–48 hours

33. An 8-year-old child is seen in the emergency room with a broken arm. Which intervention would the nurse do to be more successful in treating pain in an 8-year-old child? *(Select all that apply.)*
    a. Assume the child is hurt and administer pain drug.
    b. Discuss the child's typical responses with the caregivers.
    c. Utilize only nonpharmacologic pain control methods.
    d. Use a pain scale appropriate for children.
    e. Utilize developmentally appropriate communication techniques.

34. A client will be discharged home with a prescription for an opioid with acetaminophen. Which drug, when taken with an opioid with acetaminophen, will the nurse question?
    a. Ampicillin
    b. Cholestyramine
    c. Furosemide
    d. Propranolol

35. The nurse is concerned that the client is experiencing side effects of opioid agonist-antagonists. Which assessment would be a priority for the nurse to monitor?
    a. Constipation
    b. Dysuria
    c. Hypertension
    d. Respiratory depression

36. A client 4-hours postoperative is requesting morphine for the third time for pain rated an 8 on the numeric pain scale. The vital signs include temperature 97.5° F, heart rate 88 beats/min, respiratory rate 12 breaths/min, blood pressure 104/60 mm Hg, and oxygen saturation 98% on room air. Assuming that a dose of the drug is due, which action would be best for the nurse to take?
    a. Administer the dose and contact the health care provider about the respiratory rate.
    b. Administer the dose and contact the health care provider about inadequate pain control.
    c. Hold the dose and contact the health care provider regarding the respiratory rate.
    d. Hold the dose and contact the health care provider about inadequate pain control.

37. The older adult client has a fentanyl patch 75 mcg for chronic pain. Which statement is correct regarding this drug for the older adult?
    a. This patient should not have a fentanyl patch for chronic pain.
    b. The dose may be too low.
    c. The dose may be too high for this patient.
    d. The dose is appropriate.

38. The client is taking a combination drug of hydrocodone and ibuprofen after reconstructive knee surgery. Which statement by the client indicates the need for more teaching?
    a. "I must take only what is prescribed for my pain."
    b. "I may need to take a laxative if I get constipated while I am taking this drug."
    c. "Having a few beers on the weekend will help me relax and ease the pain."
    d. "I should not take anything with ibuprofen in it while I am taking this drug."

39. A client was prescribed oral ketorolac for postoperative pain. Which time frame indicates the maximum length of time this drug can be taken?
    a. 24 hours
    b. 3 days
    c. 5 days
    d. 2 weeks

40. Which drug(s) would be appropriate for pain management for a client who sustained multiple abrasions to both knees after falling off a bicycle? *(Select all that apply.)*
    a. Acetaminophen
    b. Aspirin
    c. Hydrocodone
    d. Ibuprofen
    e. Morphine

CASE STUDY

Read the scenario and answer the following questions on a separate sheet of paper.

G.F., 25-years-old, presents to the emergency department with a severe headache on the left side of the head. G.F. states that the headache has been present for 24 hours and "it just won't go away." G.F. is nauseated and is vomiting. G.F. states that lights hurt the eyes and "everything sounds loud." Vital signs include temperature 98.2° F, heart rate 92 beats/min, respiratory rate 18 breaths/min, blood pressure 142/76 mm Hg, and oxygen saturation 100% on room air. Pain is rated as a "13 on a scale of 1–10." The health care provider diagnoses G.F. with a migraine headache.

1. What is the mechanism behind the pain associated with a migraine?

2. What is the difference between the two types of migraine and a cluster headache?

3. What treatment options are available for G.F.?

26 Antibacterials

PENICILLINS AND CEPHALOSPORINS

STUDY QUESTIONS

Match the antibiotic in Column I to its category in Column II.

Column I

_____ 1. Penicillin G

_____ 2. Cefaclor

_____ 3. Oxacillin

_____ 4. Ceftolozane/tazobactam

_____ 5. Cefazolin

_____ 6. Amoxicillin

_____ 7. Cefdinir

_____ 8. Cefepime

_____ 9. Piperacillin/tazobactam

Column II

a. First-generation cephalosporin
b. Second-generation cephalosporin
c. Third-generation cephalosporin
d. Fourth-generation cephalosporin
e. Fifth-generation cephalosporin
f. Basic penicillin
g. Penicillinase-resistant penicillins
h. Broad-spectrum penicillin
i. Extended-spectrum penicillins

REVIEW QUESTIONS

Select the best response.

10. A client, who recently completed five days of antibiotics, presents to the clinic with complaints of severe vaginal itching and discharge. Which mechanism will the nurse recognize as a possible cause of vaginal itching and discharge will the nurse recognize?
    a. Poor hygiene
    b. Hypersensitivity
    c. Kidney infection
    d. Superinfection

11. A client is scheduled to receive ceftriaxone for an infection due to *Klebsiella*. Which teaching will the nurse provide to the client about this drug?
    a. It is given intramuscularly (IM) or intravenously (IV).
    b. There is no cross-reaction to penicillins.
    c. Ceftriaxone is safe to take with anticoagulants.
    d. There is no effect on lab values.

12. A client with renal dysfunction and *Staphylococcus aureus* infection is prescribed cefprozil monohydrate. Which dose indicates the maximum amount the nurse will anticipate?
    a. 250 mg/d
    b. 500 mg/d
    c. 750 mg/d
    d. 1 g/d

13. A young client is admitted to the intensive care unit with a severe lower respiratory tract infection and is started on aztreonam. Which dose of aztreonam will the nurse anticipate administering?
    a. 500 mg q8h
    b. 500 mg q6h
    c. 1500 mg q8h
    d. 2000 mg daily

14. Which class of drug would increase the risk of nephrotoxicity in a client taking ceftriaxone?
    a. Angiotensin-converting enzyme (ACE) inhibitor
    b. Antidysrhythmic
    c. Loop diuretic
    d. Nonsteroidal antiinflammatory drug (NSAID)

15. A client is concerned about some weight loss while on ceftriaxone. Which information can the nurse tell the client regarding side effects of ceftriaxone?
    a. Loss of appetite is a common side effect.
    b. Gastrointestinal bleeding may occur frequently.
    c. Ceftriaxone causes nutrient absorption problems.
    d. The client will eat more when the infection is cured.

16. Which statement by a parent indicates more discharge teaching is necessary for care of a 5-year-old child who has been prescribed dicloxacillin for otitis media?
    a. "Abdominal pain can be a side effect."
    b. "She needs to drink plenty of orange juice with this medication."
    c. "My child must take all of the drug until it is gone."
    d. "If my child develops a rash, I should bring her back to the doctor."

17. Which category of drugs is known to increase the serum levels of cefotetan?
    a. Antacids
    b. Laxatives
    c. Opioids
    d. Uricosurics

18. Which mechanism of action is correct about penicillin V potassium?
    a. Alteration in membrane permeability
    b. Inhibition of cell-wall synthesis
    c. Inhibition of protein synthesis
    d. Interference with cellular metabolism

19. A client, who is allergic to dextromethorphan, is diagnosed with strep throat and is prescribed amoxicillin/clavulanate potassium. The client takes oral contraceptives, vitamin C, and fexofenadine. Which instruction will the nurse include in the discharge teaching regarding amoxicillin/clavulanate potassium?
    a. "Increase calcium intake."
    b. "Wear sunscreen at all times."
    c. "Use an alternate method of birth control."
    d. "Stop the fexofenadine."

20. A client is started on ceftazidime. Which nursing intervention(s) will the nurse perform? *(Select all that apply.)*
    a. Obtain a culture.
    b. Administer IV dose over 20 minutes every day.
    c. Assess for allergic reaction.
    d. Monitor urine output.
    e. Restrict oral fluid intake.

21. A nurse is administering morning drugs to several clients. Which client will the nurse be concerned about in administering amoxicillin?
    a. A child with skin infection
    b. A pregnant client
    c. A client with asthma
    d. A client with diabetes

22. An adult client has been prescribed cefaclor for otitis media. Which order will the nurse question?
    a. Immediate release (IR), 250 mg q8h
    b. Immediate release (IR), 500 mg q8h
    c. Immediate release (IR), 750 mg q8h
    d. Extended release (ER), 500 mg q12h

MACROLIDES, OXAZOLIDINONES, LINCOSAMIDES, GLYCOPEPTIDES, KETOLIDES, TETRACYCLINES, AND GLYCYLCYCLINES

STUDY QUESTIONS

Match the drug in Column I with the category in Column II. Categories in Column II may be used more than once.

Column I

_____ 1. Clindamycin

_____ 2. Tigecycline

_____ 3. Erythromycin

_____ 4. Telithromycin

_____ 5. Azithromycin

_____ 6. Doxycycline

_____ 7. Clarithromycin

Column II

a. Macrolides
b. Lincosamides
c. Ketolides
d. Tetracyclines
e. Glycylcyclines

REVIEW QUESTIONS

Select the best response.

8. Which laboratory test is most likely influenced by doxycycline?
   a. Serum potassium
   b. Serum calcium
   c. Platelets
   d. Hemoglobin and hematocrit

9. A client has been prescribed doxycycline. Which statement(s) by the client indicate(s) that the nurse needs to provide more discharge teaching? *(Select all that apply.)*
   a. "It is best if I take this with meals."
   b. "I should drink milk."
   c. "I have to take this drug on an empty stomach."
   d. "I should wait a half-hour after meals to take the medication."
   e. "I cannot eat eggs when I take this drug."

10. Which information will the nurse include in the teaching for a client taking tetracycline for a respiratory tract infection? *(Select all that apply.)*
    a. Outdated tetracycline breaks down into toxic by-products and must be discarded.
    b. Observe for superinfection like vaginitis.
    c. Avoid tetracycline during first and third trimesters of pregnancy.
    d. Anticipate urinary urgency.
    e. Wear sunscreen and limit outdoor exposure during peak daylight hours.

11. Which drug(s), if prescribed for a client taking oral doxycycline, will the nurse question? *(Select all that apply.)*
    a. Prenatal vitamins
    b. Antacids
    c. Warfarin
    d. Morphine
    e. Omeprazole

12. Which specific nursing intervention(s) would the nurse implement for a client taking doxycycline for chlamydia? *(Select all that apply.)*
    a. Restricting fluids
    b. Storing the drug away from light
    c. Ordering renal and liver profiles
    d. Obtaining a specimen for culture and sensitivity
    e. Advising the patient to use additional contraceptives when taking this drug

13. The nurse is performing a morning assessment on a client who is receiving gentamicin. The client reports tinnitus all night. Which information is correct about gentamicin and tinnitus?
    a. Only low-pitched sounds are affected by gentamicin.
    b. Tinnitus is a sign of gentamicin allergy.
    c. Ototoxicity is caused by damage to cranial nerve VIII.
    d. Only female clients have ringing in their ears.

14. The nurse is noting the urine output has decreased to 500 mL/day in an older adult client receiving vancomycin. Which action would be best by the nurse?
    a. Increase the client's oral fluid intake.
    b. Increase the rate on client's intravenous fluid.
    c. Contact the health care provider.
    d. Document this in the client's chart.

15. The client has been prescribed azithromycin for an upper respiratory tract infection. Which statement by the client indicates understanding of drug's side effects?
    a. "I need to stay out of the sun or wear sunscreen."
    b. "I have to take it on an empty stomach to prevent nausea."
    c. "If my eyes get red and itchy, I shouldn't wear my contacts."
    d. "I cannot take anything for pain if I get a headache."

16. For which bacteria is quinupristin-dalfopristin appropriate for life-threatening infection?
    a. Vancomycin-resistant *Enterococcus faecium*
    b. *Escherichia coli*
    c. *Proteus mirabilis*
    d. *Klebsiella pneumoniae*

AMINOGLYCOSIDES, FLUOROQUINOLONES, AND LIPOPEPTIDES

Complete the following.

1. Streptomycin sulfate was the first _____ available against the bacterium *Streptomyces griseus*.

2. Aminoglycosides cross the blood-brain barrier in (adults/children) but not in (adults/children). *(Circle the correct answers.)*

3. An increased risk for ototoxicity can occur when taking aminoglycosides concurrently with _____.

4. Fluoroquinolones interfere with the enzyme _____ _____, which is needed to synthesize bacterial _____.

5. Patients taking fluoroquinolones should (increase/decrease) fluid intake. *(Circle the correct answer.)*

Match the drug in Column I with its category in Column II. Categories in Column II may be used more than once.

Column I

_____ 6. Amikacin

_____ 7. Moxifloxacin

_____ 8. Gentamicin

_____ 9. Ciprofloxacin

_____ 10. Daptomycin

_____ 11. Tobramycin

Column II

a. Aminoglycosides
b. Fluoroquinolones
c. Lipopeptides

REVIEW QUESTIONS

12. Which fluoroquinolone order will the nurse question?
    a. Levofloxacin 750 mg IV q12h
    b. Ofloxacin 200 mg PO q12h
    c. Moxifloxacin 400 mg PO q day
    d. Ciprofloxacin 250 mg PO bid

13. The nurse assesses a client who is taking gentamicin. Which assessment finding(s) should be cause for serious concern? *(Select all that apply.)*
    a. Nausea
    b. Ototoxicity
    c. Headache
    d. Photosensitivity
    e. Elevated renal function tests

14. A client is taking gentamicin intravenously for a postsurgical infection at 9:00 am and 9:00 pm. Which time is most correct for the nurse to check drug peak level?
    a. 9:15 am
    b. 10:00 am
    c. 9:15 pm
    d. 10:30 pm

15. The trough level that the nurse drew for a client taking gentamicin is 3.5 mcg/mL. Which action would be taken by the nurse?
    a. Administer the medication at the correct time.
    b. Hold the drug and contact the health care provider.
    c. Repeat the trough level after the next dose of medication.
    d. Give the client diphenhydramine to decrease the risk of a reaction.

16. The client has developed vaginal discharge since beginning gentamicin. Which cause does the nurse suspect may have occurred?
    a. The client has been exposed to other infectious agents.
    b. The client is experiencing an allergic reaction.
    c. A superinfection has developed.
    d. A drug-drug interaction is taking place.

17. Which finding will the nurse routinely monitor for in a client receiving gentamicin? (Select all that apply.)
    a. Hearing loss
    b. Color and clarity of urine
    c. AST/ALT
    d. Blood glucose
    e. Visual acuity

18. A trough level is obtained in a client receiving daptomycin. Which trough level will the nurse know is appropriate?
    a. 5 mcg/mL by the second dose
    b. 5.9 mcg/mL by the third dose
    c. 6 mg/mL by the third dose
    d. 6.5 mg/mL by the fourth dose

SULFONAMIDES AND NITROIMIDAZOLES

STUDY QUESTIONS

Complete the following.

1. Sulfonamides inhibit bacterial synthesis of _____ _____.

2. Clinical use of sulfonamides has decreased because of the availability and effectiveness of _____.

3. The antibacterial drug that has a synergistic effect with sulfonamides is _____.

4. Sulfonamides (are/are not) effective against viruses and fungi. (Circle correct answer.)

5. Anaphylaxis (is/is not) common with the use of sulfonamides. (Circle correct answer.)

6. Sulfonamide drugs are metabolized in the _____ and excreted by the _____.

7. Sulfonamides are (bacteriostatic/bactericidal). (Circle correct answer.)

8. The use of warfarin with sulfonamides (increases/decreases) the anticoagulant effect. (Circle correct answer.)

Match the drug in Column I with its duration of action in Column II. Duration of action in Column II may be used more than once.

Column I
_____ 9. Trimethoprim-sulfamethoxazole

_____ 10. Sulfasalazine

_____ 11. Sulfadiazine

Column II
a. Short-acting
b. Intermediate-acting

Select the best response.

12. A client has sustained partial-thickness and full-thickness burns over 20% of the body. Which drug would be useful for this client?
    a. Sulfadiazine
    b. Sulfasalazine
    c. Sulfacetamide sodium
    d. Silver sulfadiazine

13. A recent postpartum client was prescribed TMP-SMZ for urinary tract infection (UTI). Which important question(s) will the nurse ask? *(Select all that apply.)*
    a. "What kind of juice do you like to drink?"
    b. "Are you breastfeeding?"
    c. "Are you allergic to any medications?"
    d. "Do you have a history of kidney stones?"
    e. "What drugs do you take regularly?"

14. Which intervention(s) will the nurse implement in a client with bronchitis who is receiving TMP-SMZ and lisinopril? *(Select all that apply.)*
    a. Encourage fluids.
    b. Monitor urinary output.
    c. Observe for undesired side effects.
    d. Assess lung sounds.
    e. Administer laxatives.

15. Which dose is the usual adult dose of TMP-SMZ?
    a. 160 mg TMP/800 mg SMZ q6h
    b. 160 mg TMP/800 mg SMZ q12h
    c. 40 mg TMP/60 mg SMZ q6h
    d. 40 mg TMP/60 mg SMZ q12h

16. For which reason are sulfonamides not classified as antibiotics?
    a. They do not inhibit cell-wall growth.
    b. They are only bacteriostatic, not bactericidal.
    c. They were not obtained from biological sources.
    d. They are only effective against viruses and fungi.

17. A client has been started on TMP-SMZ for otitis. The nurse will advise the client about which side effect?
    a. Confusion
    b. Constipation
    c. Fever
    d. Insomnia

18. Which amount is the maintenance dose for sulfasalazine in the treatment of an inflammatory bowel disease, such as ulcerative colitis?
    a. 500 mg q6h
    b. 1000 mg q6h
    c. 1250 mg per day
    d. 1500 mg per day

CASE STUDY

Read the scenario and answer the following questions on a separate sheet of paper.

D.T., 72-years-old, presents to the emergency department from a long-term acute care facility (LTAC) with complaints of fever, shaking chills, flank pain, and burning on urination. Vital signs are temperature 100.3° F, heart rate 94 beats/min, respiratory rate 16 breaths/min, and blood pressure 102/70 mm Hg. D.T.'s medical history includes adult-onset diabetes and cerebrovascular accident with residual left-sided weakness. Current drugs include glyburide, warfarin, and a daily multivitamin. D.T. is allergic to all cephalosporins. D.T. is diagnosed with an *E. coli* urinary tract infection and was prescribed oral trimethoprim-sulfamethoxazole (TMP-SMZ).

1. What is the mechanism of action and standard dosage for oral TMP-SMZ?

2. What will the nurse discuss with the client and/or caregivers regarding the plan of care as it relates to TMP-SMZ?

3. For what adverse reactions will the nurse monitor?

27 Antituberculars, Antifungals, and Antivirals

Complete the following.

1. *Mycobacterium* species is a/an _____ bacillus that can cause _____.

2. Multidrug-resistant tuberculosis (MDRTB) continues to be a problem because people (do/do not) complete the drug regimen. *(Circle correct answer.)*

3. Tuberculosis is transmitted by droplets when people _____, _____, or _____ and people in close contact _____ the particles.

4. A person who had _____ _____ _____ can develop TB disease.

5. Since isoniazid is metabolized through the liver and excreted by the kidneys, isoniazid is contraindicated in persons with severe _____ and _____ disease. List the other contraindications for receiving isoniazid.

6. Psychotic behavior (is/is not) a side effect of isoniazid. *(Circle correct answer.)*

7. (Single/Combination) therapy against TB disease is more effective in eradicating infection. *(Circle correct answer.)*

8. A common adverse effect with isoniazid is peripheral neuropathy. A supplement with _____ is usually taken concomitantly to prevent neuropathy.

9. Children who have latent TB infection should be treated with _____ for _____ months.

Match the drug in Column I with its type in Column II. Answers may be used more than once.

Column I

_____ 10. Ethambutol

_____ 11. Rifapentin

_____ 12. Pyrazinamide

_____ 13. Capreomycin

_____ 14. Isoniazid

_____ 15. Aminosalicylate

_____ 16. Ethionamide

_____ 17. Streptomycin

_____ 18. Rifampin

Column II

a. First-line drug
b. Drug-resistant TB medication

Complete the following.

19. Overgrowth of fungus usually occurs in persons who are immunocompromised and is classified as an _____ infection.

20. Rapid IV infusion of echinocandins can cause _____ reactions.

21. Herpes virus type 1 (HSV-1) is usually associated with _____, and herpes virus type 2 (HSV-2) is associated with _____.

22. Varicella-zoster virus that has lain dormant in nerve root ganglia can be reactivated as _____. Painful vesicular rash occurs along the _____.

23. Currently, hepatitis _____ and hepatitis _____ are vaccine preventable.

24. Specific therapy (does/does not) exist for acute hepatitis B. *(Circle correct answer.)*

25. Hepatitis _____ and hepatitis _____ can develop into chronic hepatitis.

REVIEW QUESTIONS

Select the best response.

26. Which outcome is a life-threatening adverse effect of isoniazid?
    a. Crystalluria
    b. Hepatotoxicity
    c. Ototoxicity
    d. Palpitations

27. Which person should not receive prophylactic treatment for tuberculosis with isoniazid?
    a. 29-year-old concurrently taking theophylline
    b. 46-year-old with alcoholism
    c. 57-year-old taking warfarin
    d. 65-year-old with parkinsonism

28. The client has just started taking rifapentine for active tuberculosis. The nurse knows that this drug will be taken how often?
    a. Twice per day
    b. Daily
    c. Twice per week
    d. Every other day

29. An immunocompromised client has recently been diagnosed with histoplasmosis. The client has been started on amphotericin B. The nurse will anticipate administering which drug to alleviate side effects? *(Select all that apply.)*
    a. Diphenhydramine
    b. Acetaminophen
    c. Diazepam
    d. Hydrocortisone

30. Which drug would be ordered for a client with hepatitis C viral infection?

a.

b.

c.

d.

31. During the admission interview, which information will the nurse seek to obtain from a client taking isoniazid? *(Select all that apply.)*
    a. Blood glucose level
    b. Drug allergies
    c. History of tuberculosis exposure
    d. Date of last purified protein derivative (PPD) and chest x-ray

32. The 28-year-old client has been diagnosed with tuberculosis (TB) disease. The client weighs 80 kg. Which dose of isoniazid (INH) would the nurse anticipate administering initially?
    a. 2 mg/kg/day
    b. 5 mg/kg/day
    c. 7.5 mg/kg/day
    d. 10 mg/kg/day

33. A client with active tuberculosis (TB) is prescribed isoniazid (INH). The nurse will teach the client that frequent laboratory test to monitor liver function is needed for which reason?
    a. INH is excreted by the liver.
    b. INH causes liver cancer.
    c. INH can be hepatotoxic.
    d. INH cannot be metabolized by patients who have liver disease.

34. The client has just been prescribed isoniazid (INH) for active tuberculosis. Which drug taken by the client would be of concern to the nurse?
    a. Cetirizine
    b. Lisinopril
    c. Maalox
    d. Metformin

35. Which priority health teaching would the nurse include for the client who has just started a course of isoniazid (INH)? *(Select all that apply.)*
    a. The patient may need to take vitamin B_6 supplements.
    b. Alcohol should be avoided.
    c. Fluid intake should be restricted.
    d. Body fluids including urine and tears may turn a brownish-orange color.
    e. Daily weights should be monitored.

36. Which instruction would rifampin be taken to decrease the incidence of resistance?
    a. Daily
    b. In conjunction with another antitubercular drug
    c. Once a week
    d. Only if patient is symptomatic

37. An immunocompromised client has aspergillosis and has been prescribed amphotericin B. Which route will the nurse administer this drug?
    a. Intramuscularly
    b. Intravenously
    c. Orally
    d. Rectally

38. A client with coccidioidomycosis is in the intensive care unit and has been prescribed amphotericin B. Which administration instruction would the nurse anticipate?
    a. Dilute and infuse over 30 minutes while monitoring vital signs every 5 minutes.
    b. Dilute, protect from light, and infuse slowly using an in-line filter.
    c. Prepare to administer undiluted by intravenous push slowly over 15 minutes.
    d. Prepare the drug in a solution and have the patient drink it slowly.

39. A client is being treated with amphotericin B for histoplasmosis. Which statement by the client would be concerning to the nurse?
    a. "I know I can only get this drug by having an intravenous site."
    b. "This drug may make me feel flushed."
    c. "I should not eat for 12 hours before receiving the drug."
    d. "I should let my health care provider know if I am not urinating as much."

40. A client has been prescribed acyclovir. Which information should be part of the teaching plan for a client who has been prescribed acyclovir? *(Select all that apply.)*
    a. Be sure to drink plenty of water to maintain hydration.
    b. Be sure to use spermicide to prevent infecting others.
    c. Drug can be taken at mealtime.
    d. Arise slowly because of the risk for orthostatic hypotension.
    e. Report any decreased urinary output, dizziness, or confusion.

41. Which symptom(s) will the nurse advise the client taking peginterferon to report to the health care provider? *(Select all that apply.)*
    a. Mood changes
    b. Fever
    c. Vision changes
    d. Photophobia
    e. Urinary urgency

42. Available:

The patient's prescription is for a maintenance dose of fluconazole, 150 mg/day. How many tablets should the client take per dose?
a. 1 tablet
b. 1.5 tablets
c. 2 tablets
d. 2.5 tablets

43. Which laboratory value(s) must be frequently monitored in the client taking fluconazole? *(Select all that apply.)*
a. AST
b. ALT
c. BUN
d. Glucose
e. Potassium
f. PT

CASE STUDY

Read the scenario and answer the following questions on a separate sheet of paper.

C.J. has presented to the clinic complaining of "white spots in my mouth." C.J. has been taking multiple antibiotics during the past month for a severe lower respiratory tract infection. Nystatin suspension is ordered, 5 mL oral swish and swallow four times daily.

1. What questions should the nurse ask in the assessment?

2. What is the likely source of the client's symptoms?

3. What specific instructions will the nurse include in health teaching regarding nystatin?

28 Antimalarials, Anthelmintics, and Peptides

STUDY QUESTIONS

Match the term in Column I with the appropriate definition in Column II.

Column I

_____ 1. Tissue phase

_____ 2. Erythrocyte phase

_____ 3. Prophylaxis

_____ 4. Helminthiasis

_____ 5. Trichinosis

_____ 6. Drug-resistant infection

_____ 7. Peptides

Column II

a. Prevention
b. Worm infection
c. Invasion of the body tissue
d. Infection caused by eating raw or undercooked pork
e. Invasion of the blood cells
f. Provides the ability to kill a range of parasites and viruses
g. When microbes are not sensitive to antimicrobials

REVIEW QUESTIONS

8. Which site is common for helminthiasis?
    a. Blood
    b. Intestines
    c. Liver
    d. Urinary tract

9. Which pathogen is the causative species for malaria?
    a. Bacterium
    b. Fungus
    c. Protozoan
    d. Virus

10. A client who recently returned from an archeology dig overseas presents to the emergency department with complaints of fever, chills, and body aches. Which drug will the nurse anticipate in giving for a client diagnosed with malaria?
    a. Acyclovir
    b. Chloroquine HCl
    c. Delavirdine
    d. Tobramycin

11. Which laboratory value(s) is/are affected by chloroquine usage? *(Select all that apply.)*
    a. Creatinine
    b. Glucose
    c. Hemoglobin
    d. Hematocrit
    e. Red blood cell count
    f. Aspartate aminotransferase (AST)

12. The client is planning an oversea mission trip to a mosquito infested area and was prescribed chloroquine as prophylaxis for malaria. Which statement by the client indicates the need for more health education by the nurse?
    a. "I may have some abdominal cramping and nausea."
    b. "I only need to take my medication before my trip."
    c. "If my ears start ringing, I should contact my health care provider."
    d. "I should avoid taking any antacid while I am taking this drug."

13. A client returns to the clinic complaining of not getting better after completing treatment with chloroquine for malaria. Vital signs are temperature 104.5° F, heart rate 120 beats/min, respiratory rate 22 breaths/min, blood pressure 138/82 mm Hg, and oxygen saturation 99% on room air. Which treatment will the nurse anticipate the next?
    a. Continue 5 more days of chloroquine.
    b. Change medication to artemether/lumefantrine.
    c. Start thiabendazole.
    d. Start zidovudine.

14. Which instruction priority(ies) would be included in the teaching for anthelmintics? *(Select all that apply.)*
    a. Bathing in hot water instead of showering
    b. Changing clothing, linen, and towels daily
    c. Taking the drug on an empty stomach to aid in absorption
    d. Understanding the importance of hand hygiene
    e. Thoroughly cooking all foods containing pork

15. The client diagnosed with taeniasis is being treated with praziquantel. Which possible side effect(s) should the nurse include in client teaching? *(Select all that apply.)*
    a. Blurred vision
    b. Difficulty hearing
    c. Dizziness
    d. Headache
    e. Weakness

16. Which statement(s) by a client who is being treated with an antibiotic would concern the nurse about a potential risk for antibiotic resistance? *(Select all that apply.)*
    a. "If I run out of my antibiotic, I can use my left-overs from a previous infection."
    b. "I will take the antibiotics as prescribed."
    c. "Sometimes my friends ask me if I have any antibiotics. If I feel better, I will give my friends my leftovers."
    d. "When I stop having a fever I can stop taking the drug."

CASE STUDY

Read the scenario and answer the following questions on a separate sheet of paper.

J.C. started having abdominal pain and anal itching after working on a farm and ranch. J.C. was diagnosed with helminths.

1. What are helminths?

2. What are the common helminths causing infection in humans and how do they infect humans?

3. How are helminths treated?

29 HIV- and AIDS-Related Drugs

STUDY QUESTIONS

Match the drug in Column I to its drug classification of antiretroviral therapy in Column II. Answers may be used more than once.

Column I

_____ 1. Didanosine

_____ 2. Enfuvirtide

_____ 3. Raltegravir

_____ 4. Maraviroc

_____ 5. Idinavir

_____ 6. Ritonavir

_____ 7. Efavirenz

_____ 8. Tenofovir

_____ 9. Nevirapine

_____ 10. Zidovudine

Column II

a. Nucleoside/nucleotide reverse transcriptase inhibitors

b. Protease inhibitors

c. Integrase strand transfer inhibitors

d. Fusion inhibitors

e. Nonnucleoside reverse transcriptase inhibitors

f. CCR5 antagonists

Complete the following.

11. The phases of the HIV life cycle include _____, _____, reverse transcription, integration, _____, _____, and budding.

12. Individuals who fail antiretroviral therapy (ART) (should/should not) be tested for drug-resistance. (Circle correct answer.)

13. Patients on HIV medication therapy should strive for _____ percent adherence.

14. Drug-drug interactions can occur when drugs are metabolized by the _____ system.

15. _____ is the only NNRTI that penetrates cerebrospinal fluid.

16. Selection of a protease inhibitor–based regimen should consider _____. (List at least three considerations.)

17. _____ is a syndrome that is related to a disease- or pathogen-specific inflammatory response in patients on antiretroviral therapy.

Select the best response.

18. A nurse is teaching a client who is positive for HIV. Which statements by the client indicates a need for further teaching on HIV transmission? *(Select all that apply.)*
    a. "It is okay to share my razor."
    b. "I need to wear a condom with any type of sexual intercourse."
    c. "I can spread HIV by sharing my toothbrush."
    d. "I can donate my sperm."

19. Which laboratory tests is used to monitor the efficacy of HIV drug therapy?
    a. White blood cell count
    b. CD4+ T-cell count
    c. Plasma B-cells
    d. Complete blood count

20. Which statement is correct on the goal of combination antiretroviral therapy?
    a. Decrease the viral load and decrease the CD4+ count
    b. Decrease the CD4+ count and increase the viral load
    c. Increase the CD4+ count and decrease the viral load
    d. Replace the memory cells within the immune system

21. If therapy is to be initiated, the selection of antiretroviral therapy (ART) should be based on which client status? *(Select all that apply.)*
    a. Client's other comorbid conditions
    b. Client's age and support system
    c. Client's willingness to accept therapy
    d. Probability of adherence to therapy
    e. Pregnancy status

22. Drug adherence has improved since the advent of antiretroviral therapy (ART). Which advancements to ART helped in increasing adherence?
    a. More pill burden
    b. Increased potency of newer ART
    c. Improved side effect profile
    d. Decreased potency of newer ART to reduce side effects

23. An adult client is scheduled to begin taking zidovudine 300 mg by mouth. Which time frame is zidovudine generally scheduled to be taken?
    a. Daily
    b. Every 12 hours
    c. Every 6 hours
    d. Every 8 hours

24. An 8-week-old neonate has been diagnosed with HIV and will be receiving zidovudine orally. The child weighs 4.5 kg. Which dose would the nurse anticipate for this child?
    a. 9 mg/kg/dose bid
    b. 12 mg/kg/dose bid
    c. 120 mg/kg/dose bid
    d. 300 mg/kg/dose bid

25. During the time that a client is taking zidovudine, frequent monitoring of which laboratory value(s) is required? *(Select all that apply.)*
    a. Liver enzymes ALT/AST
    b. Complete blood count (CBC) with differential
    c. Creatinine
    d. Serum sodium
    e. Urine sedimentation rate

26. The nurse is assessing a client taking zidovudine. Which side effects are common? *(Select all that apply.)*
    a. Constipation
    b. Headache
    c. Myalgia
    d. Rash
    e. Seizures

27. Which nonnucleoside reverse transcriptase inhibitor (NNRTI) penetrates the blood-brain barrier?
    a. Rilpivirine
    b. Delavirdine
    c. Efavirenz
    d. Nevirapine

28. Efavirenz is initially scheduled to be taken at which intervals?
    a. 600 mg q6h
    b. 600 mg q8h
    c. 600 mg q12h
    d. 600 mg daily

29. During the time that a client is taking efavirenz, periodic monitoring of which laboratory value is required?
    a. BUN/creatinine
    b. CBC
    c. Electrolytes
    d. Liver panel

30. Which side effects would be common in a client taking efavirenz? *(Select all that apply.)*
    a. Diarrhea
    b. Difficulty swallowing
    c. Dizziness
    d. Rash
    e. Seizures

31. A client is being discharged on efavirenz. Which priority teaching point(s) will the nurse provide? *(Select all that apply.)*
   a. "Avoid alcohol while taking this drug."
   b. "Be sure to drink 2500 mL of fluid a day."
   c. "Don't take St. John's wort with this drug, as it will decrease its effectiveness."
   d. "This drug can cause convulsions and possibly liver failure."
   e. "Vomiting is a serious adverse reaction to efavirenz."

32. Which laboratory value(s) is/are high priority for the nurse to monitor in a client taking tenofovir? *(Select all that apply.)*
   a. Blood glucose
   b. Cholesterol
   c. Liver enzymes
   d. Triglycerides
   e. Potassium

33. A client is being discharged on tenofovir. Which teaching information should this client receive? *(Select all that apply.)*
   a. "You cannot take St. John's wort while taking this drug."
   b. "You can take this drug with or without food."
   c. "You will need to learn to measure your blood glucose level."
   d. "Side effects may include nausea, vomiting, and diarrhea."
   e. "You will not be able to drive until you stop taking this drug."

34. Which treatment is the standard of care for prophylactic therapy of a pregnant client who is HIV positive and asymptomatic?
   a. Combination drug therapy
   b. No therapy since all ART is contraindicated during pregnancy
   c. Single drug therapy with zidovudine only
   d. No therapy since the patient is asymptomatic

35. Which side effect(s) would the nurse expect to see in a client taking atazanavir? *(Select all that apply.)*
   a. Diarrhea
   b. Nausea
   c. Rash
   d. Urinary retention
   e. Vomiting

36. Which modalities can help increase HIV drug adherence? *(Select all that apply.)*
   a. Pill organizers
   b. Drug charts
   c. Scheduled pill holidays
   d. Alarms on cell phone or watch
   e. Taking drugs at the same time each day, such as after brushing teeth.

CASE STUDY

Read the scenario and answer the following questions on a separate sheet of paper.

D.D. works as a nurse in a trauma unit. D.D. sustains a needle stick from a client with HIV.

1. What should the nurse do first?

2. What is involved in postexposure prophylaxis (PEP), and how long does treatment last?

3. What are potential side effects associated with PEP?

30 Transplant Drugs

Complete the following.

1. Transplantation of a healthy organ at the time of the donor's death is called _____.

2. A critical component of the cellular immune response is the activation of _____.

3. Clients on belatacept are at increased risk for _____ _____ _____ if they do not have immunity to _____ _____.

4. Sirolimus is in the class of _____ drugs that block _____ and _____ activation.

5. Combining corticosteroids with potassium-wasting diuretics increases the risk of _____.

6. Clients taking trimethoprim-sulfamethoxazole should protect their _____ from the _____.

Make the following false statements into true statements.

7. Induction therapy includes transplant drugs that provide improved immunity.

8. An example of a living-donor transplantation is when a kidney donated by a living person is transplanted into the body with severe kidney disease.

9. Transplant recipients receiving immunosuppressive drugs can receive live vaccines.

10. Sirolimus is primarily excreted by the kidneys.

11. Antithymocyte globulin alters B-cell function and prolongs T-cell addition.

Match the drug in Column I to the correct drug classes in Column II. Answers may be used more than once.

Column I

_____ 12. Tacrolimus

_____ 13. Everolimus

_____ 14. Basiliximab

_____ 15. Cyclosporine

_____ 16. Belatacept

_____ 17. Sirolimus

_____ 18. Azathioprine

_____ 19. Mycophenolate mofetil

_____ 20. Prednisone

Column II

a. Purine antimetabolites
b. Corticosteroids
c. Calcineurin inhibitors
d. Inosine monophosphate dehydrogenase inhibitors
e. Mammalian target of rapamycin inhibitors
f. T-cell co-stimulation blocker
g. Monoclonal antibody

21. A nurse believes cytokine release syndrome is occurring in a client receiving basiliximab before renal transplant surgery. Which signs and symptoms are related to cytokine release syndrome? *(Select all that apply.)*
    a. Hypotension
    b. Bradycardia
    c. Dyspnea
    d. Hypothermia
    e. Headache

22. A nurse would anticipate administering which drug to reduce the symptoms from cytokine release syndrome?
    a. Corticosteroid
    b. Diltiazem
    c. Furosemide
    d. Naloxone

23. Cyclosporine oral solution should not be mixed in which type of fluid?
    a. Apple juice
    b. Orange juice
    c. Grape juice
    d. Grapefruit juice

24. Which statement by the client demonstrates an understanding of cyclosporine?
    a. "If I get an infection, I can take any antibiotics."
    b. "I can take cimetidine if I get an upset stomach."
    c. "If I have a fever, I need to call my doctor."
    d. "If I get mild muscle aches, I can take ibuprofen."

25. A client is scheduled to receive a maintenance dose of belatacept post renal transplant. The provider ordered belatacept 10 mg/kg IV starting at week 10. Which action would be correct by the nurse?
    a. Call the provider who ordered the drug.
    b. Give the drug since the order is correct.
    c. Give the drug; the provider wanted the lower dose.
    d. Give the drug but at the correct recommended dose.

26. Which client is appropriate to treat with mammalian target of rapamycin (mTOR) inhibitors?
    a. A client who had a lung transplant
    b. A client who had a heart transplant
    c. A client who had a liver transplant
    d. A client who had a kidney transplant

27. Which organ transplant(s) is/are appropriate for mycophenolate mofetil? *(Select all that apply.)*
    a. Heart transplant
    b. Pancreas transplant
    c. Liver transplant
    d. Kidney transplant
    e. Corneal transplant

28. A client is taking high doses of corticosteroids for acute transplant rejection. For which reason would a nurse teach the client to avoid abrupt discontinuation of corticosteroids?
    a. Corticosteroids prevent infections by promoting leukocytes.
    b. Corticosteroids promote the inflammatory response that suppresses the immune system.
    c. Corticosteroids suppress adrenal function.
    d. Corticosteroids promote leukocyte activation.

29. Before receiving antithymocyte globulin, the client would receive which drugs to decrease the incidence and severity of adverse reactions?
    a. Corticosteroid and antibiotic
    b. Antihistamine and antibiotic
    c. Antibiotic and diuretic
    d. Corticosteroid and antihistamine

30. A client who had a heart transplant is to receive immunosuppressive drugs to prevent rejection. Which nursing intervention is a priority in this patient?
    a. Advise the client to avoid anyone with an active infection.
    b. Instruct the client to take blood pressure and temperature measurements each day.
    c. Instruct the client that exercising places undue stress on the body, further suppressing the immune system.
    d. Promote proper nutrition by cooking all foods, including fruits and vegetables.

CASE STUDY

Read the scenario and answer the following questions on a separate sheet of paper.

J.R. is scheduled to receive a liver transplant. Several hours before the surgery, J.R. is to receive cyclosporine and methylprednisolone sodium succinate.

1. What types of drugs are cyclosporine and methylprednisolone sodium succinate, and what are their general mechanisms of action?

2. What are some of the common side effects and adverse effects of cyclosporine and methylprednisolone sodium succinate?

3. Explain why clients receiving immunosuppressive drugs should not receive live vaccines.

31 | Vaccines

Match the term in Column I to its definition in Column II.

Column I

_____ 1. Seroconversion

_____ 2. Pathogen

_____ 3. Vaccine

_____ 4. Antibody

_____ 5. Attenuated viruses

_____ 6. Passive immunity

_____ 7. Toxoids

Column II

a. Immediate and short-lived
b. Weakened microorganisms
c. Another term for immunoglobulins
d. Acquisition of detectable levels of antibodies
e. A small amount of antigen that is administered to stimulate the immune response
f. Microorganisms, such as bacteria, viruses, and fungi that invade the body
g. Inactivated toxins to stimulate antitoxins

Complete the following.

8. In the United States, there are more than _____ infectious diseases that may be prevented with vaccination.

9. The Advisory Committee on Immunizations identified recommended _____, _____ to vaccinate, _____, and _____.

10. Yellow fever is transmitted by _____.

11. Adverse effects to vaccines must be reported through a surveillance system called _____.

12. _____ zoster is the reactivation of _____ zoster, usually settling in a dorsal root ganglion and causing severe pain.

REVIEW QUESTIONS

13. Which term is used for vaccines made from the inactivated toxic substances produced by some microorganisms?
    a. Attenuated vaccines
    b. Conjugate vaccines
    c. Recombinant subunit vaccines
    d. Toxoids

14. In which situation(s) would persons receive immunoglobulin for acquired passive immunity? *(Select all that apply.)*
    a. Fetuses in utero
    b. When time does not permit active vaccination alone
    c. When the exposed individual is at high risk for complications of the disease
    d. During pregnancy
    e. Someone who is immunosuppressed

15. By which process are antibodies received by an individual, used for protection against a particular pathogen, and acquired from another source?
    a. Active immunity
    b. Childhood immunity
    c. Passive immunity
    d. Toxoids

16. Which action occurs when there is an acquisition of detectable levels of antibodies in the bloodstream after receiving vaccines?
    a. Passive immunity
    b. Acquired natural immunity
    c. Immunization
    d. Seroconversion

17. When a parent asks about vaccine's action, which statement is the nurse's correct response?
    a. "Vaccines are perceived by the body as antibodies."
    b. "Vaccines cause an allergic reaction."
    c. "Vaccines produce a mild form of the disease."
    d. "Vaccines stimulate an immune response."

18. Which type of immunity develops that usually persists for the remainder of the individual's life after being infected with a disease?
    a. Natural acquired
    b. Humoral
    c. Active acquired artificial
    d. Passive natural

19. Which age is a child's first vaccine usually administered?
    a. At birth
    b. 2 months of age
    c. 4 months of age
    d. 6 months of age

20. Which condition is rubella commonly known as?
    a. German measles
    b. Hard measles
    c. Herpes zoster
    d. Smallpox

21. Susceptible individuals age 13 years or older receive two doses of varicella vaccine spaced how long apart?
    a. At least 4 weeks
    b. 3 months
    c. 6 months
    d. 1 year

22. Which organization would a health care provider report the details of an adverse reaction to a vaccine?
    a. Centers for Disease Control and Prevention (CDC)
    b. National Vaccine Injury Compensation Program (NVICP)
    c. Vaccine Adverse Events Reporting System (VAERS)
    d. Vaccine manufacturer

23. Which type of immunity is conferred by the Td vaccine?
    a. Active
    b. Inactive
    c. Natural
    d. Passive

24. Which immunizations are examples of live, attenuated vaccines?
    a. Influenza and hepatitis B
    b. Measles-mumps-rubella (MMR) and poliomyelitis
    c. MMR and varicella
    d. Varicella and Td

25. A client presents to a health care provider and states, "I think I have the flu." Which signs and symptoms are indicative of influenza?
    a. Abdominal pain, cough, and nasal congestion
    b. Fever, diarrhea, and dizziness
    c. Fever, myalgia, and cough
    d. Vomiting, diarrhea, and headache

26. When the MMR vaccine is not given the same day as the varicella vaccine, which time frame should be the minimum interval between administrations?
    a. 1 week
    b. 2 weeks
    c. 3 weeks
    d. 4 weeks

27. A parent reports their child developed some redness and tenderness at the injection site after the first dost of DTaP. Which action would the nurse take?
    a. Administer DTaP again, because these are common side effects, not contraindications
    b. Provide DT in the right thigh
    c. Give DTaP subcutaneously instead of intramuscularly to prevent muscle soreness
    d. Inject half the usual dose of DTaP to reduce the likelihood of a reaction

28. Which information would the nurse provide the parent of a 4-month-old child who just received immunizations? *(Select all that apply.)*
   a. Appointment card for the next immunization clinic visit
   b. Immunization record
   c. List of side effects to observe
   d. Report of adverse reaction form
   e. Vaccine Information Statements (VIS) for all vaccines administered

29. Which health and immunization information would be a good source for nurses assisting clients before international travel?
   a. Centers for Disease Control and Prevention
   b. No source is necessary because there are no special immunization needs for travelers
   c. The patient's travel agent
   d. U.S. embassy in the destination country

30. In the case of an anaphylactic reaction to a vaccine, which drug should the nurse have readily available?
   a. Acetaminophen
   b. Diphenhydramine
   c. Epinephrine
   d. Ranitidine

CASE STUDY

Read the scenario and answer the following questions on a separate sheet of paper.

M.E., an older adult, sustained a deep puncture wound to the right foot from a gardening tool. The nurse observes localized redness and swelling to the injured foot. Client has no known drug allergy and takes "only aspirin for my arthritis because I don't really like coming to the doctor much." Prior immunization includes annual influenza vaccine at a local flu shot clinic but has received no other vaccinations in more than 20 years. Vital signs are blood pressure 118/80 mm Hg, heart rate 70 beats/min, respiratory rate 16 breaths/min, and temperature 37.8° C. M.E. weighs 53 kg.

1. What is the concern for a client who has sustained a puncture wound?

2. What are the signs and symptoms of this disease process?

3. Which vaccines should be administered to the client at this time?

32 Anticancer Drugs

Match the chemotherapy drugs/terms in Column I with the most appropriate description in Column II.

Column I

_____ 1. Alkylating drugs

_____ 2. Aromatase inhibitors

_____ 3. Cyclophosphamide

_____ 4. Doxorubicin

_____ 5. Palliative chemotherapy

_____ 6. Fluorouracil

_____ 7. Hormonal agents

_____ 8. Methotrexate

_____ 9. Personal protective equipment (PPE)

_____ 10. Vincristine

Column II

a. Associated with hemorrhagic cystitis
b. Leucovorin rescue
c. Stomatitis is early sign of toxicity
d. Associated with cardiotoxicity
e. Associated with neurotoxicity
f. Powder-free gloves, mask, impermeable gown
g. Mask cancer cells and prevent them from using hormones
h. Cause cross-linking of DNA strands, abnormal base pairing, or DNA strand breaks
i. Used to relieve symptoms associated with advanced disease
j. Block conversion of androgens to estrogen

Identify the environmental influences on cancer.

11. _____ Benzene

12. _____ Ultraviolet rays

13. _____ Epstein-Barr virus

14. _____ Animal fat

15. _____ Alcohol

REVIEW QUESTIONS

16. The nurse is caring for a client receiving combination chemotherapy. The client asks why more than one drug is prescribed. Which response by the nurse would be correct?
    a. "It has better response rates than single-drug chemotherapy."
    b. "It has fewer side effects than when given alone."
    c. "It is always more effective than surgery or radiation."
    d. "Survival rates are always better."

17. The nurse is teaching a community group about factors that influence the development of cancer in humans. Which information will the nurse include in this teaching?
    a. Aflatoxin is associated with cancer of the lung.
    b. Benzene is associated with cancer of the tongue.
    c. Epstein-Barr virus is associated with cancer of the stomach.
    d. Human papillomavirus is associated with cancer of the cervix.

18. Which information will the nurse tell the client concerning the side effects of chemotherapy?
    a. They are minimal because chemotherapy drugs are highly selective.
    b. Side effects usually occur during the first cycle of treatment.
    c. Toxicities to normal cells cause the side effects.
    d. Side effects of chemotherapy are usually permanent.

19. An older adult client is diagnosed with advanced metastatic cancer and is scheduled to receive palliative chemotherapy. Which response by the nurse is appropriate when the client questions the benefits of palliative chemotherapy if it will not kill the cancer cells?
    a. "Quality of life is improved."
    b. "Limits further growth of the cancer."
    c. "Growth of cancer will be slower."
    d. "Tumors will shrink throughout your body."

20. The client will be receiving chemotherapy that will lower white blood cell count. Monitoring for which finding will be a nursing priority?
    a. Change in temperature
    b. Evidence of petechiae
    c. Increase in diarrhea
    d. Taste changes

21. The client has thrombocytopenia secondary to chemotherapy. Which nursing actions would be most appropriate?
    a. Apply pressure to the injection site and assess for occult bleeding.
    b. Help the patient conserve energy by scheduling care.
    c. Monitor breath sounds and vital signs.
    d. Provide small, frequent meals and monitor loss of fluids from diarrhea.

22. The client has diarrhea secondary to chemotherapy. Which important information should be included in client teaching about chemotherapy-related diarrhea?
    a. Eat only very hot or very cold foods.
    b. Increase intake of fresh fruits and vegetables.
    c. Increase intake of high-fiber foods.
    d. Limit caffeine intake.

23. An older adult client is to receive cyclophosphamide for treatment of lymphoma. Medical history includes atrial fibrillation, arthritis, and cataracts. Digoxin 0.125 mg daily and naproxen 500 mg at bedtime are the current drugs the client is on. Which information will the nurse need to be aware of when giving these drugs?
    a. Cyclophosphamide increases digoxin levels.
    b. Cyclophosphamide decreases digoxin levels.
    c. Digoxin increases cyclophosphamide levels.
    d. These drugs cannot be given together.

24. The client is in the outpatient oncology clinic for treatment with fluorouracil (5-FU) for colon cancer. The client has recently been started on metronidazole for treatment of trichomoniasis. Which drug-drug interactions will concern the nurse about administering 5-FU?
    a. 5-FU may decrease the effectiveness of metronidazole.
    b. 5-FU cannot be given with metronidazole.
    c. Metronidazole may increase the side effects of 5-FU.
    d. Metronidazole may increase 5-FU toxicity.

25. An older adult client is receiving acetaminophen, cyclophosphamide, doxorubicin, and methotrexate (CAM) for the treatment of prostate cancer. During morning rounds, the client complains of feeling short of breath. Physical assessment reveals crackles in both lungs. Which drug most likely caused this clinical manifestation?
    a. Acetaminophen
    b. Cyclophosphamide
    c. Doxorubicin
    d. Methotrexate

26. A client is to receive an antiemetic and fluorouracil (5-FU) intravenously as part of a treatment protocol for colon cancer. Which time frame would the nurse administer the antiemetic?
    a. 1 day after administering 5-FU
    b. 1 day before administering 5-FU
    c. 30–60 minutes before administering 5-FU
    d. 4 hours before administering 5-FU

27. Which nursing outcome would be most appropriate as part of the planning for a client scheduled to receive cyclophosphamide?
    a. Patient will be free from symptoms of stomatitis.
    b. Patient will maintain cardiac output.
    c. Patient will show no signs of hemorrhagic cystitis.
    d. Patient will show no signs of syndrome of inappropriate antidiuretic hormone secretion (SIADH).

28. The client is to receive cyclophosphamide as part of cancer treatment. Which nursing intervention should the nurse expect to complete?
    a. Assess for signs of hematuria, urinary frequency, or dysuria.
    b. Decrease fluids to reduce the risk of calculus formation.
    c. Hydrate the client with intravenous (IV) fluids only after administration of cyclophosphamide.
    d. Medicate with an antiemetic only after the client complains of nausea.

29. The nurse is administering doxorubicin to a client diagnosed with cancer. Which time frame will the nurse assess for tissue necrosis due to doxorubicin?
    a. 3–4 weeks after administration.
    b. Immediately after administration.
    c. 2–4 days after administration.
    d. Tissue necrosis rarely occurs with this drug.

30. The nurse is preparing IV vinblastine, bleomycin, and cisplatin (VBP) for administration to a client on the nursing unit. Which precaution should the nurse take when hanging IV chemotherapy?
    a. Wear a clean cotton gown.
    b. Wear shoe covers.
    c. Wear a hair net.
    d. Wear two pairs of gloves.

31. A client is being discharged after receiving IV chemotherapy. Which statement made by the patient indicates a need for additional teaching?
    a. "Chemotherapy is excreted in my bodily fluids."
    b. "I will not need to know how to check my temperature."
    c. "My spouse should wear gloves when emptying my urinal."
    d. "The chemotherapy will remain in my body for 2–3 days."

32. A client with breast cancer is scheduled to receive anastrozole, an aromatase inhibitor. Which information will the nurse include in the teaching?
    a. Peripheral conversion of androgens to estrogens is blocked.
    b. Tumors that are not hormonally sensitive are treated with aromatase inhibitors.
    c. Premenopausal women with breast cancer are treated with aromatase inhibitors.
    d. Postmenopausal women with breast cancer are treated with aromatase inhibitors.

33. A client is scheduled to receive vincristine as part of treatment for cancer. The medication record for the client indicates that phenytoin is taken to control a seizure disorder. Which medical contidion will the nurse monitor in this client?
    a. Headaches
    b. Increased blood pressure
    c. Renal failure
    d. Seizures

34. A client in the outpatient oncology clinic has developed stomatitis secondary to cancer therapy. Which statement made by the client would indicate that additional teaching about stomatitis is needed?
    a. "I will rinse my mouth out frequently with normal saline."
    b. "I will try using ice pops or ice chips to help relieve mouth pain."
    c. "I will use a mouthwash that has an alcohol base."
    d. "I will use a soft toothbrush."

CASE STUDY

Read the scenario and answer the following questions on a separate sheet of paper.

C.Z. is being treated for multiple myeloma with cyclophosphamide.

1. To which class of drugs does cyclophosphamide belong, and how does it work?

2. What are the major side effects of cyclophosphamide?

3. What are key factors in the nursing assessment for C.Z. receiving cyclophosphamide?

4. What are priority teaching points for C.Z. with regard to the drug regimen?

33 Targeted Therapies to Treat Cancer

STUDY QUESTIONS

Complete the following.

1. The _____ _____ binding to cell receptors on the cell membrane can activate tyrosine kinases, which then turn on signal transduction pathways promoting cell division.

2. _____ are multienzyme complexes that degrade proteins intracellularly.

3. Targeted therapies block the _____ and _____ of cancer cells.

4. The largest class of targeted therapy drugs that attack one particular molecular target is _____ inhibitor.

5. _____ are enzymes that activate other proteins, including signal transduction pathways.

Match the class of targeted therapy drug in Column I to the mechanism of action in Column II.

Column I	Column II
_____ 6. mTOR kinase inhibitor	a. Prevents formation of new blood vessels
_____ 7. EGFR inhibitor	b. Binds to different areas of EGFR, blocking its activity
_____ 8. Angiogenesis inhibitor	c. Primarily affects BCR-ABL kinase enzyme
_____ 9. Monoclonal antibody	d. Leads to G_1 arrest and cell death
_____ 10. Tyrosine kinase inhibitor	e. Targets cell-membrane surface antigens

REVIEW QUESTIONS

11. During the first dose of trastuzumab, the client complains of shortness of breath and pruritus. What is the best action by the nurse?
    a. Decrease the infusion rate by 50% and notify the health care provider.
    b. Disconnect the IV and attach a 0.22-micron filter.
    c. Review the pretreatment multigated acquisition (MUGA) scan.
    d. Stop the infusion and manage the reaction.

12. What is the rationale for administering bevacizumab in a client with metastatic colon cancer?
    a. To enhance the client's immune response
    b. To increase apoptosis
    c. To inhibit tumor's microvascular growth
    d. To modulate an inflammatory response

13. Gefitinib most frequently causes which side/adverse effect?
    a. Hypocalcemia
    b. Diarrhea
    c. Myelosuppression
    d. Seizures

14. Which antibodies are types of monoclonal antibodies? *(Select all that apply.)*
    a. Fully human antibodies
    b. Chimeric antibodies
    c. Equine antibodies
    d. Porcine antibodies
    e. Murine antibodies

15. An oncology client is to begin treatment for non–small-cell lung cancer (NSCLC) with administration of gefitinib. The nurse notes on the medical record that the client is also taking warfarin daily for atrial fibrillation. Which genfitinib action would concern the nurse about the client taking gefitinib and warfarin?
    a. Gefitinib increases the effects of warfarin.
    b. Gefitinib may require a dose increase when taken with warfarin.
    c. Gefitinib should not be given to a patient taking anticoagulants.
    d. Gefitinib may reach toxic levels when given concurrently with warfarin.

16. A client in the outpatient oncology clinic is receiving sunitinib as part of the treatment for gastrointestinal stromal tumors (GIST). The health care provider prescribes ketoconazole to treat a fungal infection. Which drug-drug interaction would concern the nurse about taking these drugs concurrently?
    a. Ketoconazole may decrease the effectiveness of sunitinib.
    b. Ketoconazole may potentiate sunitinib toxicity.
    c. Sunitinib may decrease the effectiveness of ketoconazole.
    d. Sunitinib may lead to toxic levels of ketoconazole.

17. A client is beginning therapy with the epidermal growth factor/receptor inhibitor (EGFRI) erlotinib for non-small cell lung cancer (NSCLC). Which status would be important for the nurse to assess before beginning therapy with this targeted drug?
    a. Cardiac status
    b. Hearing function
    c. Lung sounds
    d. Mental status

18. A client is admitted to the hospital 1 week after receiving imatinib. On physical assessment, the nurse notes the presence of petechiae, ecchymoses, and bleeding gums. Which nursing diagnosis would be most appropriate?
    a. Bleeding
    b. Falls
    c. Fatigue
    d. Altered nutrition

19. A client is to start ziv-aflibercept, in addition to the already prescribed 5-fluorouracil (5-FU), leucovorin, and irinotecan. Which statements made by the client indicates a lack of understanding for receiving ziv-aflibercept?
    a. "The new drug is going to starve cancer cells."
    b. "I will need to stay indoors because medicine will make my skin more sensitive to the sun."
    c. "The drug will allow my good cells to grow new vessels."
    d. "The drug will prevent the cells from dividing."

20. A client who is to receive rituximab has a blood pressure of 90/52 mm Hg and a heart rate of 82 beats/min. Upon reviewing the client's routine drugs, the nurse notes antihypertensives. Which action would be best for the nurse to take?
    a. Start the infusion. The blood pressure and heart rate are within the parameters.
    b. Notify the health care provider.
    c. Infuse 250 mL of 0.9% sodium chloride over 2 hours before infusing rituximab.
    d. Retake the blood pressure in the other arm.

CASE STUDY

Read the scenario and answer the following questions on a separate sheet of paper.

S.M. has been diagnosed with ovarian cancer and presents to the outpatient oncology clinic for treatment. S.M. is being treated with bevacizumab for metastatic disease.

1. How is bevacizumab administered?

2. What is the mechanism of action?

3. What are potential side effects and adverse effects?

4. What teaching should be provided by the nurse in relation to bevacizumab therapy?

34 Biologic Response Modifiers

Complete the following.

1. Immunotherapies, also called _____ _____ _____, enhance, direct, or _____ the body's immune system.

2. Two advances in biologic therapies include _____ _____ and _____ _____.

3. Biologic response modifiers assist the immune system through _____ and prevent cancer cells from _____.

4. Macrophages are considered mature _____.

5. Erythropoietin stimulates the production of _____ _____ _____ in the bone marrow.

6. Granulocyte colony–stimulating factor is produced by macrophages, _____, and other immune cells and stimulates the synthesis of _____.

7. Many adverse effects of exogenous interleukins are due to _____ _____ _____.

Match the appropriate term in Column I with the description in Column II.

Column I	Column II
_____ 8. Colony-stimulating factors (CSFs)	a. Glycoprotein that stimulates the production of neutrophils
_____ 9. Erythropoietin	b. Proteins that stimulate growth and maturation of bone marrow stem cells
_____ 10. Granulocyte colony–stimulating factor (G-CSF)	c. Glycoprotein produced by the kidneys in response to low oxygen (hypoxia)
_____ 11. Granulocyte-macrophage colony–stimulating factor (GM-CSF)	d. Supports survival, proliferation, and differentiation of hematopoietic progenitor cells

REVIEW QUESTIONS

12. Which mechanism of action is/are the primary function(s) of biologic response modifiers (BRMs)? *(Select all that apply.)*
    a. Slow spread of tumor cells
    b. Enhance host's normal immunologic function
    c. Improve liver functioning
    d. Change cancers cells to behave more like healthy cells
    e. Replicate red blood cells

13. A client is receiving GM-CSF therapy. Which system will the nurse focus attention on, both during and after these infusions?
    a. Cardiac system
    b. Central nervous system
    c. Musculoskeletal system
    d. Respiratory system

14. Before administering erythropoietin, which assessment would the nurse conduct?
    a. Renal function
    b. Hemoglobin level
    c. Liver function
    d. Chest x-ray

15. A client is being treated with interferon for chronic myelogenous leukemia. Which drug effect would the nurse anticipate stopping treatment? *(Select all that apply.)*
    a. Severe depression
    b. Hepatic decompensation
    c. Absolute neutrophil count $<500/mm^3$
    d. Platelets $>140,000/mm^3$

16. A client with hairy cell leukemia is being treated with interferon. The client reports neurologic side effects. Which information will the nurse tell the client about the side effects?
    a. "These side effects are common and will subside after the drug is stopped."
    b. "These side effects rarely occur."
    c. "These side effects will diminish as treatment goes on."
    d. "The worst effect is mild confusion."

17. For which dermatologic effect(s) would the nurse assess in a client taking interferon? *(Select all that apply.)*
    a. Alopecia
    b. Bruising
    c. Xerostomia
    d. Rash

18. Which statements are appropriate health teaching information for a client who has hairy cell leukemia and is being treated with interferon alpha? *(Select all that apply.)*
    a. Report any unusual weight loss.
    b. Teach information on the effect of BRM-related fatigue on activities of daily living
    c. Side effects from a BRM disappear within 12–24 hours after discontinuation of therapy.
    d. Persistent headache or blurred vision should be reported to the health care provider.

19. For which condition(s) may GM-CSF be administered to clients? *(Select all that apply.)*
    a. Absolute neutrophil count $>1500/mm^3$
    b. Autologous bone marrow transplant (BMT) recipient
    c. Allogeneic BMT recipient
    d. 12 hours after high-dose chemotherapy administration
    e. Kaposi sarcoma

20. A client is to start aldesleukin for metastatic renal cell cancer. Which potential drug effects would the nurse monitor to determine dose interruption or discontinuation? *(Select all that apply).*
    a. New irregular cardiac rhythm
    b. Oxygen saturation less than 95%
    c. Stool positive for blood
    d. Existing skin rash that was present before starting aldesleukin
    e. Hypoglycemia

CASE STUDY

Read the scenario, and answer the following questions on a separate sheet of paper.

K.U. has been diagnosed with acute myelogenous leukemia (AML) and will be undergoing treatment. K.U. is scheduled to receive granulocyte colony-stimulating factors (G-CSF) and wants to know what this drug will do to cure the cancer. K.U. will be receiving 75 mcg/kg/day IV.

1. What type of medication is G-CSF, and how does it work?

2. What are the potential side effects K.U. may experience with this drug?

3. What priority teaching will the nurse provide to the patient and her significant others?

35 Upper Respiratory Disorders

Match the drug class in Column I to the description in Column II.

Column I

_____ 1. Antihistamines

_____ 2. Antitussives

_____ 3. Decongestants

_____ 4. Expectorants

Column II

a. Act on the cough-control center in the medulla

b. Loosen bronchial secretions so they can be removed by coughing

c. H_1 blockers or H_1 antagonists

d. Stimulate the alpha-adrenergic receptors, producing vascular constriction in the nasal capillaries

Complete the following.

5. Antihistamines are ____ antagonists that have effects on the _____ muscles.

6. Many over-the-counter (OTC) cold remedies contain a _____ _____ antihistamine that can cause side effects such as ____ _____ and _____.

7. Second-generation antihistamines are considered _____ and have fewer _____ side effects.

8. Frequent use of nasal decongestants can result in _____ and _____ _____ _____, which can occur in as little as ___ _____.

9. Nasal decongestants stimulate the _____ receptors that cause _____, which can also cause _____.

Match the antihistamine in Column I to the correct generation in Column II. The generation in Column II may be used more than once.

Column I

_____ 10. Diphenhydramine

_____ 11. Cetirizine

_____ 12. Loratadine

_____ 13. Chlorpheniramine

_____ 14. Azelastine

_____ 15. Clemastine fumarate

Column II

a. First generation

b. Second generation

16. Antihistamines are another group of drugs used for the relief of cold symptoms. Which properties of these drugs result in decreased secretions?
    a. Analgesic
    b. Anticholinergic
    c. Antitussive
    d. Cholinergic

17. Compared to first-generation antihistamines, second-generation antihistamines have a lower incidence of which side effect?
    a. Drowsiness
    b. Headache
    c. Tinnitus
    d. Vomiting

18. The U.S. Food and Drug Administration has ordered removal of all cold remedies containing which drug?
    a. Dextromethorphan
    b. Guaifenesin
    c. Histamine
    d. Phenylpropanolamine

19. The client has seasonal allergies and asks the student health nurse about the appropriate dose of diphenhydramine. Which amount is the recommended dosage of diphenhydramine?
    a. 25–50 mg q6–8h
    b. 25–50 mg daily
    c. 50–100 mg q4–6h
    d. 100 mg daily

20. Which effects of diphenhydramine is a therapeutic effect?
    a. Anticoagulant
    b. Anticonvulsant
    c. Antihypertensive
    d. Antitussive

21. Which advice will the nurse give to the breastfeeding client who is also taking diphenhydramine?
    a. Breastfeeding provides allergy relief to the infant.
    b. Large amounts of the drug pass into breast milk; breastfeeding is not recommended.
    c. Small amounts of the drug pass into breast milk; breastfeeding is not recommended.
    d. The drug does not affect breastfeeding.

22. Which statement indicates an advantage of systemic decongestants over nasal sprays and drops?
    a. Fewer side effects
    b. Less costly
    c. Preferred by older patients
    d. Provide longer relief

23. Which expectorant is frequently an ingredient in cold remedies?
    a. Dextromethorphan
    b. Ephedrine
    c. Guaifenesin
    d. Promethazine

24. Which group(s) of drugs is/are used to treat cold symptoms? *(Select all that apply.)*
    a. Antihistamines
    b. Antitussives
    c. Decongestants
    d. Expectorants
    e. Xanthines

25. Decongestants are contraindicated or to be used with extreme caution for clients with which condition(s)? *(Select all that apply.)*
    a. Cardiac disease
    b. Diabetes mellitus
    c. Hypertension
    d. Hyperthyroidism
    e. Obesity

26. Which priority information should be included in teaching a client who is taking drugs for a common cold and has a history of atrial fibrillation and depression? *(Select all that apply.)*
    a. Administer 4 puffs of nasal spray for a full 10 days.
    b. Antibiotics are also needed to fight a common cold virus.
    c. Do not drive during initial use of a cold remedy containing an antihistamine.
    d. Read labels of over-the-counter drugs for any interactions with current drugs.
    e. Take cold remedies with a decongestant for a better night's sleep.

CASE STUDY

Read the scenario and answer the following questions on a separate sheet of paper.

G.H., who is preparing to fly across the country for a conference, presents to the health care provider with nasal stuffiness. G.H. tells the provider "I hate to fly when my nose is this way. It just makes the trip all that much longer." A decongestant, oxymetazoline, is ordered.

1. What is the purpose of oxymetazoline, and how does it work?

2. What is the standard dosage for this drug?

3. What is rebound congestion? What other side effects might be expected, and how can they be prevented? Are there any other options for a decongestant?

36 Lower Respiratory Disorders

Match the drug in Column I with its category in Column II. Drugs may belong to more than one category.

Column I

_____ 1. Acetylcysteine

_____ 2. Zafirlukast

_____ 3. Albuterol

_____ 4. Ipratropium bromide

_____ 5. Dexamethasone

_____ 6. Epinephrine

_____ 7. Arformoterol tartrate

_____ 8. Tiotropium

Column II

a. Alpha-adrenergic agonist
b. Beta-adrenergic agonist
c. Glucocorticoid
d. Mucolytic
e. Leukotriene receptor antagonist
f. Anticholinergic

Complete the following.

9. The substance responsible for maintaining bronchodilation is _____ _____.

10. In an acute bronchospasm caused by anaphylaxis, the nonselective sympathomimetic drug administered subcutaneously to promote bronchodilation and elevate the blood pressure is _____.

11. The first line of defense in an acute asthmatic attack are the drugs categorized as _____ _____.

12. Sympathomimetics cause dilation of the bronchioles by increasing _____.

13. Theophylline (increases/decreases) the risk of digitalis toxicity. *(Circle correct answer.)*

14. When theophylline and beta$_2$-adrenergic agonists are given together, a(n) _____ effect can occur.

15. The half-life of theophylline is (shorter/longer) for smokers than for nonsmokers. *(Circle correct answer.)*

16. Aminophylline, theophylline, and caffeine are _____ derivatives used to treat _____.

17. The drugs commonly prescribed to treat unresponsive asthma are _____.

18. Cromolyn is used as a _____ treatment for bronchial asthma. It acts by inhibiting the release of _____.

19. A serious side effect of cromolyn is _____ _____.

20. The newer drugs for asthma are more selective for _____ receptors.

21. The leukotriene receptor antagonist (is/is not) considered safe for use in children 6 years and older. *(Circle correct answer.)*

22. The preferred time of day for the administration of leukotriene receptor antagonists is _____.

23. The usual dose of montelukast for an adult is _____.

24. A group of drugs used to liquefy and loosen thick mucous secretions is _____.

25. With infection resulting from retained mucous secretions, a(n) _____ may be prescribed.

REVIEW QUESTIONS

26. A client is being treated for chronic obstructive pulmonary disease (COPD) with a drug that is delivered via a metered-dose inhaler. Related health teaching would include which priority information?
    a. Hold the inhaler upside down.
    b. Refrigerate the inhaler.
    c. Shake the inhaler well just before use.
    d. Test the inhaler each time to see if the spray works.

27. When compared to oral drugs for asthma, which information regarding a drug administered by a metered-dose inhaler will the nurse be aware? *(Select all that apply.)*
    a. Inhaled dose will deliver more of the drug directly to the lungs.
    b. There are fewer side effects with an inhaled drug.
    c. Inhaled drug is longer-lasting.
    d. Inhaled drug has a more rapid onset.
    e. Some oral and inhaled drugs can be taken together.

28. A client expresses not having the time to wait between taking an inhaled beta agonist and an inhaled steroid for asthma. Which response would be appropriate by the nurse?
    a. "The inhaled drug will allow the bronchioles to dilate so the steroid works better."
    b. "This is done so you remember which one comes first."
    c. "The inhaled medication will make your heart circulate the steroid faster."
    d. "The steroid may make your nose stuffy, so you take the inhaled drug first."

29. What is/are the side effect(s) of long-term use of glucocorticoids? *(Select all that apply.)*
    a. Impaired immune response
    b. Insomnia
    c. Hyperglycemia
    d. Vomiting
    e. Weight loss

30. Which anticholinergic drug has few systemic effects and is administered by aerosol?
    a. Albuterol
    b. Ipratropium
    c. Isoproterenol
    d. Tiotropium

31. A client who has been taking theophylline for asthma has also been taking ephedra to stay alert while finishing a project at work. Heart rate is 124 beats/min, respiratory rate 18 breaths/min, blood pressure 170/90 mm Hg, and oxygen saturation 99% on room air. Fingerstick blood glucose is 210 mg/dL and the theophylline level is 26 mcg/mL. Which side effect or reaction would the nurse suspect may be the cause of the client's symptoms?
    a. Acute allergic reaction
    b. Asthma attack
    c. Stevens-Johnson syndrome
    d. Theophylline toxicity

32. The client has exercise-induced bronchospasm and is being treated with a short-acting beta$_2$ agonist. Which priority information will the nurse include in a review of inhaler administration for this client? *(Select all that apply.)*
    a. "Cleanse all washable parts of inhaler equipment daily."
    b. "Hold your breath for a few seconds, remove mouthpiece, and exhale slowly."
    c. "Keep your lips secure around the mouthpiece and inhale while pushing the top of the canister once."
    d. "Monitor your heart rate while taking this medication."
    e. "Wait 5 minutes and repeat the procedure if a second inhalation is needed."

33. Which medication(s) when prescribed with theophylline will concern the nurse? *(Select all that apply.)*
    a. Beta blockers
    b. Digitalis
    c. Lithium
    d. Stool softeners
    e. Phenytoin

34. Which statement by a patient prescribed cromolyn indicates the need for more education?
    a. "I must take this drug every day."
    b. "It will stop an asthma attack when taken immediately."
    c. "I can rinse my mouth out with water to get rid of the taste."
    d. "It is important for me to take this exactly as directed."

35. A client is taking theophylline, and the nurse is reviewing the lab results. Which level of theophylline would fall in the therapeutic range?
    a. 2 mcg/mL
    b. 8 mcg/mL
    c. 14 mcg/mL
    d. 23 mcg/mL

CASE STUDY

Read the scenario, and answer the following questions on a separate sheet of paper.

H.K. has recently been diagnosed with asthma and has been prescribed albuterol, montelukast sodium, and fluticasone propionate/salmeterol 100/50 mcg.

1. To which classifications do each of these drugs belong?

2. What are the mechanisms of action for each drug?

3. What are priority teaching points for this client with a new diagnosis of asthma?

37 Cardiac Glycosides, Antianginals, and Antidysrhythmics

Match the ECG waveform in Column I to its definition in Column II.

Column I

_____ 1.   P wave

_____ 2.   QRS complex

_____ 3.   T wave

_____ 4.   PR interval

_____ 5.   QT interval

Column II

a.   Ventricular action potential duration
b.   Atrial activation (depolarization)
c.   Ventricular repolarization
d.   trioventricular (AV) conduction time
e.   Ventricular depolarization

Complete the following.

6.   Heart failure occurs when the myocardium (strengthens/weakens) and (shrinks/enlarges), which causes the heart to lose its ability to pump blood through the heart and circulatory system. *(Circle correct answers.)*

7.   With heart failure there is a(n) (increase/decrease) in preload and afterload. *(Circle correct answer.)*

8.   Cardiac glycosides are also called _____ _____ which _____ the sodium-potassium pump.

9.   The action of antianginal drugs is to increase blood flow and to (increase/decrease) oxygen supply or to (increase/decrease) oxygen demand by the myocardium. *(Circle correct answers.)*

10.   Name three of the four effects digitalis preparations have on the heart muscle (myocardium): _____, _____, and _____.

11.   Beta blockers and calcium channel blockers (decrease/increase) the workload of the heart. *(Circle correct answer.)*

12.   To prevent thromboembolus in patients with atrial dysrhythmias, _____ is prescribed concurrently with antidysrhythmics.

13.   Electrolyte imbalances such as _____, _____, and _____ can increase digitalis toxicity.

14.   Angiotensin converting enzyme (ACE) inhibitors help patients with heart failure by _____ venules and _____, which improves _____ blood flow and _____ blood fluid volume.

15.   Short-acting nitroglycerin (NTG) is not swallowed because it undergoes _____, thereby decreasing its effectiveness.

16.   NTG acts directly on the _____, causing relaxation and dilation.

17.   NTG sublingually acts within _____ minutes. Administration may be repeated _____ times.

18.   The most common side effect of NTG is _____.

19. The two drug groups that may be used as an antianginal, antidysrhythmic, and antihypertensive are _____ _____ and _____ _____ _____.

20. Calcium channel blockers that are effective in the long-term treatment of angina, dysrhythmia, and hypertension and have the side effect of bradycardia are _____ and _____.

21. Beta blockers and calcium channel blockers should not be discontinued without health care provider approval. Withdrawal symptoms may include _____ _____ and _____.

22. Classic angina occurs when the patient is _____.

23. Unstable angina (preinfarction) has the following pattern of occurrence: Occurs _____, is _____, and manifests with _____ severity.

24. Variant angina (Prinzmetal's angina) occurs when the patient _____.

25. Prinzmetal's angina is due to _____ of the vessels.

26. The major systemic effect of nitrates is _____.

27. Cardiac dysrhythmias can result from (hypoxia/hyperoxia) and (hypocapnia/hypercapnia). *(Circle correct answers.)*

28. Examples of antidysrhythmics include _____, _____, and _____.

29. Patients with heart failure should avoid _____ and _____.

Match the herbs in Column I with their effects on digoxin in Column II. Answers may be used more than once.

Column I

_____30. St. John's wort

_____31. Ephedra

_____32. Aloe

_____33. Goldenseal

_____34. Ginseng

Column II

a. Increased risk of digitalis toxicity
b. Decreased digoxin absorption
c. Decreased effects of digoxin
d. Falsely elevated digoxin levels

REVIEW QUESTIONS

35. Phosphodiesterase inhibitors promote which actions in treating heart failure?
   a. Increase serum sodium and potassium levels
   b. Promote negative inotropic action
   c. Promote positive inotropic action
   d. Promote vasoconstriction

36. A client with a history of atrial flutter is prescribed quinidine. What is the nurse's best response when answering a patient who asks how the drug helps the heart?
   a. "It will help your heart pump stronger."
   b. "It will prevent you from having chest pain."
   c. "It will decrease myocardial oxygen consumption."
   d. "It will slow down the speed of your heart so that it will work more effectively."

37. Which is more effective when other drugs are ineffective in treating ventricular fibrillation.
   a. Amiodarone
   b. Atropine
   c. Acebutolol HCl
   d. Propafenone HCl

38. What is lidocaine primarily used to treat?
   a. Atrial fibrillation
   b. Bradycardia
   c. Complete heart block
   d. Ventricular dysrhythmias

39. A client with angina has been prescribed verapamil. Which priority teaching point(s) will the nurse include regarding this drug? *(Select all that apply.)*
    a. "Eat lots of fiber to avoid constipation."
    b. "High blood pressure can be caused by verapamil."
    c. "This drug is taken three times per day."
    d. "Wear sunscreen due to photosensitivity."
    e. "You should not take this drug if you are diabetic."

40. A client has been prescribed amlodipine to help control hypertension. Which laboratory values must be monitored carefully when on amlodipine?
    a. Arterial blood gasses
    b. Blood glucose
    c. Complete blood count
    d. Liver enzymes

41. Abnormal levels of atrial natriuretic peptide (ANP) and brain natriuretic peptide (BNP) indicate which disease process?
    a. Aneurysm
    b. Cerebrovascular accident
    c. Heart failure
    d. Myocardial infarction

42. A client taking digoxin daily along with several other drugs has a brain natriuretic peptide (BNP) level of 630 pg/mL. What concerns the nurse about this level?
    a. It is below the normal/reference range for her age.
    b. Nothing. It is within the normal range.
    c. It is slightly elevated.
    d. It is markedly elevated.

43. The nurse knows that digitalis is usually prescribed for which abnormal rhythm?
    a. Atrial fibrillation
    b. Paroxysmal atrial tachycardia
    c. Second-degree heart block
    d. Ventricular tachycardia

44. What is the usual maintenance dose of digoxin?
    a. 0.125-5 mg/d
    b. 0.025-1 mg/d
    c. 0.05-1.75 mg/d
    d. 6–10 mg/d

45. A client, who has been on digoxin, presents to the clinic complaining of nausea, malaise, and "just not feeling well." The nurse suspects digoxin toxicity. What is a therapeutic digitalis level?
    a. 0.15–0.5 ng/mL
    b. 0.8–2 ng/mL
    c. 2–3.5 ng/mL
    d. 3.5–4 ng/mL

46. What is the antidote for digitalis toxicity?
    a. Cardizem
    b. Digoxin immune Fab
    c. Gamma globulin
    d. Protamine

47. The nurse is reviewing the patient's medication administration record (MAR). Which drug(s) on the MAR will concern the nurse, given that the patient is taking digitalis? *(Select all that apply.)*
    a. Cortisone
    b. Furosemide
    c. Hydrochlorothiazide
    d. Nitroglycerin
    e. Potassium supplement

48. The nurse is providing health teaching to a client prescribed digoxin for heart failure. Which food(s) will the nurse tell the client to avoid? *(Select all that apply.)*
    a. Apples
    b. Celery
    c. Hot dogs
    d. Lettuce
    e. Potatoes

49. Which priority health teaching should be given to a client taking sublingual (SL) nitroglycerin (NTG)? *(Select all that apply.)*
    a. Sips of water may be taken before placing NTG SL to aid in absorption.
    b. NTG should be stored in its original container and away from light.
    c. The tablet is to be chewed and swallowed.
    d. Call your health care provider if chest pain is not relieved after three tablets.
    e. Clients should not take vitamin C supplements while taking NTG.

50. What is the duration of action of a nitroglycerin transdermal patch?
    a. 6–8 hours
    b. 10–12 hours
    c. 18–24 hours
    d. 36–48 hours

51. Which priority teaching should the nurse provide to a client who has just started taking acebutolol?
    a. "Do not abruptly stop this drug, or you risk your heart rate beating very fast or irregularly."
    b. "Drowsiness is a common side effect."
    c. "No laboratory work will be required while taking this drug."
    d. "Fluid intake should be increased to prevent dehydration."

52. Which herbal preparation(s) must be avoided when taking digitalis preparations? *(Select all that apply.)*
    a. Aloe
    b. Feverfew
    c. *Ginkgo biloba*
    d. Ginseng
    e. Ma-huang

53. Which condition(s) can directly lead to cardiac dysrhythmias? *(Select all that apply.)*
    a. Electrolyte imbalances
    b. Excess catecholamines
    c. Hepatitis
    d. Hypocapnia
    e. Hypoxia

CASE STUDY

Read the scenario and answer the following questions on a separate sheet of paper.

P.E., with a history of hypertension, diet-controlled diabetes, and vasospastic angina, presents to the emergency department with severe left-sided chest pain, nausea, shortness of breath, and diaphoresis. Vital signs include the following: temperature 97.7° F, heart rate 102 beats/min, respiratory rate 20 breaths/min, blood pressure 164/100 mm Hg, and oxygen saturation on room air of 99%. After administering one sublingual nitroglycerin tablet, vital signs are heart rate 120 beats/min, respiratory rate 22 breaths/min, and blood pressure 110/60 mm Hg. P.E. now feels lightheaded and nauseated, but the chest pain persists. A nitroglycerin drip is started, and the client is admitted to critical care.

1. What are the three different types of angina?

2. Describe nonpharmacologic and pharmacologic treatments for vasospastic angina.

3. What drugs other than nitroglycerin can be used to treat angina?

4. Why did this client's blood pressure drop?

38 Diuretics

Labeling Diagram

1. **Label the different segments of the renal tubules, the major class of diuretics for each, and the primary electrolytes influenced by the diuretic.**

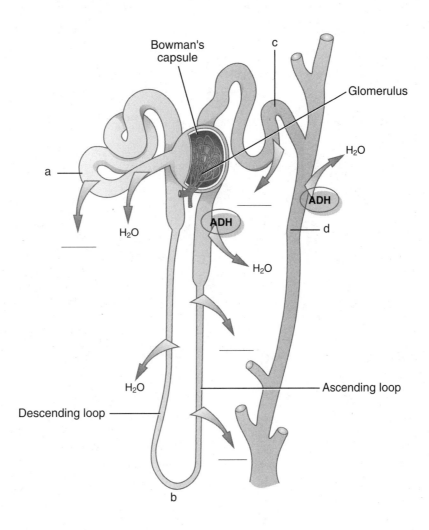

Identify the normal levels of the chemistry panel, and list the possible abnormal results (hypo- or hyper-) associated with thiazide diuretics.

Laboratory Test	Normal Levels	Abnormal Results
2. Potassium		
3. Magnesium		
4. Ionized calcium		
5. Chloride		
6. Bicarbonate		
7. Uric acid		
8. Blood sugar		
9. Blood lipids		

SHORT ANSWER QUESTIONS

Answer the following in one to two sentences.

10. What are the two main purposes for diuretics?

11. How do diuretics have antihypertensive properties?

REVIEW QUESTIONS

12. Which group(s) of diuretics is/are frequently prescribed to treat hypertension and congestive heart failure? *(Select all that apply.)*
    a. Carbonic anhydrase inhibitors
    b. Loop diuretics
    c. Osmotic diuretics
    d. Potassium-sparing diuretics
    e. Thiazide diuretics

13. What is the pharmacologic action of spironolactone?
    a. Increase potassium and sodium excretion
    b. Promote potassium retention
    c. Promote potassium and calcium retention
    d. Promote potassium excretion and sodium retention

14. What is the classification of furosemide?
    a. Loop diuretic
    b. Osmotic diuretic
    c. Potassium-sparing diuretic
    d. Thiazide diuretic

15. A client has been prescribed spironolactone 100 mg/day to treat an irregular heart rhythm. Which statement by the client indicates an understanding of the drug teaching the nurse provided?
    a. "I need sodium so my heart beats regularly."
    b. "This drug is dangerous if you have had a heart attack."
    c. "It helps keep potassium so my heart does not get irregular."
    d. "I need to take it with lots of bananas to keep my potassium up."

16. The nurse has received an order to administer 40 mg of furosemide intravenously (IV) to the client. What does the nurse know about how this drug should be administered?
    a. It must be mixed in 50 mL of normal saline.
    b. It can only be given in a central line.
    c. The patient must be on a cardiac monitor.
    d. It should be given over 1–2 minutes.

17. Which lab value(s) should a nurse monitor in a client receiving chlorothiazide? *(Select all that apply.)*
    a. Potassium
    b. Sodium
    c. Bicarbonate
    d. Calcium
    e. AST/ALT

18. A client who has had an acute myocardial infarction has been started on spironolactone 50 mg/day. When evaluating routine laboratory work, the nurse discovers the client has a potassium level of 5.8 mEq/L. What is the priority intervention to be implemented?
    a. The spironolactone dose should be held and the intake of foods rich in potassium should be restricted.
    b. The spironolactone dose should be continued and the patient should be encouraged to eat fruits and vegetables.
    c. The spironolactone dose should be increased and the patient instructed to decrease foods rich in potassium.
    d. Instruct the patient to continue with the current dose of spironolactone and report any signs or symptoms of hypokalemia.

19. Which type of acid-base imbalance could occur if a patient is taking high doses of acetazolamide or uses the drug constantly?
    a. Metabolic acidosis
    b. Metabolic alkalosis
    c. Respiratory acidosis
    d. Respiratory alkalosis

20. The client with heart failure has been prescribed hydrochlorothiazide. Which statement by the client indicates understanding of the dosing regimen?
    a. "I need to take it on an empty stomach for it to work."
    b. "I really only need to take my medicine when I am having a hard time breathing."
    c. "It may take several weeks before it starts to work."
    d. "I should take it in the morning so I don't have to go to the bathroom at night."

21. The client with a complicated medical history including heart failure, cardiac arrhythmias, arthritis, and depression was started on furosemide for heart failure. Which drug would be of major concern to the nurse?
    a. Amiodarone
    b. Acetaminophen
    c. Amitriptyline
    d. Zolpidem

22. A client taking furosemide reports being weak, having severe leg cramps, and unable to ambulate. Knowing the mechanism of action of furosemide, the nurse is concerned about which electrolyte imbalance?
    a. Hyponatremia
    b. Hypermagnesemia
    c. Hypokalemia
    d. Hyperchloremia

23. In which client are loop diuretics contraindicated?
    a. The client with anuria
    b. The client with asthma
    c. The client with allergy to ceftriaxone
    d. The client with gastric ulcers

24. A client diagnosed with hypertension and diabetes was started on hydrochlorothiazide. Which statement by the client indicates understanding of the drug teaching the nurse has provided?
    a. "It will start working within minutes."
    b. "I don't need to monitor my blood sugar."
    c. "I should take my drug on an empty stomach so it works better."
    d. "I need to keep track of my weight and blood pressure at home."

CASE STUDY

Read the scenario, and answer the following questions on a separate sheet of paper.

J.S. was involved in a motorcycle collision and has a severe traumatic brain injury. While preparing to take the client to surgery, the neurosurgeon orders mannitol to be administered. Client's weight is 80 kg. Vital signs include temperature 97.9° F, heart rate 62 beats/min, respiratory rate controlled on a ventilator at 18 breaths/min, and blood pressure 194/132 mm Hg. The client has an increased intracranial pressure (ICP) of 36 mm Hg.

1. What class of diuretic is mannitol, and how does it work?

2. What is the standard dosage range for mannitol? How is mannitol administered?

3. What would the correct dose be for this client?

39 Antihypertensives

STUDY QUESTIONS

Complete the following.

1. When hypertension cannot be controlled nonpharmacologically, antihypertensive drugs may be prescribed. Three of the five sympatholytic groups are _____, _____, and _____.

2. Two categories of antihypertensives in addition to the sympatholytics are _____ and _____.

3. Thiazide diuretics may be combined with other antihypertensive drugs. Examples of other antihypertensives include _____ and _____.

4. Many antihypertensive drugs can cause fluid retention. To decrease body fluid, the drug group often administered with antihypertensive drugs is _____.

5. Beta-adrenergic blockers reduce cardiac output by diminishing the sympathetic nervous system response. With continued use of beta blockers, vascular resistance is (increased/diminished) and blood pressure is (lowered/increased). *(Circle correct answers.)*

6. Atenolol and metoprolol are examples of (cardioselective/noncardioselective) antihypertensive drugs. *(Circle correct answer.)*

7. The alpha blockers are useful in treating hypertensive patients with lipid abnormalities. The effects they have on lipoproteins include (decreased/increased) VLDL and LDL; and (decreased/increased) HDL. *(Circle correct answers.)*

Match the generic drug name in Column I with the category of antihypertensive in Column II.

Column I

_____ 8. Captopril

_____ 9. Verapamil

_____10. Prazosin

_____11. Atenolol

_____12. Methyldopa

_____13. Hydralazine

_____14. Candesartan

_____15. Carvedilol

Column II

a. Cardioselective beta blocker

b. Selective alpha blocker

c. Angiotensin-converting enzyme (ACE) inhibitor

d. Calcium channel blocker

e. Centrally acting alpha$_2$ agonist

f. Direct-acting vasodilator

g. Angiotensin II–receptor antagonist (A-II blocker)

h. Nonselective beta$_1$ and beta$_2$ blocker

16. Which client would be most suited for treatment with a nonselective alpha-adrenergic blocker?
    a. A client with mild to moderate renal failure
    b. A client with hypertension associated with pheochromocytoma
    c. A client with hyperlipidemia
    d. A client with type 2 diabetes

17. Where in the body do direct-acting vasodilators act to decrease blood pressure?
    a. Cardiac valves
    b. Dopaminergic receptors in kidneys
    c. Renal tubules
    d. Smooth muscles of the blood vessels

18. With use of direct-acting vasodilators, sodium and water are retained and peripheral edema occurs. Which category of drugs should be given to avoid fluid retention?
    a. Anticoagulants
    b. Antidysrhythmics
    c. Cardiac glycosides
    d. Diuretics

19. Which is/are action(s) of angiotensin II–receptor blockers (ARBs)? (Select all that apply.)
    a. Block angiotensin II
    b. Cause vasodilation
    c. Decrease peripheral resistance
    d. Increase sodium retention
    e. Slow heart rate

20. An angiotensin II–receptor blocker (ARB) can be combined with the thiazide diuretic hydrochlorothiazide. What is the purpose of combining these two drugs?
    a. To decrease rapid blood pressure drop
    b. To enhance the antihypertensive effect by promoting sodium and water loss
    c. To increase sodium and water retention for controlling blood pressure
    d. To promote potassium retention

21. Angiotensin II–receptor blockers (ARBs) may be prescribed for hypertensive clients instead of an angiotensin-converting enzyme (ACE) inhibitor. What is the most limiting factor in the use of ACE inhibitors?
    a. Coughing
    b. Dizziness
    c. Shortness of breath
    d. Sneezing

22. A nurse is preparing to administer cardiac drugs to several clients. The nurse would be concerned about administering an ACE inhibitor as a monotherapy to which client?
    a. A Hispanic client
    b. An Asian client
    c. A Caucasian client
    d. A African American client

23. A African American client presents to a health care provider for continued high blood pressure. Which group of drugs would be more effective for this client?
    a. Angiotensin II blockers
    b. Beta blockers
    c. Calcium blockers
    d. Direct renin inhibitor

24. Which drug-herb interaction can occur when ma-huang (ephedra) is taken concomitantly with an antihypertensive drug?
    a. A decrease or counteraction of the effects of the antihypertensive drug
    b. A decrease in the hypertensive state
    c. An increase in the hypotensive effects of the antihypertensive drug
    d. No effect on the action of the antihypertensive drug

25. If a client takes captopril with nitrates, diuretics, or adrenergic blockers, which effect will the nurse assess in this client?
    a. Hypoglycemic reaction
    b. Hypotensive reaction
    c. Hyperkalemic reaction
    d. Hypertensive reaction

26. If a client takes captopril with a potassium-sparing diuretic, which electrolyte imbalance might occur?
    a. Hypokalemia
    b. Hyperkalemia
    c. Hypocalcemia
    d. Hypercalcemia

27. A client wishes to stop taking captopril for the treatment of hypertension. What is the nurse's best response?
    a. "Blood pressure can be controlled by diet and exercise, so you don't have to take drug."
    b. "It is important to keep taking your drug as directed until you speak with your health care provider."
    c. "Once your blood pressure is normal for one month, you can stop taking your drug."
    d. "Wean yourself off of the drug over a 10-day period."

28. What is the protein-binding power of amlodipine?
    a. Highly protein-bound
    b. Moderately to highly protein-bound
    c. Moderately protein-bound
    d. Low protein-bound

29. What will the nurse assess in a client experiencing side effects from metoprolol? *(Select all that apply.)*
    a. Dizziness
    b. Headache
    c. Increased blood pressure
    d. Nausea
    e. Paranoia

30. A client taking amlodipine complains of swelling in the ankles. What is the nurse's best response to the client's concern?
    a. "Swelling is common when taking amlodipine. You should cut the tablet in half to reduce your dosage."
    b. "Swelling may occur with amlodipine. I will contact your health care provider to determine if the drug should be changed."
    c. "You should not be taking that drug because of your age. I will see what other antihypertensive drug you can take."
    d. "You should stop taking the drug for several days and check that the swelling has decreased."

31. What is/are the advantage(s) of using cardioselective beta-adrenergic blockers as an antihypertensive? *(Select all that apply.)*
    a. They can be abruptly discontinued without causing rebound symptoms.
    b. They help prevent bronchodilation.
    c. They increase serum electrolyte levels.
    d. They maintain renal blood flow.
    e. They minimize the hypoglycemic effect.

32. Which statement best describes the direct renin inhibitor aliskiren?
    a. It is effective for treating severe hypertension.
    b. It can be combined with another antihypertensive drug.
    c. It can cause hypokalemia when taken as a monotherapy drug.
    d. It is more effective than calcium channel blockers in treating hypertension in Black patients.

CASE STUDY

Read the scenario and answer the following questions on a separate sheet of paper.

J.H., who has a history of hypertension, presents to the clinic with complaints of headache, epistaxis, and dizziness. Vital signs are blood pressure 232/146 mm Hg, heart rate 62 beats/min, respiratory rate 16 breaths/min, and temperature 98.3° F. J.H.'s electrocardiogram (ECG) reveals normal sinus rhythm with an occasional premature ventricular contraction. The health care provider calls for emergency medical services (EMS) to transport J.H. to the hospital for treatment of a hypertensive emergency. While waiting for EMS, the nurse reviews the client's drug list and finds that J.H. takes chlorthalidone with clonidine daily but "sometimes forgets a dose or two."

1. How does chlorthalidone work with clonidine to lower blood pressure?

2. What are the options for J.H. for treatment of a hypertensive emergency?

3. What priority teaching should the nurse provide to J.H. at time of discharge from the hospital?

40 Anticoagulants, Antiplatelets, and Thrombolytics

Complete the following.

1. A thrombus can form in a(n) _____ or in a(n) _____.

2. Anticoagulants are used to inhibit _____ _____. They (do/do not) dissolve clots (*Circle correct answer*).

3. Anticoagulants and thrombolytics (have/do not have) the same action. (*Circle correct answer.*)

4. The most frequent use of heparin is to prevent _____ _____ that may lead to _____ _____.

5. Heparin can be given (orally/subcutaneously/intravenously). (*Circle all the correct answers.*)

6. The low–molecular-weight heparins (LMWHs) are derivatives of _____ heparin. The advantage of LMWHs is that they lower the risk of _____.

7. The international normalized ratio (INR) is a laboratory test to monitor the therapeutic effect of (warfarin/heparin). (*Circle correct answer.*)

8. Heparin can (decrease/increase) the platelet count, causing thrombocytopenia. (*Circle correct answer.*)

9. A thrombus disintegrates when a thrombolytic drug is administered within _____ hours following an acute myocardial infarction.

10. The action of the thrombolytic drugs streptokinase and urokinase is the conversion of _____ to _____.

11. The major complication with the use of thrombolytic drugs is _____.

12. A synthetic anticoagulant, _____, indirectly inhibits thrombin production and is closely related in structure to heparin and LMWH.

13. **Number the following steps of heparin activity in correct order.**

    _____ a. Inhibits conversion of fibrinogen to fibrin

    _____ b. Inactivates antithrombin III to prevent the formation of thrombin

    _____ c. Clot prevented

    _____ d. Heparin binds with antithrombin III

Match the drug in Column I with its drug group in Column II. The drug group in Column II may be used more than once.

Column I

_____14. Warfarin

_____15. Aspirin

_____16. Enoxaparin

_____17. Dalteparin sodium

_____18. Protamine sulfate

_____19. Clopidogrel

_____20. Streptokinase

_____21. Bivalirudin

_____22. Alteplase (tissue plasminogen activator [tPA])

Column II

a. Anticoagulant: LMWH

b. Direct thrombin inhibitor (parenteral)

c. Oral anticoagulant

d. Antiplatelet

e. Anticoagulant antagonist

f. Thrombolytic

REVIEW QUESTIONS

23. A client on warfarin for a deep vein thrombosis asks the nurse how warfarin works. What is the nurse's best response?
    a. "Warfarin will help dissolve the blood clots."
    b. "Warfarin is given with thrombolytics to help break up clots."
    c. "Warfarin prevents new clots from forming."
    d. "Warfarin dilates the veins to improve blood flow."

24. The nurse has several clients receiving warfarin. Which INR(s) would concern the nurse? *(Select all that apply.)*
    a. 1.2
    b. 1.4
    c. 1.8
    d. 2.0
    e. 2.4

25. Which drug is not considered a LMWH? *(Select all that apply.)*
    a. Enoxaparin sodium
    b. Clopidogrel
    c. Dalteparin
    d. Apixaban

26. A client with unstable angina is having an emergent percutaneous transluminal coronary angioplasty (PTCA). The nurse is completing preprocedural teaching and explains a drug will be given right before the procedure and then for the next 12 hours by an intravenous (IV) drip to prevent ischemia. Which drug is the nurse teaching the client about?
    a. Abciximab
    b. Aminocaproic acid
    c. Protamine sulfate
    d. Warfarin

27. A client weighs 168 pounds and is going to receive abciximab for unstable angina. What is the correct dosage for a continuous infusion?
    a. 9.5 mcg/min
    b. 19 mcg/min
    c. 25 mg/min
    d. 42 mg/min

28. Which statement best describes clopidogrel?
    a. It is the most effective anticoagulant when used with ibuprofen.
    b. It is most effective when prescribed as a single drug to prevent stroke.
    c. It is an inexpensive alternative to warfarin.
    d. It can be used together with aspirin after myocardial infarction (MI) or cerebrovascular accident (CVA) to prevent platelet aggregation.

29. A client with a history of atrial fibrillation is being discharged from the hospital on warfarin. What is a priority teaching intervention?
    a. "INR will be monitored closely."
    b. "Periodic evaluation of your electrolytes is very important."
    c. "Your blood must be monitored for BUN/creatinine values to evaluate for new renal failure."
    d. "You will not need any further lab work while taking this medication."

30. A client on warfarin has an international normalized ratio of 10.3 seconds. Physical assessment reveals the client with multiple petechiae to the body. Which drug will the nurse prepare to administer?
    a. Anagrelide
    b. Protamine sulfate
    c. Ticagrelor
    d. Vitamin K (phytonadione)

31. The client is given heparin for early treatment of deep vein thrombosis. Later, warfarin is prescribed. If the client is also taking fluoxetine, which is highly protein-bound, which drug-drug interaction can occur?
    a. Drug displacement of the highly protein-bound drug but not displacement of warfarin
    b. Drug displacement of warfarin
    c. Drug displacement varies from patient to patient
    d. No drug displacement of either drug

32. A client, who has been on fondaparinux at home, presents to the emergency department with complaints of gastrointestinal bleeding. What does the nurse anticipate is occurring?
    a. Adverse reaction
    b. Allergic reaction
    c. Insufficient dose of fondaparinux
    d. Stevens-Johnson syndrome

33. A client who received alteplase for treatment of cerebrovascular accident (CVA) begins to hemorrhage. Which drug will the nurse anticipate administering?
    a. Reteplase
    b. Aminocaproic acid
    c. Calcium gluconate
    d. Protamine sulfate

34. Which action(s) will the nurse perform when caring for a client who is receiving tenecteplase? *(Select all that apply.)*
    a. Assess for reperfusion arrhythmias.
    b. Monitor liver panel.
    c. Observe for signs and symptoms of bleeding.
    d. Obtain a type and crossmatch.
    e. Record vital signs and report changes.

35. Which client(s) would be candidate(s) for anticoagulant? *(Select all that apply.)*
    a. A client with deep vein thrombosis (DVT)
    b. A client with an artificial heart valve
    c. A client with migraines
    d. A client who has had a knee replacement
    e. A client with a cerebrovascular accident (CVA)

CASE STUDY

Read the scenario, and answer the following questions on a separate sheet of paper.

R.K. has been diagnosed with a pulmonary embolus after having laparoscopic surgery. R.K. is admitted to the intensive care unit and started on a heparin drip. The client will be discharged home on warfarin and will receive therapy for 3–6 months.

1. How does heparin work in a client who already has a pulmonary embolus?

2. How does warfarin work to prevent further development of deep vein thrombosis that may lead to pulmonary embolism?

3. What priority teaching information will the nurse need to provide for this client before discharge?

41 Antihyperlipidemics and Drugs to Improve Peripheral Blood Flow

STUDY QUESTIONS

Complete the following.

1. The four major categories of lipoprotein are _____, _____, _____, and _____.

2. High-density lipoproteins (HDLs) are the densest lipoproteins and contain more _____ and less _____ than the other lipoproteins.

3. Persons with elevated low-density lipoproteins (LDLs) have the risk of developing _____ _____ and _____ _____.

4. In addition to LDL, _____ (a lipoprotein) is a better indicator of risk for coronary artery disease (CAD).

5. Statin drugs inhibit _____ _____ in cholesterol biosynthesis and are called _____ _____ _____.

6. B vitamins and folic acid can lower serum _____ levels.

7. Primary causes of peripheral arterial disease include _____ and _____.

Match the drug in Column I with its drug group in Column II. Drug group in Column II may be used more than once.

Column I

_____ 8. Colestipol hydrochloride

_____ 9. Gemfibrozil

_____ 10. Atorvastatin

_____ 11. Simvastatin

_____ 12. Cholestyramine resin

_____ 13. Niacin

_____ 14. Ezetimibe

Column II

a. Statins
b. Bile-acid sequestrants
c. Fibrates
d. Cholesterol absorption inhibitors
e. Nicotinic acid

15. Which elevated apolipoprotein can be an indication of risk for coronary artery disease (CAD)?
    a. apoA-1
    b. apoA-2
    c. apoB-100
    d. apoC-4

16. A client who was prescribed atorvastatin 80 mg/day presented to the emergency department feeling weak and complaining of muscle pain. What severe side effect of statins does the nurse suspect?
    a. Stevens-Johnson syndrome
    b. Pseudomembranous colitis
    c. Gastric ulcers
    d. Rhabdomyolysis

17. Homocysteine is a protein in the blood that has been linked to cardiovascular disease and stroke. What other negative action can it also promote?
    a. Flushing of skin
    b. Loss of blood vessel flexibility
    c. Photosensitivity and sunburn
    d. Lowering of low-density lipoprotein levels

18. A client who has intermittent claudication and leg pain tells the nurse, "I don't believe in taking all of that medicine stuff. I prefer to use only natural drugs." What herb does the nurse recognize as being used by some clients with intermittent claudication?
    a. Ginger
    b. Ginseng
    c. Ginkgo
    d. Goldenseal

19. Low-density lipoproteins (LDLs) are the so-called "bad" lipoproteins. Why are high levels of LDL considered unhealthy?
    a. There is an increased risk of hyperthyroidism.
    b. There is the possibility of digestive problems.
    c. There is an increased risk of rhabdomyolysis.
    d. There is an increased risk of heart disease.

20. The client with hyperlipidemia has a high-density lipoprotein (HDL) of 22 mg/dL. What will the nurse conclude about this client's HDL level?
    a. An HDL level of 22 mg/dL puts the patient in a high-risk category.
    b. An HDL level of 22 mg/dL places the patient in a moderate-risk category.
    c. The HDL level must be compared with all other levels before a decision can be made.
    d. An HDL level of 22 mg/dL is within the standard preferred range.

21. A client with a total cholesterol level of 228 mg/dL has been on a low-fat, low-cholesterol diet for 2 months. A follow-up total cholesterol level is 212 mg/dL. What will the nurse tell the client on the reason of the level not being lower?
    a. The client most likely did not adhere to the diet.
    b. Diet modification usually decreases cholesterol levels by only 10–30%.
    c. The client lost less than 10 pounds on the diet.
    d. The client's exercise program was not rigorous enough.

22. A client who is prescribed simvastatin asks if dietary modification is still needed. What is the nurse's best response?
    a. "Yes, you may eat whatever you want as long as you are taking simvastatin."
    b. "Diet is not an important factor if you are compliant with your drugs."
    c. "You should maintain a low-fat, low-cholesterol diet and exercise as well."
    d. "With simvastatin, you must lose weight as well as exercise."

23. What priority information should the nurse include in the health teaching plan for a client taking cilostazol? *(Select all that apply.)*
    a. Take medications with meals.
    b. Avoid drinking grapefruit juice.
    c. Do not take acetaminophen.
    d. Monitor for side effects such as headache and abdominal pain.
    e. Monitor blood pressure.

CASE STUDY

Read the scenario and answer the following questions on a separate sheet of paper.

S.S. has a family history of coronary artery disease and has recently been having intermittent chest pain. S.S.'s cholesterol level is 267 mg/dL; LDL level is 146 mg/dL; and HDL level is 44 mg/dL. S.S. was initially prescribed atorvastatin 10 mg/day. The dosage has now been increased to 20 mg/day. S.S.'s medical history is positive for type 2 diabetes. S.S. has no allergies and plans on "getting pregnant."

1. Discuss the mode of action for atorvastatin and the purpose of this drug.

2. What are the implications of atorvastatin and pregnancy?

3. What should be monitored during drug therapy, and how long will the drug therapy last?

4. What teaching points should be included in patient education for S.S.?

42 Gastrointestinal Tract Disorders

STUDY QUESTIONS

Match the words in Column I with the description they are most associated with in Column II.

Column I

_____ 1. Adsorbents

_____ 2. Cannabinoids

_____ 3. Chemoreceptor trigger zone (CTZ)

_____ 4. Emetics

_____ 5. Opiates

_____ 6. Osmotics

_____ 7. Purgatives

Column II

a. Harsh cathartics that cause a watery stool with abdominal cramping

b. Induce vomiting (used after poisoning)

c. Hyperosmolar laxatives

d. Relieve chemotherapy-induced nausea/vomiting

e. Lies near the medulla

f. Adsorb bacteria or toxins that cause diarrhea

g. Decrease intestinal motility, thereby decreasing peristalsis

Complete the following.

8. The _____ lies near the medulla, and the vomiting center is in the _____.

9. Nonprescription drugs for emesis include _____, _____, and _____ solution.

10. Antihistamine antiemetics have similar side effects to those of _____.

11. Antiemetic drugs in the classes of anticholinergics and antihistamines should not be used in clients with _____ because of their side effects.

12. Phenothiazines and benzodiazepines are classified as _____ _____ that suppress emesis by blocking dopamine receptors in the chemoreceptor trigger zone.

13. Serotonin antagonists suppress _____ and _____ by blocking the _____ receptors.

14. A drug to alleviate nausea and vomiting, such as a _____, can also be used as an appetite stimulant.

15. _____ promote a soft stool, whereas _____ result in a soft to watery stool.

16. Saline osmotic laxative products consist of _____ or _____.

17. Laxative abuse can cause fluid volume _____ and _____ losses.

SHORT ANSWER

18. List the eight classes of prescription antiemetics.

19. List at least five common causes of constipation.

20. Which instructions would be given to a client who is prescribed psyllium, a bulk-forming laxative?

_____ 21. Prescription or nonprescription antiemetics are safe for pregnant women to take.

_____ 22. A person should have one bowel movement per day to be "normal."

_____ 23. Chronic use of laxatives can cause laxative dependence.

_____ 24. Because castor oil is a natural substance, it is safe for woman in early pregnancy to use castor oil for occasional constipation.

REVIEW QUESTIONS

25. Which class of drugs can be used as antiemetics? *(Select all that apply.)*
    a. Anticholinergics
    b. Antihistamines
    c. Cannabinoids
    d. Opioids
    e. Phenothiazines

26. A client with severe nausea and vomiting asks how promethazine works. Which response by the nurse would be correct?
    a. "It stimulates the dopamine receptors in the brain associated with vomiting."
    b. "It blocks the histamine receptor sites and inhibits the CTZ."
    c. "It blocks the acetylcholine receptors associated with vomiting."
    d. "It prohibits the muscle contraction in the abdominal wall, preventing vomiting."

27. Which nonpharmacologic method(s) can the nurse suggest to a client who has been vomiting for 18 hours to decrease nausea and vomiting? *(Select all that apply.)*
    a. "Drink weak tea."
    b. "Takes sips of flat soda."
    c. "Eat small amounts of gelatin if tolerated."
    d. "Crackers may be helpful."
    e. "Breathe deeply in and out through your nose."

28. A client overdosed on prescription drugs is given activated charcoal orally. Which action is a goal behind giving activated charcoal?
    a. Absorb poison
    b. Cause diarrhea
    c. Promote vomiting
    d. Stop nausea

29. The client is receiving diphenoxylate with atropine for diarrhea. Which side effect(s) might the nurse expect to see during treatment? *(Select all that apply.)*
    a. Headache
    b. Drowsiness
    c. Hypertension
    d. Hypoglycemia
    e. Urinary retention

30. Which substances is/are a type of laxative/cathartic? *(Select all that apply.)*
    a. Adsorbents
    b. Bulk-forming
    c. Emetics
    d. Emollients
    e. Stimulants

31. The client who is scheduled for a barium enema is prescribed bisacodyl the day before the procedure. Which response by the nurse would be appropriate when the client asks how bisacodyl works?
    a. "Bisacodyl increases peristalsis by irritating the lining of the intestines."
    b. "By stimulating more smooth muscle contraction, bisacodyl will cause your bowel to empty."
    c. "Bisacodyl increases water in the gut."
    d. "Bisacodyl is an emetic, so you will vomit, and your stomach will be empty for the test."

32. The client who is on several vitamins is taking mineral oil as a laxative. Which side effect will the nurse tell the client?
    a. Abdominal bloating and flatulence
    b. Decreased absorption of fat-soluble vitamins A, D, E, and K
    c. Dependence on the drug
    d. Excessive fluid loss attributable to diarrhea

33. Which client would not use a laxative/cathartic?
    a. A client with cirrhosis
    b. A client with parkinsonism
    c. A client with stable angina
    d. A client with bowel obstruction

34. The client with migraines has been prescribed promethazine 25 mg PO for nausea. Which side effect(s) should be included in the teaching? *(Select all that apply.)*
    a. Blurred vision
    b. Diarrhea
    c. Drowsiness
    d. Dry mouth
    e. Hypotension

35. The client is experiencing diarrhea. Which food(s) will the nurse advise the client to avoid? *(Select all that apply.)*
   a. Bottled water
   b. Clear liquids
   c. Fried foods
   d. Milk products
   e. Gelatin

CASE STUDY

Read the scenario and answer the following questions on a separate sheet of paper.

L.B., who lives independently at a senior living center, presents to the clinic with complaints of constipation. Approximately 2 months ago, L.B. fell and broke the left hip. The client had surgery to fix the left hip, received physical therapy, and has returned home. Current drugs L.B. is taking include digoxin, a calcium supplement, omeprazole, and hydrocodone as needed (PRN) for pain. L.B. is prescribed bisacodyl 5 mg orally (PO) for the constipation.

1. What are the potential causes of constipation in L.B.?

2. How does bisacodyl work to treat constipation?

3. Are there any contraindications with any of L.B.'s other drugs? If so, what?

4. What priority teaching instructions are important for L.B. regarding bisacodyl?

43 Antiulcer Drugs

Match the descriptor in Column I with the drug/factor in Column II. Drug/factor in Column II may be used more than once.

Column I

_____ 1. Risk factor for the development of peptic ulcer disease (PUD)

_____ 2. Two drug/factor that neutralizes gastric acid

_____ 3. The first proton pump inhibitor marketed

_____ 4. Associated with the development of PUD

_____ 5. Prostaglandin analogue for prevention of NSAID-induced ulcer

_____ 6. Binds with protein to form a protective viscous coat covering the ulcer

_____ 7. Eradication of *H. pylori* requires addition of this antimicrobial

_____ 8. An antacid that can have a diarrheal effect

_____ 9. Over-the-counter (OTC) proton pump inhibitor used in combination to eradicate *H. pylori*

_____ 10. H_2 antagonist with multiple drug interactions

Column II

a. Magnesium hydroxide
b. *Helicobacter pylori*
c. Sucralfate
d. Cimetidine
e. Omeprazole
f. Misoprostol
g. Smoking
h. Antacids
i. Metronidazole

Match the drug in Column I with the category to which it belongs in Column II. Category in Column II may be used more than once.

Column I

_____ 11. Rabeprazole

_____ 12. Ranitidine

_____ 13. Glycopyrrolate

_____ 14. Nizatidine

_____ 15. Esomeprazole magnesium

_____ 16. Sucralfate

_____ 17. Calcium carbonate

_____ 18. Famotidine

_____ 19. Sodium bicarbonate

Column II

a. Anticholinergics
b. Antacid
c. Proton pump inhibitor
d. Histamine$_2$ blocker
e. Pepsin inhibitors

20. A client asks the nurse when would be the best time to take an over-the-counter (OTC) antacid for "heartburn." Which time frame will the nurse provide?
    1. 1 hour before meals
    2. 1–3 hours after meals and at bedtime
    3. With meals and at bedtime
    4. With meals and 1 hour after

21. Which drug(s) may be used to prevent ulcers? *(Select all that apply.)*
    a. Antibiotics
    b. Anticholinergics
    c. Antacids
    d. Histamine$_2$ blockers
    e. Opiates
    f. Proton pump inhibitors

22. Which drug(s) does the nurse know is/are most commonly used to treat gastroesophageal reflux disease (GERD)? *(Select all that apply.)*
    a. Antacids
    b. Anticholinergics
    c. Histamine$_2$ blockers
    d. Pepsin inhibitors
    e. Proton pump inhibitors

23. A client with peptic ulcer disease has been on propantheline bromide 15 mg 30 minutes before meals and 30 mg at bedtime. Which action describes propantheline bromide?
    a. It blocks H$_2$ receptors.
    b. It coats the lining of the stomach.
    c. It increases gastric motility.
    d. It inhibits gastric secretions.

24. A client diagnosed with an ulcer was prescribed nizatidine. Which information will the nurse include in the teaching plan? *(Select all that apply.)*
    a. "Antacids should not be taken within 1 hour of taking your nizatidine."
    b. "Avoid alcoholic beverages and caffeine."
    c. "Eating small, frequent meals may be helpful."
    d. "This drug should be taken with meals and at bedtime."
    e. "You will need to take this for the rest of your life."

25. A client is taking ranitidine for gastroesophageal reflux disease (GERD). Which side effect(s) of ranitidine will the nurse monitor in this client? *(Select all that apply.)*
    a. Confusion
    b. Headache
    c. Hypertension
    d. Erectile dysfunction
    e. Nausea

26. Which drug(s) will concern the nurse if prescribed to a client who is taking esomeprazole? *(Select all that apply.)*
    a. Ampicillin
    b. Digoxin
    c. Ketoconazole
    d. Lisinopril
    e. Propranolol

27. A client who is taking high-dose nonsteroidal anti-inflammatory drug (NSAID) for arthritis is also taking sucralfate. Which laboratory value would concern the nurse?
    a. Hgb 14.1 gm/dL
    b. Potassium 4.2 mEq/L
    c. Blood glucose 185 mg/dL
    d. INR 1.1

CASE STUDY

Read the scenario and answer the following questions on a separate sheet of paper.

S.S., who has a high-stress job as a county judge, complains of abdominal distress after eating. S.S. is currently taking aluminum hydroxide 10 mL with meals and at bedtime for an "ulcer."

1. What are the various classes of drugs used to treat ulcers?

2. Aluminum hydroxide belongs to which drug class, and how does it work?

3. Is this the proper dose for S.S.?

4. What priority health teaching should the nurse provide for S.S.?

44 Eye and Ear Disorders

Complete the following.

1. Topical anesthetics (locally/systemically) block the pain signals during selected or ophthalmologic procedures. *(Circle the correct answer.)*

2. Lubricants are used to moisten contact lenses and _____ _____.

3. Classes of ophthalmic antiinflammatories include immunomodulators, _____, and _____.

4. Ophthalmic cyclosporine, an antiinflammatory, allows _____ production.

5. Miotics are used to lower _____ pressure by widening the _____ network to improve drainage of aqueous humor.

6. Ocular decongestants are contraindicated in patients with _____ _____.

7. Carbonic anhydrase inhibitors were developed as _____. They are effective in treating _____.

8. The drug group used to paralyze the muscles of accommodation is _____.

9. Instruct patients with glaucoma to avoid anticholinergic drugs because they (decrease/increase) intraocular pressure. *(Circle the correct answer.)*

10. Antiinfectives are used to treat infections of the eye, including inflammation of the membrane covering the eyeball and inner eyelid known as _____.

11. Drugs that interfere with production of carbonic acid, leading to decreased aqueous humor formation and decreased intraocular pressure, belong to the group _____ _____ _____.

12. Cholinesterase inhibitors can produce systemic _____ effects that include cardiac dysrhythmias, diarrhea, and respiratory depression.

Match the term in Column I with its definition in Column II.

Column I

_____ 13. Otalgia

_____ 14. Optic

_____ 15. Cerumen

_____ 16. Lacrimal duct

_____ 17. Ceruminolytics

_____ 18. Otic

_____ 19. Chalazion

_____ 20. Keratitis

_____ 21. Hordeolum

_____ 22. Acute otitis externa

Column II

a. Also known as tear ducts
b. Drugs that soften or break up earwax
c. Infection of the meibomian glands of the eyelids
d. Ear
e. Swimmer's ear
f. Eye
g. Also known as stye
h. Ear pain
i. Earwax
j. Corneal infection and inflammation

REVIEW QUESTIONS

23. The client presents to an ophthalmologist for a routine eye examination. Before the exam, eye-drops are used to dilate the eyes. Such drug belongs to which class of drugs?
    a. Carbonic anhydrase inhibitors
    b. Cerumenolytics
    c. Mydriatics
    d. Osmotics

24. A client is taking acetazolamide for acute angle-closure glaucoma. The nurse will assess for which side effect associated with this drug class?
    a. Agitation
    b. Constipation
    c. Electrolyte imbalances
    d. Urinary retention

25. The client has frequent cerumen buildup. Which drug will the nurse anticipate in administering?
    a. Bimatoprost
    b. Carbamide peroxide
    c. Echothiophate
    d. Proparacaine

26. The client is receiving pilocarpine eyedrops for treatment of glaucoma. Which side effect(s) will the nurse teach the client to monitor? *(Select all that apply.)*
    a. Blurred vision
    b. Cardiac dysrhythmias
    c. Eye pain
    d. Headache
    e. Respiratory depression
    f. Vomiting

27. A client has been diagnosed with dry age-related macular degeneration (AMD). Which drug(s) is/are available for treatment? *(Select all that apply.)*
    a. Aflibercept
    b. Bevacizumab
    c. Pegaptanib
    d. Ranibizumab
    e. There is no treatment for dry AMD.

28. A client, who works as a landscaper, presents to an ophthalmologist with complaints of dry, itching eyes. Which treatment option(s) does the client have? *(Select all that apply.)*
    a. Azelastine
    b. Olopatadine
    c. Epinastine
    d. Ketotifen
    e. Tetracaine HCl

29. A client with a painful and swollen ear is prescribed ofloxacin otic solution. Before discharge, the nurse inserts a cotton wick into the right external canal. Which statement describes the purpose of the wick?
    a. To keep the external auditory canal dry
    b. To allow the drug to reach the external auditory canal
    c. To protect the tympanic membrane from infection
    d. To keep the external auditory canal free of cerumen

Read the scenario and answer the following questions on a separate sheet of paper.

Y.G., who has chronic open-angle glaucoma and ocular hypertension, presents to the health care provider for a follow-up appointment. Current drug for the glaucoma is timolol solution 2 drops every 8 hours. Y.G.'s medical history includes hypertension, depression, arthritis, and atrial fibrillation. Y.G. denies any specific complaints except for blurred vision.

1. What is open-angle glaucoma?

2. What kind of a drug is timolol, and how does it work?

3. How are these eyedrops administered?

4. Is this the appropriate dose for this client? Why or why not?

45 Dermatologic Disorders

Match the term in Column I with the correct description in Column II.

Column I

_____ 1. Macule

_____ 2. Vesicle

_____ 3. Plaque

_____ 4. Papule

Column II

a. Raised, palpable lesion 10 mm in diameter
b. Hard, rough, raised lesion; flat on top, usually >10 mm in diameter
c. Flat, nonpalpable lesion with varying color
d. Raised lesion filled with clear fluid and <1 cm in diameter

Match the condition in Column I to the drug that treats it in Column II. Multiple drugs in Column II may be used for a condition.

Column I

_____ 5. Psoriasis

_____ 6. Burns

_____ 7. Acne vulgaris

_____ 8. Verruca vulgaris

_____ 9. Rosacea

Column II

a. Cantharidin
b. Tetracycline
c. Isotretinoin
d. Azelaic acid
e. Adapalene
f. Methotrexate
g. Silver sulfadiazine
h. Calcineurin inhibitors

COMPLETE THE FOLLOWING

10. Tinea pedis is also called _____ _____, and tinea capitis is called _____.

11. _____ are noninflammatory acne lesions that may be _____ (closed) or _____ (open).

12. Isotretinoin is a known _____ and should not be used during pregnancy. Any person started on isotretinoin must be enrolled in a risk-management program called _____.

13. Psoriasis is a _____ disease affecting predominantly the _____ and _____.

14. Worsening psoriasis with the use of topical corticosteroids is called a/an _____ effect.

15. Cyclosporine inhibits _____ activation.

16. Salicylic acid promotes _____ when used for verruca vulgaris.

17. Prolonged use of topical corticosteroids is discouraged because it can cause _____ of the skin and _____ of the dermis and epidermis.

18. Which class(s) of drug(s) is/are used to treat acne vulgaris? *(Select all that apply.)*
    a. Antibiotics
    b. Antifungals
    c. Glucocorticoids
    d. Keratolytics
    e. Nonsteroidal antiinflammatories
    f. T-cell antagonists

19. The health care provider orders calcipotriene to treat psoriasis. When the client asks how this drug will work, which statement would be the nurse's best answer?
    a. "This medication will help stop the proliferation of cells."
    b. "It will be very effective against the itching that goes with psoriasis."
    c. "Calcipotriene will cure psoriasis."
    d. "It can be used like makeup to cover up the scales."

20. The client with psoriasis is started on a course of infliximab. Which response will the nurse tell the client about the dosing regimen?
    a. "Infliximab is a gel that you will use after bathing."
    b. "Infliximab is a drug that is administered by IV at prescribed intervals."
    c. "You will be able to give yourself an injection once per week."
    d. "This is an oral drug that you will be on for the rest of your life."

21. Which substance is/are common cause(s) of contact dermatitis? *(Select all that apply.)*
    a. Anesthetics
    b. Cosmetics
    c. Dyes
    d. Peanuts
    e. Sumac

22. A client with acne vulgaris has been prescribed tetracycline. Which range is the initial standard dose?
    a. 125–250 mg q6h
    b. 250–500 mg bid
    c. 500–750 mg q6h
    d. 750–1000 mg daily

23. Which priority information would be provided to the client taking tetracycline for acne? *(Select all that apply.)*
    a. Alert the health care provider if pregnant or possibly pregnant.
    b. Avoid the use of harsh cleansers.
    c. Eat a high-fiber diet.
    d. It should not be used with isotretinoin.
    e. Use a sunscreen with SPF 2.

24. Which drug can be utilized to treat male pattern baldness?
    a. Acitretin
    b. Methotrexate
    c. Minoxidil
    d. Tretinoin

25. A client has been diagnosed with contact dermatitis from poison ivy. Which antipruritic agent(s) can be utilized for this client? *(Select all that apply.)*
    a. Triamcinolone
    b. Dexamethasone
    c. Diphenhydramine
    d. Fluconazole
    e. Salicylic acid

CASE STUDY

Read the scenario and answer the following questions on a separate sheet of paper.

C.S. has sustained full-thickness burns over the anterior chest and partial-thickness burns over the forearms bilaterally. Mafenide acetate is ordered to be applied to the burns.

1. What is the difference between full- and partial-thickness burns?

2. What type of drug is mafenide acetate?

3. What other options are available for a topical burn preparation?

4. What are priority nursing interventions for this client?

46 Pituitary, Thyroid, Parathyroid, and Adrenal Disorders

STUDY QUESTIONS

Match the information in Column I with the correct term in Column II.

Column I

_____ 1. Growth hormone hypersecretion causing excessive growth after puberty

_____ 2. Another name for the anterior pituitary gland

_____ 3. Adrenocorticotropic hormone released by the anterior pituitary gland

_____ 4. A hormone secreted by the posterior pituitary gland to resorb water

_____ 5. Severe hypothyroidism in children causing delayed physical and mental growth

_____ 6. Growth hormone hypersecretion causing excessive growth during childhood

_____ 7. Cortisol hormone secreted from the adrenal cortex affecting inflammatory response

_____ 8. Another name for the pituitary gland

_____ 9. Aldosterone hormone secreted from the adrenal cortex that regulates sodium, potassium, and hydrogen ions

_____ 10. Severe hypothyroidism in adults causing physical, emotional, and mental changes

_____ 11. Another name for the posterior pituitary gland

_____ 12. Also called Graves' disease; caused by hyperfunction of the thyroid gland

_____ 13. T_4 hormone secreted by the thyroid gland

_____ 14. T_3 hormone secreted by the thyroid gland

Column II

a. ADH
b. Gigantism
c. Mineralocorticoid
d. Neurohypophysis
e. Triiodothyronine
f. Acromegaly
g. Myxedema
h. Adenohypophysis
i. ACTH
j. Thyrotoxicosis
k. Thyroxine
l. Glucocorticoid
m. Cretinism
n. Hypophysis

15. **Place the following conditions in the appropriate column on the next page.**

hypernatremia	anemia	edema
hypoglycemia	weight loss	delayed wound healing
weight gain	hyperlipidemia	hyperglycemia
fatigue	hirsutism	hyperpigmentation
tachycardia	hypotension	hypokalemia
diarrhea	peptic ulcers	hypertension
buffalo hump	hyponatremia	hyperkalemia

Addison Disease: Adrenal Hyposecretion	Cushing Syndrome: Adrenal Hypersecretion

Match the nursing intervention in Column I with the correct rationale related to glucocorticoid drug administration in Column II.

Column I

_____ 16. Monitor vital signs.

_____ 17. Monitor weight after taking a cortisone preparation for more than 10 days.

_____ 18. Monitor laboratory values, especially blood glucose and electrolytes.

_____ 19. Instruct the patient to take the cortisone with food.

_____ 20. Advise the patient to eat foods rich in potassium.

_____ 21. Instruct the patient not to abruptly discontinue the cortisone preparation.

_____ 22. Teach the patient to report signs and symptoms of potential drug toxicity.

Column II

a. Corticosteroids increase sodium and water retention and increase blood pressure.

b. Adrenal crisis may occur if cortisone is abruptly stopped.

c. Glucocorticoid drugs promote loss of potassium.

d. Weight gain occurs with cortisone use as a result of water retention.

e. Glucocorticoid drugs promote sodium retention, potassium loss, and increased blood glucose.

f. Glucocorticoid drugs may cause moon face, puffy eyelids, edema in the feet, dizziness, and menstrual irregularity at high doses.

g. Glucocorticoid drugs can irritate the gastric mucosa and may cause peptic ulcers.

REVIEW QUESTIONS

23. A client with hypothyroidism is taking levothyroxine 100 mcg/day. What concern by the nurse would be appropriate about the patient's dose of levothyroxine?
    a. The dose is too low
    b. The dose is too high
    c. Nothing; it is within the normal maintenance dosage range.
    d. Nothing; dose should start at a low dose.

24. Which time frame after starting levothyroxine should the client report feeling its effects?
    a. 3–4 days
    b. 4–7 days
    c. 1–2 weeks
    d. 2–4 weeks

25. The nurse assesses the client for symptoms of hyperthyroidism. Which symptom(s) can indicate hyperthyroidism? *(Select all that apply.)*
    a. Palpitations
    b. Constipation
    c. Excessive sweating
    d. Tachycardia
    e. Tinnitus

26. What should the nurse teach the client regarding the time of day to take levothyroxine?
    a. Before breakfast
    b. With breakfast
    c. After breakfast
    d. With lunch

27. What information would be a priority to include in the health teaching plan for the client with hypothyroidism? *(Select all that apply.)*
    a. Avoid over-the-counter (OTC) drugs.
    b. Report numbness and tingling of the hands to the health care provider.
    c. Increase food and fluid intake.
    d. Take the drug with food.
    e. Wear a medical alert identification information device.

28. While a client is taking prednisone, which laboratory value would be closely monitored?
    a. Hematocrit
    b. Hemoglobin
    c. Magnesium
    d. Sodium

29. The client has been started on prednisone for bronchitis to decrease inflammation. Which time frame would be best to take prednisone?
    a. Before meals
    b. With meals
    c. 1 hour after meals
    d. At bedtime

30. Which drug(s) should be used with caution when taking a glucocorticoid? *(Select all that apply.)*
    a. Acetaminophen
    b. Nonsteroidal antiinflammatory drugs (NSAIDs), including aspirin
    c. Digitalis preparations
    d. Phenytoin
    e. Potassium-wasting diuretics

31. Which nursing intervention(s) would be a priority to implement in the care of a client taking prednisone? *(Select all that apply.)*
    a. Follow the physical therapy regimen.
    b. Monitor for signs and symptoms of hyponatremia.
    c. Monitor vital signs.
    d. Obtain a complete medication history.
    e. Record daily weight.

32. Which statement by a client taking prednisone indicates a need for more teaching?
    a. "I should wear a medical alert identification device or carry a card."
    b. "I will make sure I force fluids daily."
    c. "I will not abruptly stop taking my drug."
    d. "I will take glucocorticoids only as ordered."

33. When an herbal laxative such as cascara or senna and herbal diuretics such as celery seed are taken with a corticosteroid, which imbalance may occur?
    a. Hypoglycemia
    b. Hypokalemia
    c. Hyponatremia
    d. Hypophosphatemia

34. Which changes can occur when ginseng is taken with a corticosteroid?
    a. Central nervous system (CNS) depression
    b. CNS stimulation and insomnia
    c. Counteraction of the effects of the corticosteroid
    d. Electrolyte imbalance

35. Which drug(s) is/are known to interact with levothyroxine? *(Select all that apply.)*
    a. Anticoagulants
    b. Digitalis
    c. Diuretics
    d. NSAIDs
    e. Oral antidiabetics

CASE STUDY

Read the scenario and answer the following questions on a separate sheet of paper.

R.K. has been diagnosed with adrenal insufficiency and is scheduled to start treatment with hydrocortisone.

1. What signs and symptoms are associated with adrenal insufficiency?

2. What is the dosage of hydrocortisone, and how is it administered?

3. What priority teaching is important for this client?

47 Antidiabetics

STUDY QUESTIONS

Match the term in Column I with its definition in Column II.

Column I

_____ 1. Diabetes mellitus

_____ 2. Insulin

_____ 3. Hypoglycemic reaction

_____ 4. Ketoacidosis

_____ 5. Lipodystrophy

_____ 6. Polydipsia

_____ 7. Polyphagia

_____ 8. Polyuria

Column II

a. Increased hunger
b. Increased urine output
c. Use of ketones for energy in diabetics
d. Disease resulting from deficient glucose metabolism
e. Increased thirst
f. Protein secreted from the beta cells of the pancreas
g. Changes to tissue from frequent insulin injections
h. Occurs when more insulin is administered than is needed for glucose metabolism

Complete the following.

9. Hemoglobin A1c (HbA1c) has a life span of approximately _____ or _____ months.

10. Some patients may need higher doses of insulin because of _____, _____, or _____.

11. Subcutaneous injections to the _____ absorb insulin faster than other body sites.

12. Insulin is not administered orally because _____ _____ destroy insulin.

13. Lipoatrophy and lipohypertrophy are terms used to indicate _____ due to not _____ injection sites.

14. Antibody development can cause _____ _____ and _____.

Match the terms in Column I with their definitions in Column II.

Column I

_____15. NPH insulin

_____16. Sulfonylureas

_____17. Regular insulin

_____18. Glucagon

_____19. Insulin lispro

_____20. Insulin glargine

Column II

a. Oral hypoglycemic drug group
b. Hyperglycemic hormone that stimulates glycogenolysis
c. Intermediate-acting insulin
d. Long-acting insulin
e. Rapid-acting insulin
f. Short-acting insulin

Complete the following.

21. All insulins can be administered subcutaneously, but only _____ insulin can be given intravenously.

22. A hypoglycemic event that usually occurs between 2:00 am and 4:00 am followed by an increase in blood glucose

    level by lipolysis, gluconeogenesis, and glycogenolysis is called the _____.

23. _____ on awakening or the _____ phenomenon is usually controlled by increasing the
    bedtime dose of insulin.

24. A major side effect of any oral antidiabetic drug is _____.

25. Metformin, an oral antidiabetic drug in the _____ class, decreases hepatic production of

    _____, decreases the _____ from the small intestine, increases insulin _____

    sensitivity, and increases _____ glucose uptake at the cellular level.

26. Metformin should be held for _____ _____ before and after administration of IV con-

    trast because _____ _____ or acute renal failure can develop.

27. Incretin mimetics improve glucose control in people with _____ diabetes; they should not be given
    to people with type 1 diabetes.

REVIEW QUESTIONS

28. Which major symptom(s) characterize diabetes?
    (Select all that apply.)
    a. Polydipsia
    b. Polyphagia
    c. Polyposia
    d. Polyrrhea
    e. Polyuria

29. Which drug(s) may cause hyperglycemia? *(Select all that apply.)*
    a. Epinephrine
    b. Hydrochlorothiazide
    c. Doxepin
    d. Prednisone
    e. Thiazolidinediones

30. Which clinical manifestation(s) may be seen in a client experiencing a hypoglycemic (insulin) reaction? *(Select all that apply.)*
    a. Abdominal pain
    b. Headache
    c. Excessive perspiration
    d. Nervousness
    e. Tremor
    f. Vomiting

31. Which clinical manifestation(s) may be seen in a client experiencing diabetic ketoacidosis (hyperglycemia)? *(Select all that apply.)*
    a. Bradycardia
    b. Dry mucous membranes
    c. Fruity breath odor
    d. Kussmaul respirations
    e. Polyuria
    f. Thirst

32. A client has type 1 diabetes. Which medication would the client not use to control diabetes?
    a. Insulin glulisine
    b. Insulin lispro
    c. Insulin aspart
    d. Tolazamide

33. Which information would be included in health teaching for patients taking oral antidiabetic (hypoglycemic) drugs? *(Select all that apply.)*
    a. Adhere to prescribed diet.
    b. Monitor blood glucose levels.
    c. Monitor weight.
    d. Participate in regular exercise.
    e. Take the drugs based on blood glucose level.

34. In which location would the client who takes insulin daily be taught to store the opened insulin?
   a. In a cool place
   b. In the light
   c. In the freezer
   d. Wrapped in aluminum

35. Which action would be appropriate when preparing cloudy insulin before administration?
   a. Add diluent to the bottle.
   b. Allow air to escape from the bottle.
   c. Roll the bottle in the hands.
   d. Shake the bottle well.

36. The patient needs to develop a "site rotation pattern" for insulin injections. The American Diabetes Association suggests which action(s)? *(Select all that apply.)*
   a. Choose an injection site for a week.
   b. Change the injection area of the body every day.
   c. Inject insulin each day at the injection site at 1½ inches apart.
   d. Inject insulin IM in the morning and subcut at night.
   e. With two daily injection times, use the right side in the morning and the left side in the evening.

37. Which time frame would the nurse expect the client to experience a hypoglycemic reaction to regular insulin if administration occurs at 0700 and the client does not eat?
   a. 0800–0900
   b. 0900–1300
   c. 1300–1500
   d. 1500–1700

38. Insulin glargine is a long-acting insulin. Which statement(s) best describe(s) insulin glargine? *(Select all that apply.)*
   a. Always combine it with regular insulin for good coverage.
   b. It is given in the evening.
   c. It is safe because hypoglycemia cannot occur.
   d. It is available in a prefilled cartridge insulin pen.
   e. Some patients complain of pain at the injection site.

39. The insulin pump, though expensive, has become popular in the management of insulin. Which statement is true about this method of insulin delivery?
   a. It can be used with intermediate insulin as well as regular insulin.
   b. It can be used with the needle inserted at the same site for weeks.
   c. It is more effective in decreasing the number of hypoglycemic reactions.
   d. It is more effective for use by the type 2 diabetic patient.

40. Which action is correct of an oral hypoglycemic drug?
   a. It increases the number of insulin cell receptors.
   b. It increases the number of insulin-producing cells.
   c. It replaces receptor sites.
   d. It replaces insulin.

41. The nonsulfonylureas are used to control serum glucose levels after a meal. Which statement describes their action?
   a. Nonsulfonylureas cause a hypoglycemic reaction.
   b. Nonsulfonylureas decrease hepatic production of glucose from stored glycogen.
   c. Nonsulfonylureas increase the absorption of glucose from the small intestine.
   d. Nonsulfonylureas raise the serum glucose level following a meal.

42. Herb-drug interaction must be assessed in clients taking herbs and antidiabetic agents. Which drug-herb interaction is correct on how ginseng and garlic affect insulin or oral antidiabetic drugs?
   a. They can be taken with insulin without any effect, but they can cause a hypoglycemic reaction with oral antidiabetic drugs.
   b. Ginseng and garlic can lower the blood glucose level.
   c. They decrease the effect of insulin and antidiabetic drugs, causing a hyperglycemic effect.
   d. They may decrease insulin requirements.

43. Which drug(s) or category(ies) of drug(s) will interact with a sulfonylurea? *(Select all that apply.)*
   a. Antacids
   b. Anticoagulants
   c. Anticonvulsants
   d. Aspirin
   e. Cimetidine

CASE STUDY

Read the scenario and answer the following questions on a separate sheet of paper.

K.C. has type 1 diabetes, which is normally well controlled with daily insulin. K.C. has been under increased stress recently because of needing to prepare for major exams in three classes. K.C.'s friends bring the client into the emergency department because of "acting funny." Before the triage nurse can ask the friends any further questions, they leave. Initially, K.C. is confused, complains of a headache, and has slurred speech. Glucose level in triage reads "low" on the glucometer. While waiting to be taken to a treatment room, K.C. becomes unresponsive.

1. What is a possible cause of K.C.'s symptoms?

2. How will this be treated before K.C. becomes unconscious?

3. What are the treatment options after K.C. loses consciousness?

48 Urinary Disorders

STUDY QUESTIONS

Match the drug class in Column I to the appropriate therapeutic effect in Column II. Therapeutic effect in Column II may be used more than once.

Column I

_____ 1. Urinary stimulants

_____ 2. Anticholinergics

_____ 3. Urinary antiseptics

_____ 4. Bactericidal

_____ 5. Antimuscarinics

_____ 6. Antiinfectives

_____ 7. Urinary analgesics

_____ 8. Bacteriostatic

_____ 9. Antispasmodics

Column II

a. Inhibits bacterial growth
b. Increases urinary muscle tone
c. Relieves pain and burning
d. Prevents bacterial growth
e. Decreases urgency and urinary incontinence
f. Kills bacteria

Note what parts of the genitourinary tract are considered upper tract and what parts are considered lower tract. Label the infectious processes to the appropriate urinary structures.

10.

a._____

b._____

c._____

Select the best response.

11. Which complication can occur when methenamine is given with a sulfonamide?
    a. Bleeding
    b. Chest pain
    c. Crystalluria
    d. Intestinal distention

12. A client with a urinary tract infection has been advised to increase fluids to decrease urine pH. Which information would the nurse include in discharge teaching to help the client meet this goal?
    a. "Drinking whole milk will help."
    b. "Cranberry juice can help acidify the urine."
    c. "Be sure to drink 12–14 8-oz glasses of water per day."
    d. "Drink prune juice four times per day to make urine alkaline."

13. A 72-year-old client has been prescribed flavoxate for urinary spasms. Which client's medical history would be of highest concern to the nurse?
    a. Dementia
    b. Glaucoma
    c. Hypoglycemia
    d. Migraines

14. A client will be receiving ertapenem to prevent recurring urinary tract infections (UTIs). Which side effect(s) will the nurse include in client teaching? *(Select all that apply.)*
    a. Visual disturbances
    b. Back pain
    c. Diarrhea
    d. Headache
    e. Nausea

15. Which oral urinary antiseptic drug–drug interaction(s) is/are correct? *(Select all that apply.)*
    a. Trimethoprim can be combined with sulfamethoxazole.
    b. Antacids increase absorption of ciprofloxacin.
    c. Sodium bicarbonate inhibits the action of methenamine.
    d. Antacids can decrease the absorption of nitrofurantoin.

16. A client, who is being discharged from the emergency department after being diagnosed with a urinary tract infection (UTI), is prescribed nitrofurantoin 100 mg qid with meals and at bedtime. The nurse will advise the client to contact the health care provider immediately for which side effect?
    a. Brown urine
    b. Frequency in urination
    c. Diarrhea
    d. Tingling or numbness of extremities

17. For which condition(s) would the nurse expect to see urinary analgesics prescribed? *(Select all that apply.)*
    a. Burning sensation
    b. Frequency
    c. Hesitation
    d. Retention
    e. Urgency

18. Which drug is commonly prescribed as a urinary analgesic?
    a. Bethanechol
    b. Flavoxate
    c. Phenazopyridine hydrochloride
    d. Trimethoprim

19. A client who was prescribed an antiinfective and phenazopyridine for a urinary tract infection (UTI), calls the clinic reporting urine color has turned reddish orange. After reviewing the client's chart and current list of drugs, which information will the nurse tell the client?
    a. "If you do not take the antibiotic with food in your stomach, your urine will turn orange."
    b. "Inadequate liquid intake will cause your urine to turn bright orange."
    c. "This is an indication of an allergic reaction. You need to come back to the clinic."
    d. "Bright reddish-orange urine is to be expected when taking phenazopyridine."

20. Which urinary antispasmodic is commonly used to treat urinary tract spasms?
    a. Bethanechol
    b. Oxybutynin
    c. Phenazopyridine
    d. Trimethoprim

21. An older adult client has a history of environmental allergies, narrow-angle glaucoma, depression, and overactive bladder. Which drug(s), if prescribed to this client, will concern the nurse? *(Select all that apply.)*
    a. Bethanechol
    b. Dimethyl sulfoxide (DMSO)
    c. Nitrofurantoin
    d. Oxybutynin
    e. Tolterodine tartrate

22. Which client is more likely to benefit from bethanechol chloride?
    a. A 44-year-old patient with prostatitis
    b. A 53-year-old patient with paraplegia
    c. A 65-year-old patient with pyelonephritis
    d. A 70-year-old patient with overactive bladder

CASE STUDY

Read the scenario and answer the following questions on a separate sheet of paper.

G.H. sustained an injury to the urinary tract while playing football and has been prescribed oxybutynin chloride 5 mg bid for spasms.

1. What is the mechanism of action of oxybutynin?

2. Which persons should not take this drug, and why?

3. What are the side effects that can be expected?

4. What dose adjustments, if any, need to be made for this client?

49 Pregnancy and Preterm Labor

Match the terms in Column I with the definitions in Column II.

Column I

_____ 1. Preeclampsia

_____ 2. Gestational hypertension

_____ 3. HELLP

_____ 4. L/S (lecithin/sphingomyelin) ratio

_____ 5. Eclampsia

_____ 6. Preterm birth

_____ 7. Hyperemesis gravidarum

_____ 8. Surfactant

_____ 9. Teratogens

_____ 10. Tocolytic therapy

Column II

a. New onset of seizures with preeclampsia

b. Prior to 37 gestational weeks

c. Drug therapy to decrease uterine muscle contractions

d. Severe nausea and vomiting during pregnancy

e. Decreases the incidence of respiratory distress syndrome (RDS)

f. Hypertension during pregnancy without proteinuria

g. Gestational hypertension with proteinuria

h. Substances that cause developmental abnormalities

i. Predictor of fetal lung maturity and risk for neonatal RDS

j. Hemolysis, Elevated Liver enzymes, and Low Platelet count

REVIEW QUESTIONS

11. Which maternal physiologic change(s) is/are seen during pregnancy that affect(s) drug dosing? *(Select all that apply.)*
    a. Decreased urine output
    b. Gastric motility is more rapid, resulting in faster absorption
    c. Increased fluid volume
    d. Increased glomerular filtration rate and rapid elimination of drugs
    e. Increased liver metabolism of drugs

12. The mechanism drugs cross the placenta is similar to the way drugs infiltrate which type of body tissue?
    a. Breast
    b. Liver
    c. Subcutaneous
    d. Uterine

13. Which important factor(s) determine(s) the teratogenicity of any drug ingested during pregnancy? *(Select all that apply.)*
    a. Dosage
    b. Duration of exposure
    c. Gastric motility
    d. Timing
    e. Urinary clearance

14. A client in preterm labor at 28 weeks is prescribed betamethasone 12 mg intramuscularly (IM) every 24 hours for 2 doses. The client wants to know why she has to receive the drug. Which response should the nurse provide?
    a. "Betamethasone will stop your labor."
    b. "It will help the fetus' lungs mature more quickly."
    c. "It will promote closure of a patent ductus arteriosus."
    d. "This drug will promote fetal adrenal maturity."

15. The client has been diagnosed with gestational hypertension. Which treatment goal(s) is appropriate for this client? *(Select all that apply.)*
    a. Decrease the incidence of preterm labor (PTL)
    b. Delivery of an uncompromised infant
    c. Ensure future ability to conceive
    d. Prevention of HELLP syndrome
    e. Prevention of seizures

199

Chapter **49** Pregnancy and Preterm Labor

16. The nurse works in a prenatal clinic. Which side effect(s) is/are common complaint(s) during pregnancy? *(Select all that apply.)*
    a. Heartburn
    b. Headaches
    c. Nausea
    d. Vomiting
    e. Weakness

17. A pregnant client with iron-deficiency anemia was prescribed ferrous sulfate 325 mg bid. Which laboratory value will show the first indication that the client is responding to the iron supplement?
    a. Increased blood urea nitrogen
    b. Increased hemoglobin
    c. Increased reticulocyte count
    d. Increased international normalized ratio

18. A pregnant client presents to her health care provider with complaints of morning sickness. "I didn't have it with my first. I'm just not sure what to do." Which nonpharmacologic measure(s) can the nurse suggest? *(Select all that apply.)*
    a. Avoid fatty or spicy foods.
    b. Avoid fluids before arising.
    c. Drink flat soda between meals.
    d. Eat crackers, dry toast, cereal, or complex carbohydrates.
    e. Eat a high-protein snack at bedtime.

19. A pregnant client in her first trimester of pregnancy was started on a prenatal vitamin with iron. Which teaching will the nurse provide for this client? *(Select all that apply.)*
    a. Antacids can be taken with the iron tablet to help with epigastric discomfort.
    b. Ensure adequate fluid and fiber intake to assist with constipation.
    c. Iron can be taken with food if necessary to prevent nausea.
    d. Jaundice is a common side effect of iron supplements.
    e. Orange juice enhances iron absorption.

20. Which food(s) should the nurse recommend a pregnant woman eat to increase her iron intake?
    a. Broccoli
    b. Cabbage
    c. Apples
    d. Potatoes
    e. Salmon

21. Which range of folic acid is the recommended daily allowance for a pregnant woman?
    a. 100–400 mcg
    b. 400–800 mcg
    c. 800–1200 mcg
    d. 1200–1600 mcg

22. Which drug is the most commonly ingested non-prescription drug for pain during pregnancy?
    a. Acetaminophen
    b. Aspirin
    c. Diphenhydramine
    d. Ibuprofen

23. Which priority intervention would the nurse implement for the patient receiving a beta-sympathomimetic drug?
    a. Auscultate breath sounds every 4 hours.
    b. Encourage patient to sleep on her back.
    c. Have atropine available as a reversal agent.
    d. Monitor maternal vital signs every 5 minutes when receiving IV dose.

24. Which nursing intervention(s) would a patient receiving magnesium sulfate for preeclampsia require? *(Select all that apply.)*
    a. Administer the loading dose as a bolus given IVP.
    b. Continuously monitor vital signs and fetal monitor.
    c. Encourage patient to ambulate in room to prevent blood clots.
    d. Have calcium gluconate available at the bedside.
    e. Monitor deep tendon reflexes (DTRs).

25. A client who is 38 weeks pregnant and complaining of a sinus headache takes a combination drug that contains aspirin, acetaminophen, and caffeine. Which event can occur with the use of aspirin late in pregnancy? *(Select all that apply.)*
    a. Decreased hemostasis in the newborn
    b. Increased maternal blood loss at delivery
    c. Increased risk of anemia
    d. Low–birth-weight infant
    e. Precipitous delivery

26. The client is receiving magnesium sulfate for gestational hypertension. Which side effect(s) of this drug may be expected? *(Select all that apply.)*
    a. Dizziness
    b. Flushing
    c. Hyperreflexia
    d. Slurred speech
    e. Urinary incontinence

Read the scenario and answer the following questions on a separate sheet of paper.

K.R., 40 years old, is pregnant with her fourth child. She is at 33 weeks' gestation. She has had one miscarriage and has two living children, ages 15 and 9 years. It is 2100 on Friday night, and her health care provider's office is closed, so she has left a message with the answering service. She contacts OB triage and states, "I think I may be having contractions, but I know I'm too early. My 15-year-old was born at 30 weeks, and I am so scared that this is happening again." She complains of lower abdominal tightening and back discomfort that comes and goes about every 8 minutes. K.R. was instructed to come to the hospital.

1. What are some priority questions for the nurse to ask while on the phone?

2. What puts K.R. at high risk for preterm labor (PTL)?

3. What are some nonpharmacologic measures to treat PTL? What are some pharmacologic options to treat PTL?

4. What needs to be done for the fetus at 33 weeks' gestation?

50 Labor, Delivery, and Postpartum

Label the following areas for regional anesthesia.

1.

Match the term in Column I to its definition in Column II.

Column I

_____ 2. Somatic

_____ 3. Visceral

_____ 4. Contraction

_____ 5. Regional

_____ 6. Ripening

Column II

a. Type of anesthesia for pain relief during labor and delivery without loss of consciousness

b. Type of pain caused by pressure of the presenting part and stretching of the perineum and vagina

c. Softening of the cervix

d. Type of pain due to stretching of the cervix

e. Tightening and shortening of uterine muscles

Match the labor and delivery stage in Column I with its definition in Column II.

Column I

_____ 7. Dilating stage

_____ 8. Pelvic stage

_____ 9. Placental separation and expulsion

_____ 10. Early postpartum

Column II

a. Placental separation from the uterine wall and its delivery

b. Cervical effacement and dilation occur

c. First 4 hours after delivery of the placenta

d. Complete cervical dilation and ends with delivery of the newborn

Complete the following.

11. The three *phases* of the dilating stage include _____, _____, and _____.

12. Sedative-hypnotics should be given at the onset of uterine contractions to decrease (maternal/neonatal) drug exposure. *(Circle the correct answer.)*

13. Adverse effects of opioids depend on the responses activated by the _____ and _____ receptors.

14. Barbiturates (should/should not) be given during active labor. *(Circle the correct answer.)*

15. Spinal anesthesia, also known as a/an _____ _____, is injected in the subarachnoid space.

16. A uterotropic drug, _____ stimulate(s) uterine contraction.

17. Progesterone on the smooth muscle _____ gastrointestinal peristalsis, which can promote constipation during the postpartum period.

18. A mother with Rh-negative blood should receive _____ _____ ____ to prevent fetal hemolysis in an Rh-positive fetus.

REVIEW QUESTIONS

19. The client has received spinal anesthesia for delivery. Which alteration would the nurse monitor in this client?
    a. Decreased hemoglobin and hematocrit
    b. Palpitations
    c. Pedal edema
    d. Postdural headache

20. Which action(s) is/are treatment(s) for postdural headaches after spinal anesthesia? *(Select all that apply.)*
    a. Analgesics
    b. Bed rest
    c. Blood patch
    d. Caffeine
    e. Decreased fluids

21. A baby with respiratory depression was born within 15 minutes after the mother received opioids for pain. Which drug will the nurse anticipate administering to provide reversal of neonatal respiratory depression?
    a. Calcium gluconate
    b. Calcium carbonate
    c. Flumazenil
    d. Naloxone

22. Before administration of general anesthesia, a laboring woman is given an antacid. Which purpose of giving this drug is correct?
    a. Decrease gastric acidity
    b. Enhance anesthesia induction
    c. Maintain a patent airway
    d. Prevent nausea and vomiting

23. A client is receiving an epidural, and her blood pressure is beginning to decrease. Which action would be correct for the nurse to initially take?
    a. Administer oxygen.
    b. Expect an order to administer 5–15 mg of ephedrine IV.
    c. Expect an order to transfuse with 1 unit of packed red cells.
    d. Turn her on her left side.

24. Which value on the Bishop score is associated with the most successful labor induction?
    a. 5
    b. 6
    c. 8
    d. 10

25. During which stage of labor are ergot alkaloids administered?
    a. First
    b. Second
    c. Third
    d. Fourth

26. Before administering methylergonovine, which baseline value should be measured?
    a. Blood pressure
    b. Fetal heart rate
    c. Maternal hourly urinary output
    d. Respiratory rate

27. The nurse assesses a client receiving a regional anesthesia for side effects. Which side effect(s) would the nurse monitor in this client? *(Select all that apply.)*
   a. Dizziness
   b. Hypertension
   c. Metallic taste in mouth
   d. Nausea
   e. Palpitations

28. Which baseline data should the nurse collect on a client who is being inducted at 41+ weeks with oxytocin intravenously? *(Select all that apply.)*
   a. Deep tendon reflexes
   b. Fetal heart rate
   c. Pulse rate and blood pressure
   d. Type and crossmatch for blood
   e. Uterine activity

29. The client is complaining of labor pain due the pressure of the presenting part and stretching of the perineum and vagina. This pain is experienced in which stage(s) of labor? *(Select all that apply.)*
   a. First
   b. Latent
   c. Second
   d. Transition
   e. Third

30. Which type(s) of anesthesia can be used for cesarean deliveries? *(Select all that apply.)*
   a. Caudal block
   b. Epidural anesthesia
   c. General anesthesia
   d. Pudendal anesthesia
   e. Spinal anesthesia

31. Which drugs is/are most commonly used for the relief of perineal pain resulting from episiotomy or laceration? *(Select all that apply.)*
   a. Benzocaine
   b. Erythromycin
   c. Mineral oil
   d. Witch hazel compresses

32. A postpartum client with a repaired fourth-degree laceration has benzocaine topical spray. She asks if she can also use a heat lamp on her perineum for additional comfort. Which response is the nurse's best answer?
   a. "No, the heat lamp will increase the incidence of bacteria growth."
   b. "No, use of a heat lamp with benzocaine may cause tissue burns."
   c. "What a good idea; it will decrease pain while improving healing."
   d. "Yes, you can use a heat lamp to augment the action of benzocaine."

33. At which time frame is the best time to administer the standard dose of $Rh_0(D)$ immune globulin?
   a. After chorionic villus sampling and at 38 weeks' gestation
   b. At 28 weeks' gestation and again within 72 hours after delivery
   c. Before amniocentesis and at 38 weeks' gestation
   d. Only at 28 weeks' gestation

CASE STUDY

Read the scenario and answer the following questions on a separate sheet of paper.

K.E., 22 years old, is at 38 weeks' gestation and has intrauterine growth retardation (IUGR). She is scheduled for an induction.

1. What drugs are used to induce labor, and what other methods may be used to induce labor?

2. What priority teaching instructions will the nurse provide on arrival to the hospital?

3. What analgesic options are available to K.E.?

51 Neonatal and Newborn

STUDY QUESTIONS

Complete the following.

1. _____ _____ _____ can occur because of immature lung development and low _____ level, which is needed to decrease surface tension.

2. A patent _____ tube is required to administer surfactant.

3. _____ is excessive oxygenation and _____ is decreased carbon dioxide concentration.

4. Hepatitis B immunization should be initiated during the _____ period.

5. Erythromycin ophthalmic ointment is administered to newborns to prevent _____ _____, an eye infection among newborns.

REVIEW QUESTIONS

6. A baby is born at 30 weeks' gestation and is having respiratory distress. Which class of drug will be given to help the baby's lungs?
   a. Antibiotics
   b. Benzodiazepines
   c. Calcium chloride
   d. Surfactant replacement

7. A nurse is preparing to assist in administering beractant intratracheally. Which action(s) is/are needed in preparing the drug?
   a. Warm for 5 seconds under hot running water.
   b. Shake the vial to mix the solution.
   c. Warm at room temperature for 20 minutes.
   d. Keep it refrigerated until immediately before administration.

8. Which drugs could be administered to a newborn to mature lung development? *(Select all that apply.)*
   a. Erythromycin
   b. Beractant
   c. Vitamin K
   d. Poractant alfa
   e. Calfactant

9. A nurse is assisting with administering exogenous surfactant via endotracheal tube. Which complications could occur with surfactant? *(Select all that apply.)*
   a. Desaturation
   b. Bradycardia
   c. Pallor
   d. Hyperoxia

10. A preterm neonate becomes cyanotic and the oxygen level decreases during surfactant administration. Which action would be most appropriate by the nurse?
    a. Gently suction through the endotracheal tube immediately to raise the oxygen level.
    b. Reposition the neonate to disperse the drug throughout the lungs.
    c. Do nothing.
    d. Increase the amount of oxygen the neonate is receiving.

11. Which substance would be administered to a neonate born to a hepatitis B carrier to provide passive protection against hepatitis B?
    a. Recombinant hepatitis B
    b. Varicella zoster
    c. Phytonadione
    d. Hepatitis B immune globulin

12. Which ophthalmic ointment is administered to the newborn immediately after birth?
    a. Bacitracin
    b. Erythromycin
    c. Gentamicin
    d. Penicillin

Read the scenario and answer the following questions on a separate sheet of paper.

J.G. is about to deliver her first baby and is anxious. Laboratory tests during one of her prenatal checkups revealed that J.G. was positive for HBs-Ag. Additional blood work was positive for active hepatitis B virus (HBV). J.G. is worried that her baby will also have hepatitis B.

1. How can HBV be transmitted to the neonate?

2. What is the nurse's best response to J.G.'s concerns?

3. What would the nurse administer to the neonate for hepatitis B? What are the rationales for the drugs?

4. What is the immunization schedule for recombinant hepatitis B?

STUDY QUESTIONS

Match the medical disorder in Column I with its definition in Column II.

Column I

_____ 1. Endometriosis

_____ 2. Dysmenorrhea

_____ 3. Dysfunctional uterine bleeding

_____ 4. Polycystic ovarian syndrome

_____ 5. Premenstrual syndrome

Column II

a. Collection of cyclic physical and mood alterations
b. Abnormal location of endometrial tissue outside the uterus
c. A disorder in the metabolism of androgens and estrogens
d. A classification of irregular bleeding
e. Also called cyclic pelvic pain

Complete the following.

6. A women's reproductive life cycle begins with _____ and continues through _____.

7. Ethinyl estradiol is a synthetic _____ found in combined hormonal contraceptives.

8. Drospirenone is an analog of _____, a potassium-sparing _____.

9. If the minipill is delayed for more than 3 hours, a back-up contraceptive method should be used for _____ hours.

10. The inhibition of both FSH and LH secretion results in _____ and _____.

11. Gonadotropin-releasing hormone agonists (GnRH) inhibit the release of GnRH creating a _____ environment.

Match the term in Column I with its definition in Column II.

Column I

_____ 12. Amenorrhea

_____ 13. Dysmenorrhea

_____ 14. Mittelschmerz

_____ 15. Breakthrough bleeding

_____ 16. Chloasma

Column II

a. Episodes of bleeding during the active pill cycle of hormonal contraceptives
b. Absence of bleeding
c. Mid-cycle pain usually associated with ovulation
d. Painful periods
e. Hyperpigmentation of the skin

REVIEW QUESTIONS

17. Which individual would be contraindicated for oral contraceptives?
    a. 20-year-old who is not sexually active
    b. 40-year-old with diabetes
    c. 38-year-old with breast cancer
    d. 48-year-old with emphysema

18. In which client(s) would combined hormone contraceptives (CHCs) be used with caution? *(Select all that apply.)*
    a. 37-year-old who smokes
    b. 45-year-old who does not exercise
    c. 38-year-old with diabetes
    d. 28-year-old with epilepsy
    e. 18-year-old with depression

19. A client who works the night shift realized that she missed a dose of combined hormonal contraceptive (CHC). She calls the on-call nurse and asks what she should do. Which response would be most appropriate by the nurse?
    a. "It isn't a big deal. Just take one tomorrow."
    b. "Stop this pack and use alternative birth control for the next month."
    c. "Take your dose now, and then get back on schedule with the next one."
    d. "Take two now and use an alternative method of birth control."

20. A client who has been taking conjugated estrogen for contraception reports a variety of side effects. Which clinical manifestation(s) is/are due primarily to an excess of estrogen? *(Select all that apply.)*
    a. Acne
    b. Breast tenderness
    c. Fluid retention
    d. Leg cramps
    e. Nausea

21. Which drug(s) will interact with oral conjugated estrogen? *(Select all that apply.)*
    a. Aspirin
    b. Fluoxetine
    c. Folic acid
    d. Phenobarbital
    e. Topiramate

22. Which laboratory value should be monitored closely in a client who has been taking drospirenone for contraception?
    a. Blood glucose
    b. Hemoglobin
    c. Potassium
    d. Thyroid-stimulating hormone

23. A client who has been using ethinyl estradiol and etonogestrel transvaginal for contraception calls and reports that the device fell out. Which response by the nurse would be most correct?
    a. "Discard the current pill pack and start a new package of pills."
    b. "Do a home pregnancy test and report the results."
    c. "Rinse it off if it has been less than 3 hours and reinsert."
    d. "Throw it away and get a new one."

24. The family planning nurse would be correct to tell a client to stop taking her combined oral contraceptive and notify her health care provider if she experiences which alteration?
    a. Increased vaginal discharge
    b. Severe headaches
    c. Lighter/shorter periods
    d. Menstrual cramping

25. Which risk factor decreases with the use of progestin in hormone therapy (HT)?
    a. Breast cancer
    b. Cervical cancer
    c. Endometrial cancer
    d. Vaginal cancer

CASE STUDY

Read the scenario and answer the following questions on a separate sheet of paper.

During her gynecology intake interview with the nurse practitioner at her company's new health care clinic, C.W., age 55 years, states, "I seem to be having more discomfort when I have sex. I don't lubricate when I want and need to; if my husband hurries me, it is downright painful. This is probably my problem, but my husband thinks that after a 35-year marriage, I just don't really want to have sex anymore."

The nurse compiles a few more facts about C.W. for review and consideration. In addition to her dyspareunia, C.W. has urinary frequency and urgency, vaginal pruritus, thinning vaginal epithelium with a glazed-looking appearance, and minimal elasticity upon speculum examination.

C.W. is Caucasian, is very thin, and reports no periods for nearly 2 years. She has no history of vaginal infections.

1. Given this history, what does the nurse suspect is occurring, and what other history would be important to obtain regarding symptoms?

2. What treatment options can be offered to this client?

3. What other health concerns should be discussed?

53 Men's Reproductive Health

STUDY QUESTIONS

Match the terms in Column I with the definitions in Column II.

Column I

_____ 1. Anabolic steroids

_____ 2. Androgen

_____ 3. Hirsutism

_____ 4. Spermatogenesis

_____ 5. Virilization

_____ 6. Antiandrogens

_____ 7. Cryptorchidism

_____ 8. Gynecomastia

_____ 9. Oligospermia

_____10. Priapism

Column II

a. Low sperm count
b. Undescended testis
c. Breast swelling or soreness
d. Ongoing painful erection
e. Growth of facial hair and vocal huskiness in women
f. Formation of spermatozoa
g. Steroid hormones related to the hormone testosterone
h. Testosterone
i. Blocks the synthesis or action of androgens
j. Increased hair growth

REVIEW QUESTIONS

11. Which client should not receive sildenafil?
     a. 56-year-old with hepatitis
     b. 58-year-old with seizure disorder
     c. 62-year-old with renal insufficiency
     d. 68-year-old with unstable angina

12. The 17-year-old client is receiving androgen therapy for hypogonadism. He asks the nurse what androgen therapy does. What is the nurse's best response?
     a. "It ensures the ability to respond sexually."
     b. "It ensures adequate sperm production."
     c. "It promotes larger stature through protein deposition."
     d. "It stimulates the development of secondary sex characteristics."

13. A 16-year-old wrestler at a local high school tells the nurse during an annual sports physical that some of the athletes at the school use hormones to "bulk up" during the season. The client wants to know if this is safe. What is the nurse's best response?
     a. "A safer way to bulk up is to eat an all-protein diet."
     b. "As long as they don't use other street drugs, this is probably safe."
     c. "This can cause serious, often irreversible, health problems even years later."
     d. "This is a safe practice as long as a health care provider adjusts the dose."

14. A client who is receiving androgen therapy takes prescribed drugs for cardiovascular disease, diabetes, and chronic obstructive pulmonary disease. Which drug-drug interactions can occur in this client?
     a. Androgens may decrease blood glucose levels, and insulin doses must be adjusted.
     b. Androgens decrease the effect of anticoagulants.
     c. Phenytoin potentiates the action of androgens.
     d. There are no interactions with steroids.

15. Which indication(s) would be appropriate for androgen therapy in women? (Select all that apply.)
     a. Advanced carcinoma of the breast
     b. Delayed development of sexual characteristics
     c. Endometriosis
     d. Infertility
     e. Severe premenstrual syndrome

16. A teenage male client is receiving androgen therapy for hypogonadism. Which side effect(s) might this client experience? (Select all that apply.)
     a. Gynecomastia
     b. Continuous erection
     c. A rise in voice pitch
     d. Urinary urgency
     e. Visual disturbances

17. Which indication(s) would be appropriate for anti-androgen drugs? *(Select all that apply.)*
    a. Advanced prostatic cancer
    b. Erectile dysfunction
    c. Male pattern baldness
    d. Menopausal symptoms
    e. Benign prostatic hypertrophy (BPH)

CASE STUDY

Read the scenario and answer the following questions on a separate sheet of paper.

H.H., 60 years old, has a history of diabetes and hypertension and presents to his health care provider for treatment of erectile dysfunction.

1. What is erectile dysfunction, and how does it relate to the client's history?

2. What class of drugs is the client referring to, and how does it work?

3. What are common side effects associated with this class of drugs?

4. What health teaching should the nurse provide for the client regarding erectile dysfunction?

54 Sexually Transmitted Infections

Match the infection in Column I to its description in Column II.

Column I

_____ 1. Gonorrhea

_____ 2. Primary syphilis

_____ 3. Secondary syphilis

_____ 4. Tertiary syphilis

_____ 5. Bacterial vaginosis

_____ 6. Chlamydia

Column II

a. Thin, white vaginal discharge with a strong fishy odor

b. Characterized by a skin rash that appears 2 to 8 weeks after the chancre

c. Second most common sexually transmitted infection (STI) that is characterized by a greenish yellow or whitish discharge and dysuria in men

d. Most common STI in young adults and is often asymptomatic

e. A chancre at the site of original infection caused by Treponema pallidum

f. Occurs as early as one year after the initial infection, causing large sores inside the body along with systemic syphilis to the cardiovascular and neurologic systems

Match the sexually transmitted infection (STI) in Column I with its appropriate drug in Column II.

Column I

_____ 7. Herpes simplex virus

_____ 8. Bacterial vaginosis

_____ 9. Chlamydia

_____ 10. Gonorrhea

_____ 11. Syphilis

_____ 12. Trichomoniasis

Column II

a. Benzathine penicillin G

b. Acyclovir

c. Ceftriaxone and azithromycin

d. Metronidazole

e. Nitroimidazole

f. Azithromycin

TRUE OR FALSE. If the statement is false, reword the sentence to make it true.

_____ 13. Scabies in adults is often transmitted sexually.

_____ 14. Washing bed linens of a client diagnosed with scabies is not necessary.

_____ 15. Nitroimidazoles and alcohol is not contraindicated.

_____ 16. Pediculosis pubis is treated with topical azole.

REVIEW QUESTIONS

17. A client presents to the clinic complaining of dysuria and yellow-green discharge. Culture confirms *Neisseria gonorrhoeae*. Which additional test should the client be counseled to consider?
    a. Fasting blood sugar
    b. Fertility workup
    c. Human immunodeficiency virus (HIV) testing
    d. Liver panel

18. Which advise would a nurse provide to a client with gonorrhea to prevent further transmission of the gonorrhea?
    a. Abstain or use condoms during sex.
    b. Ask partners to take antibiotics.
    c. Douche before intercourse.
    d. Only engage in anal intercourse.

19. The client, who has a history of repeated gonorrhea, chlamydia, and human papillomavirus (HPV), asks how long to abstain from sex. Which response by the nurse is most appropriate?
   a. "For at least two months."
   b. "Until the drugs are finished."
   c. "Until your partner finishes his treatment."
   d. "You may have sex using condoms."

20. The client asks if gonorrhea and syphilis are the same thing. Which response by the nurse is correct?
   a. "No, but if you have one, you should consider being tested for the other."
   b. "No, gonorrhea has no serious side effects."
   c. "No, only women get gonorrhea."
   d. "No, syphilis cannot be cured."

21. The client would like to know how human immunodeficiency virus (HIV) is spread. Which method(s) of transmission should be discussed with the client? *(Select all that apply.)*
   a. Breast milk
   b. Contact with infected blood
   c. Vaginal secretions
   d. Sexual contact
   e. Mosquitoes

CASE STUDY

Read the scenario and answer the following questions on a separate sheet of paper.

K.E., 21 years old, presents to her health care provider complaining of abnormal vaginal discharge and pelvic pain that worsens during intercourse. She also complains of pharyngitis. On examination, the pharynx is erythematous with whitish patches. The pelvic examination revealed odiferous, whitish discharge with adnexal tenderness. She reports being sexually active, including oral sex, with multiple partners.

1. What is the presumptive diagnosis, and what are some of its clinical manifestations?

2. How should K.E. be treated pharmacologically? What are the dosages?

3. What information should be provided to K.E.?

55 Adult and Pediatric Emergency Drugs

Match the condition in Column I with the drug of choice that treats it in Column II.

Column I

_____ 1. Anaphylactic shock

_____ 2. Angina pectoris

_____ 3. Opioid overdose

_____ 4. Extravasation of dopamine

_____ 5. Hypoxemia

_____ 6. Torsades de pointes

_____ 7. Frequent premature ventricular contractions (PVCs)

_____ 8. Atrial fibrillation

_____ 9. Increased intracranial pressure

_____ 10. Hemodynamically significant bradycardia

_____ 11. Paroxysmal supraventricular tachycardia (PSVT)

Column II

a. Magnesium sulfate
b. Diltiazem
c. Atropine sulfate
d. Mannitol
e. Phentolamine
f. Amiodarone
g. Nitroglycerin
h. Epinephrine
i. Oxygen
j. Adenosine
k. Naloxone

Match the drug in Column I with its classification in Column II. Classifications may be used more than once.

Column I

_____ 12. Nitroprusside

_____ 13. Epinephrine

_____ 14. Lidocaine

_____ 15. Norepinephrine

_____ 16. Mannitol

_____ 17. Diltiazem

_____ 18. Albuterol

_____ 19. Furosemide

Column II

a. Antidysrhythmic, class IB
b. Osmotic diuretic
c. Calcium channel blocker
d. Catecholamine
e. Beta-adrenergic agonist
f. Vasodilator
g. Loop diuretic

20. Sublingual nitroglycerin may be prescribed for chest pain. Which vital sign would be most important to assess before giving this drug?
    a. Blood pressure
    b. Heart rate
    c. Respiratory rate
    d. Temperature

21. Following administration of intravenous (IV) morphine to treat chest pain associated with acute myocardial infarction, which nursing action would be most important aspect of client monitoring?
    a. Assessment of respiratory status
    b. Documentation of neurologic function
    c. Measurement and strict recording of intake and output
    d. Measurement of central venous pressure

22. When monitoring a client with a dobutamine infusion, the nurse must be alert to the development of adverse effects. Which side or adverse effect may require slowing or discontinuing drug administration?
    a. Bradycardia
    b. Confusion
    c. Diaphoresis
    d. Myocardial ischemia

23. Procainamide 1.4 mg/minute is infusing in a client with supraventricular tachycardia (SVT). The nurse is closely monitoring the client to determine if the procainamide should be discontinued. Which side or adverse effect is an end point of procainamide administration?
    a. Headache
    b. Hypotension
    c. Respiratory depression
    d. Vomiting

24. A client post myocardial infarction complains of "heart racing" and is dyspneic. The cardiac monitor shows the patient to be in a tachyarrhythmia. Which dysrhythmia(s) is/are amiodarone intravenous (IV) used to treat? (Select all that apply.)
    a. Asystole
    b. Atrial fibrillation
    c. Bradycardia
    d. Second-degree heart block
    e. Ventricular fibrillation

25. Which acid-base imbalance is the best indication for sodium bicarbonate?
    a. Metabolic acidosis
    b. Metabolic alkalosis
    c. Respiratory acidosis
    d. Respiratory alkalosis

26. The client is admitted to the critical care unit after sustaining a severe closed head injury in a motorcycle collision. Mannitol is ordered to decrease intracranial pressure. Through which mechanism does mannitol exert its pharmacologic effects?
    a. Cerebral vasoconstriction
    b. Loop diuresis
    c. Osmotic diuresis
    d. Peripheral vasodilation

27. The client, who is allergic to shellfish, presents to the emergency department with hives after eating soup at a wedding reception. Client's tongue and lips are swollen. Which drug would be appropriate to administer to this client?
    a. Atropine
    b. Diltiazem
    c. Diphenhydramine
    d. Lidocaine

28. An unresponsive client presents to the emergency department in respiratory distress. The client's friends report the client "using a lot of those pain pills for the back." Client's pupils are pinpoint and has a respiratory rate of 4 breaths/minute. Which drug will the nurse be prepared to administer?
    a. Diltiazem 0.25 mg/kg IV piggyback
    b. Flumazenil 2.5 mg IV push
    c. Naloxone 0.4 mg IV push
    d. Magnesium 2 g IV piggyback

29. For which type(s) of shock would dopamine be administered? (Select all that apply.)
    a. Cardiogenic shock
    b. Hypovolemic shock
    c. Insulin shock
    d. Neurogenic shock
    e. Septic shock

30. Through which mechanism does dobutamine elevate blood pressure?
    a. Increasing cardiac output
    b. Positive alpha effects
    c. Vasoconstriction
    d. Vasodilation

31. The client has a diagnosis of septic shock. A norepinephrine drip is infusing through a central intravenous (IV) line. The bag of norepinephrine is almost empty. For which reason would the nurse prepare to hang another bag of norepinephrine?
    a. hypertensive crisis can result if the infusion is interrupted.
    b. profound hypotension can occur if the infusion is abruptly discontinued.
    c. the client is at high risk for bradycardia and heart block.
    d. the organisms responsible for septic shock will proliferate.

Chapter **55** **Adult and Pediatric Emergency Drugs**

32. An unconscious client was brought to the emergency department with a blood glucose level of 15 mg/dL. The nurse will prepare to administer dextrose 50% (D_{50}). For which conditions is D_{50} most commonly prescribed?
    a. As a maintenance infusion to keep a vein open
    b. To increase urine output
    c. To treat hyperglycemia
    d. To treat insulin-induced hypoglycemia

33. A client was brought into the emergency department with supraventricular tachycardia. The nurse is preparing to administer adenosine. Which method of administering adenosine is correct?
    a. Slow IV push over 2 minutes
    b. Diluted in 50 mL as IVPB over 30 minutes
    c. Rapid IV push as a bolus followed by saline flush
    d. Via a nebulizer

34. Which priority nursing action would be implemented after administering a total intravenous lidocaine dose of 3 mg/kg to an adult and the dysrhythmia has been suppressed?
    a. A continuous infusion of lidocaine must be initiated to maintain a therapeutic serum level.
    b. A therapeutic serum level will be achieved and maintained.
    c. Additional bolus doses must be administered to achieve a therapeutic serum level.
    d. 3 mg/kg is too much, and the patient has been overdosed.

35. The nurse is preparing to administer epinephrine intramuscularly (IM) to a client with an allergic reaction. Which concentration should the nurse select?
    a. 1:10,000 concentration of epinephrine
    b. 1:1000 concentration of epinephrine
    c. 1:100 concentration of epinephrine
    d. 1:1 concentration of epinephrine

36. The patient is in cardiac arrest. To administer epinephrine intravenously, which concentration should the nurse select?
    a. 1:10,000 concentration of epinephrine
    b. 1:1000 concentration of epinephrine
    c. 1:100 concentration of epinephrine
    d. 1:1 concentration of epinephrine

37. A client presents to the emergency department with hemodynamically unstable bradycardia. The nurse prepares to administer atropine 0.5 mg intravenously, knowing that lower dosages can cause which adverse effects?
    a. Paradoxical bradycardia can occur.
    b. Miosis occurs.
    c. The patient is at high risk for tachycardia.
    d. Vagal activity is completely increased.

38. A client with history of panic disorder is brought to the emergency department from an overdose of diazepam. The nurse prepares to administer flumazenil knowing that it is effective in reversing which class of drugs?
    a. Antipsychotics
    b. Benzodiazepines
    c. Opioids
    d. Paralytic agents

39. Magnesium sulfate is indicated for treatment of which medical condition(s)? *(Select all that apply.)*
    a. Atrial dysrhythmias
    b. Hypokalemia
    c. Cardiac arrest with hypomagnesemia
    d. Refractory ventricular fibrillation
    e. Torsades de pointes

40. A client with heart failure and pulmonary edema was ordered furosemide 60 mg by intravenous push (IVP). Furosemide exerts its effects on pulmonary edema through which mechanisms?
    a. Bronchodilation and diuresis
    b. Bronchodilation and antiinflammatory actions
    c. Vasoconstriction and diuresis
    d. Vasodilation and diuresis

41. Which priority nursing intervention(s) should be implemented when caring for a client with a nitroprusside infusion? *(Select all that apply.)*
    a. Always use nitroprusside with a blue or brown color to the solution.
    b. Monitor blood pressure continuously.
    c. Stop the nitroprusside immediately when blood pressure has stabilized.
    d. Protect the solution from light.
    e. Monitor thiocyanate levels.

42. Which side and/or adverse effect(s) is/are associated with intravenous (IV) atropine? *(Select all that apply.)*
    a. Dry mouth
    b. Miosis
    c. Mydriasis
    d. Urinary retention
    e. Vomiting

Read the scenario and answer the following questions on a separate sheet of paper.

M.E. calls emergency medical services (EMS) with complaints of chest pain and shortness of breath. M.E. has a history of angina, asthma, and obesity. M.E. states, "It just hit me hard. I think I'm going to die." M.E. has taken three nitroglycerin tablets, and was given oxygen, aspirin, and morphine en route to the hospital. On arrival at the hospital, an electrocardiogram is obtained. M.E. is not having a myocardial infarction but is diagnosed with unstable angina and is admitted to the coronary care unit. Vital signs on admission are temperature 97.3° F, heart rate 88 beats/min, respiratory rate 20 breaths/min, and blood pressure 214/118 mm Hg. A nitroglycerin drip is started.

1. How does nitroglycerin work to treat a client with angina?

2. Explain the benefit of M.E. receiving aspirin, oxygen, and morphine en route to the hospital? Why was the nitroglycerin drip started?

M.E. became unresponsive and developed widened QRS complex ventricular tachycardia with a ventricular rate of 190 beats/min. Code blue was called, and a crash cart was brought into the room. M.E. was shocked with 360 joules three times, without any change to the rhythm. A nurse prepares to administer emergency drugs.

3. What drug would a nurse prepare to first administer for pulseless ventricular tachycardia after unsuccessful defibrillation?

Answer Key

CHAPTER 1: THE NURSING PROCESS AND PATIENT-CENTERED CARE

1. False. "Concept" focuses on the *patient-centered model of care* instead of a disease-centered model.
2. False. Concepts are related to patient's problems, the medications, or topic of care listed within the *nursing process.*
3. False. The Nursing Alliance for Quality Care (NAQC) that supports quality patient-centered health care is partnered with the American *Nurses* Association.
4. False. NAQC believes that it is *nurse's* role to cultivate successful patient and family engagement.
5. False. The purpose of the nursing process is to *identify* a patient's problem and provide care. Nurses do not diagnose.
6. d, e, b, a, c
7. b
8. a
9. c
10. a
11. d
12. a
13. d or e
14. d
15. d
16. a
17. e
18. b
19. a
20. b
21. a
22. b
23. a
24. a
25. d. A *patient problem* is based on analysis of subjective and objective data so that patient-centered care is provided.
26. a. Data is gathered during an *assessment* of subjective and objective data to provide patient-centered care.
27. c. Goals are set during the *planning* phase after analyzing all the data that was gathered during the assessment phase. Usually, a goal statement starts with "The patient will.. . "
28. c. Goals are set during the *planning* phase after analyzing all the data that was gathered during the assessment phase. Usually, a goal statement starts with "The patient will.. . "
29. b. Nurses provide education, drug administration, patient care, and other interventions during the i*mplementation* phase.
30. b. After implementing part of the plan, the nurse must evaluate to determine whether the goals and teaching objectives have been met during the *evaluation* phase. Patient-centered care is an ongoing assessment data gathering, planning, implementing, and evaluating.
31. d. A *patient problem* is based on analysis of subjective and objective data so that patient-centered care is provided. Knowing the patient is receiving a diuretic is objective data.
32. b. Nurses provide education, drug administration, patient care, and other interventions during the *implementation* phase.
33. c. A *patient problem* is based on analysis of subjective and objective data so that patient-centered care is provided. Knowing the patient is receiving a diuretic is an objective data.
34. c. Nurses provide education, drug administration, patient care, and other interventions during the *implementation* phase.

Case Study

1. The nurse will consider the nursing process: assessment, patient problem, planning, implementation, and evaluation.

    The assessment phase of the nursing process for this client would include not only obtaining subjective and objective data, such as patient history and physical examination, but also reviewing current drugs and allergies. Physical examination should include physical reasons why the patient may not be able to administer the injection. Other items to assess include the home environment and, most importantly, the patient's readiness to learn and education level.

    The next phase in the nursing process is the development of a patient problem. These are based on actual concerns discovered in the assessment phase or potential problems attributable to risk factors that arise in the assessment. The patient's statements suggest several potential problems, including those related to anxiety, knowledge deficit, and nonadherence.

    In the planning phase, patient-centered, measurable goals are established in collaboration with the client, family, and other members of the health care team. The goals must be realistic and measurable and occur in a certain time frame. A realistic goal for this client could be *The client will prepare the prescribed dose of insulin by the second day of instruction.*

During the implementation phase, the nurse provides the education necessary for the client to be able to achieve the goal. In this situation, the teaching needs to address several areas, including the psychomotor skill of preparing and administering an insulin injection.

2. The nurse can determine the effectiveness of the teaching plan by a demo-return. Adequate time for questions must be provided, as well as contact information for the health care provider. The nurse must ensure that the client is ready to learn, the material is presented in an appropriate manner for learning to occur, and the materials are culturally appropriate.

Continue to assess the attainment of the objectives and goals and revise the plan to ensure success. Evaluation is the final step in the nursing process. The goal must be evaluated, and changes made if necessary. Was the client able to correctly demonstrate insulin preparation? Did the client have problems with anxiety surrounding the preparation? Was the client able to verbalize concerns to the health care provider?

CHAPTER 2: DRUG DEVELOPMENT AND ETHICAL CONSIDERATIONS

1. b
2. g
3. e
4. a
5. d
6. b
7. f
8. trade or brand
9. I
10. health information
11. FDA; health; innovative; safe; effective
12. nurse practice act
13. False. Schedule II drugs include cocaine, methadone, meperidine, and oxycodone.
14. True
15. True
16. True
17. False. A nurse will be prosecuted for omitting a drug dose, giving the wrong drug, or giving the drug by the wrong route.
18. b. Beneficence is the duty to protect research participants from harm. It clearly defines the research and ensures the benefits outweigh the risks. Justice involves the selection process of research participants is fair. Autonomy is the right to self-determination and the nurse must allow the research participant to make decisions. Respect for persons mean that all clients, including research participants, are treated as an independent persons who are capable of making decisions in their own best interests.
19. a. Prior to administering *any* drugs, a nurse should verify orders. When administering any controlled substances, a nurse must document all wasted amount,

keep all controlled drugs in a secure, locked area; and have a witness for *any* controlled drug wastages.

20. d. the *International Pharmacopeia* provides a basis for standards in strength and composition of drugs for use *throughout* the world. The *United States Pharacopeia/ National Formulary* sets the drug standards used in the United States. The *American Hospital Formulary Service Drug Information* provides complete drug information for both the health care provider and the consumer for drugs marketed in the United States. The *Medline Plus* provides extensive drug information and is available on the world wide web.

21. c. Federal legislation's primary purpose is to ensure safety and protect the public from drugs that are impure, toxic, ineffective, or not tested.

22. d. The Kefauver-Harris Amendment requires adverse reactions and contraindications to be included in the drug's literature.

23. d. LSD and mescaline are schedule I drugs. Schedule IV drugs include alprazolam and zolpidem. Schedule III drugs include ketamine and products containing less than 90 milligrams of codeine. Schedule II drugs include products with less than 15 milligrams of hydrocodone, cocaine, meperidine, and fentanyl.

24. d. Schedule V drugs include cough preparation containing not more than 200 mg of codeine. Schedule II drugs include products with less than 15 milligrams of hydrocodone, cocaine, meperidine, and fentanyl. Schedule III drugs include ketamine and products containing less than 90 milligrams of codeine. Schedule IV drugs include alprazolam and zolpidem.

25. d. All controlled substances must be stored in a locked, secured area.

26. c. All participants in a research study has the right to be informed. It is the responsibility of the health care provider, *not the nurse*, to explain the study. In order for the participant provide an informed consent, the person must be alert and able to comprehend the information.

27. a, c, d, e. Differences in appearance, either in the drug or in the packaging, can be an indication of a counterfeit drug. However, it is important to remember that pharmacies may change their pharmaceutical supplier, so the drug may appear as a different color or shape to the patient. This is an opportunity for the nurse and the pharmacist to work together to provide client education.

Case Study

1. The nurse will tell L.L. that the personal information will be shared with the pharmacist as it pertains to proper health care. The pharmacist will be able to discuss the drug and treatment with the client in a separate counseling area, away from other people.
2. HIPAA sets the standard for privacy of individuals of their identifiable health information. The act allows clients more control on who has access to their health records.

CHAPTER 3: PHARMACOKINETICS AND PHARMACODYNAMICS

1. absorption, distribution, metabolism, and excretion
2. half-life
3. Pharmacodynamics
4. bloodstream; administration
5. antagonists
6. receptors
7. f
8. e
9. c
10. a
11. b
12. d
13. g
14. a
15. d
16. c
17. b
18. c. Since liquid drugs do not need to dissolute and dissolve like tablets and capsules, they are absorbed more rapidly. Absorption of drugs is the movement of the drug from the gastrointestinal (GI) tract into the bloodstream after administration. Sublingual drugs enter the blood stream without having to be absorbed by the GI tract.
19. c. Disintegration of enteric-coated (EC) tablets occur in an alkaline environment of the small intestine. Drugs that are EC resist disintegration in the stomach by the gastric acid.
20. b. Food usually decrease dissolution and absorption of drugs. However, there are some drugs that are irritating to the gastric mucosa. Food can decrease the irritating effects.
21. d. Absorption, distribution, metabolism, and excretion are the correct sequence of pharmacokinetic phase. The drug must be absorbed from the GI tract into the bloodstream; drug must be distributed to the tissues; drug must be metabolized into an excretable form; the drug must be excreted.
22. b. Drugs that are lipid-soluble and nonionized can readily pass through the GI membrane. The mucous membrane lining the GI tract is composed of lipids and protein which allows lipid-soluble drugs to pass through. On the other hand, water-soluble drug needs a carrier.
23. b, c, e. The gastrointestinal tract is not considered vital to a patient in shock and hypotensive, so blood is shunted away, and drug absorption is slowed. Blood flow is also slowed because of pain and stress, resulting in a prolonged emptying time of the stomach.
24. c. Both drugs are highly protein-bound. When two or more highly protein-bound drugs are taken at the same time, they compete for the protein-binding sites. The more highly bound drug could displace the weakly bound drug; ampicillin/sulbactam could displace diazepam, which results in increase activity of diazepam.

25. b. The liver is the major site of drug metabolism. Kidneys excrete the drug.
26. b. The percentage of drug (bioavailability) for therapeutic activity is greatest after intravenous administration. Factors that affect bioavailability of drugs include drug form, route of administration, gastric mucosa and motility, food or other drugs, and liver function.
27. b. The best description is the time required for half of the drug to be eliminated. Other factors affecting drug's half-life are amount administered, amount of drug remaining from previous dose, and metabolism.
28. a. A drug that has a half-life of 24 to 30 hours will be taken once daily to maintain a steady state.
29. d. Kidneys excrete drugs that are water-soluble, drugs that are not bound, and drugs that are unchanged.
30. b. A decreased eGFR indicates renal dysfunction. Decreased eGFR is expected in older adults because of their decreased muscle mass. Many drugs, including trimethoprim, are eliminated through the kidneys. To prevent toxicity, the dose would need to be decreased.
31. a. Drug is more active if it is able to "fit" at the receptor site. The drug-receptor interactions are similar to the fit of the right key in a lock.
32. b. An antagonist prevents (inhibits) and/or blocks a response. An agonist activates receptors and/or produces a desired response. A cholinergic is a type of a receptor. Nonspecific drug can either be an antagonist or agonist; depends on the type of receptors the drug affects.
33. c. A nonspecific drug affects same type of receptors located throughout the body, producing both antagonist and agonist effects. On the other hand, a nonselective drug affects more than one type of receptors.
34. b. Therapeutic index describes the relationship between the therapeutic dose and the toxic dose.
35. a. Measurements that check a drug's concentration include peak and trough levels; peak level measures the highest serum concentration and the trough level measures the lowest serum concentration of the drug.
36. a, b, d, e. The nurse must be completely familiar with any drug being administered, such as contraindications, half-life, protein-binding effect, and therapeutic range. Information needs to be obtained not only on the drug but also on the specific patient's history. Drug reference books, drug pamphlets/inserts, or a pharmacist may be consulted with questions.
37. b. Side effects are secondary effects of all drugs and are often predictable. They may be desirable or undesirable. Adverse reactions, either mild or severe, are unintentional, unexpected reactions that occur at *normal* dosages. Synergistic effects occur when two or more drugs given together have a combined effect greater than the sum of their separate effects. Toxic effects are undesirable drug effects, often times life-threatening.

38. c. Loading dose is a larger than usual dose to obtain a therapeutic effect while waiting for the steady state to be achieved.

39. a, b, c. A time-response curve shows the dose-relationship of the drug's pharmacodynamics, which include onset, peak, and the duration of the drug's action.

40. a, b, d, e. The nurse should assess the client for side effects (both desirable and undesirable) when administering drugs. This is especially important for drugs that have nonselective actions. The nurse must be familiar with the drug, including its dose range, desired effects, side effects, and adverse effects, before administration. This information can be obtained from a variety of sources including current reference books, drug inserts, and pharmacists. If the drug has a narrow therapeutic range or requires peak/trough levels, these should be evaluated before and after administration. Side effects may occur immediately or up to several days after a dose. There is no set time to wait and see if side effects disappear. The health care provider should be notified as soon as possible after the appearance of side effects, especially if they are undesirable.

Case Study

1. The receptor theory states that drugs bind to receptor sites to activate a receptor, produce a response, or inhibit (block) a response. Some receptor sites are specific to only one drug, whereas others may accommodate several different drugs. However, some "fit better" and are more active. The drug binding sites are located on cell membranes and are primarily protein, glycoprotein, proteolipids, and enzymes in nature. The four receptor families are cell membrane–embedded enzymes, ligand-gated ion channels, G protein–coupled receptor systems, and transcription factors.

   Verapamil is a calcium channel blocker. Ligand-gated ion channels stretch across the cell membrane. If the channel is open, ions (usually calcium and sodium) can flow across the membrane. A calcium channel *blocker* prevents the flow of calcium. In the case of verapamil, this causes a decreased force of contraction, less spasm, and ultimately less anginal chest pain.

2. As with any new drug, the client should be taught about how to take the drug (with or without food, timing during the day), what effects to expect and how soon to expect to see results, what undesirable side effects or adverse effects to expect, and what to report to the health care provider. It is important to stress that the drug must be taken "as prescribed" even if the client is feeling better or not feeling any changes because some drugs work immediately and some medications may take several weeks to build up to a therapeutic level.

CHAPTER 4: PHARMACOGENETICS

1. Pharmacogenetics
2. irinotecan
3. abacavir
4. CYP2C9; VKORC1
5. False. Persons with genetic variation necessary to convert clopidogrel to the active metabolite is at risk for *clot formation*.
6. False. The CYP2D6 enzyme has 90 known variants slowing down drug metabolism.
7. False. *Not* everyone within the same ethnic group shares the same genetic variations.
8. True
9. c. Pharmacogenetics is the study of how a person's genetic makeup (genomes) affect their responses to drugs. Pharmacogenetics help personalize medicine to optimize therapy and decrease adverse drug reactions. Pharmacodynamics study how drugs affect the body as it relates to onset, peak, duration, and half-lives.
10. d. A client on multiple drugs would benefit the most in the use of pharmacogenetics. Other clients that would benefit are those who are on complex treatment regimen, such as clients on multiple antivirals to treat HIV or on combination anticancer drugs.
11. a. Clients with UGT1A1 gene variations may not be able to eliminate irinotecan. Clients with a variation to the CYP2D6 are unable to metabolize codeine and tramadol; thereby, not achieving pain relief. Clients with a variation to the CYP2C19 enzyme will not be able to convert clopidogrel to its active metabolite. Gene variation in TPMT can interfere with the metabolism of mercaptopurine.

Case Study

1. The first concern for the nurse should be whether R.J. has a variant gene for metabolizing tramadol. Persons who lack the CYP2D6 enzyme cannot metabolize opioids to the active form. Since R.J. is of Asian descent, the possibility for lacking the enzyme can occur.
2. The nurse needs to guard against genetic profiling. Determine if there is a family history of treatment failures by assessing family back three generations. Also determine client's ethnicity. If genetic variations are suspected, determine client's knowledge concerning genetics and genetic testing; explore any concerns. Consider other treatment options.

CHAPTER 5: COMPLEMENTARY AND ALTERNATIVE THERAPIES

1. e
2. b
3. a
4. d
5. c

6. plants; infusion
7. tincture
8. Extract; liniment
9. decoction
10. volatile; herb-infused oils
11. d, h
12. g
13. h
14. j
15. a, h
16. f
17. b
18. c
19. e, h
20. i
21. a. Chamomile is used for stomach or intestinal distress. It is also used for sleeplessness, and anxiety. Milk thistle is used for liver and gallbladder disorders. *Echinacea* is commonly used for virus related symptoms. St. John's wort is used to treat mental disorders and nerve pain.
22. c. *Gingko biloba* is used to improve memory, prevent Alzheimer disease and other dementias. It is also used for pulmonary distress, fatigue, and tinnitus. *Echinacea* is mostly used for virus related symptoms. Ginger is mostly used for nausea and diarrhea. Peppermint is good for nausea, indigestion, headaches, and nerve pain.
23. a, b, c, d. Bilberry, garlic, ginseng, and licorice can interfere with anticoagulants, such as warfarin.
24. a, d, e. The nurse should intervene by discussing with the patient that ginseng can interfere with the anticoagulants and increase the chance of bleeding; therefore, the patient should report any signs or symptoms of bleeding, such as bleeding of gums, black and tarry stools, and blood in the urine. Although educating the patient about the potential food-drug interactions while taking an anticoagulant, it is not appropriate in this specific scenario.
25. b, d. Large quantities of any one herbal product can lead to an "overdosage" of that product. Because specific doses and quantities are not regulated in this country, it is difficult to determine the correct amount. More is not necessarily better. Infants and children should not receive herbal preparations because of the lack of standardization and testing in a pediatric population.
26. c, d. Ginseng and milk thistle can have an additive effect when used with antidiabetic drugs causing hypoglycemia.
27. a, b, c, d. St. John's wort interacts with multiple drugs including anticoagulants and antiplatelets, anticonvulsants, antidepressants, and drugs for birth control. St. John's wort can increase bleeding time; it can cause decreased drug levels of anticonvulsants and oral contraceptives; it can increase serotonin levels, leading to serotonin syndrome.

28. a, b, d. The effects of antihypertensive medications may be decreased. Because licorice may have similar effects to aldosterone and corticosteroids, the effects of corticosteroid drugs may be increased. Taking licorice with digitalis may increase the effects of digitalis and lead to digitalis toxicity.

Case Study

1. The most commonly utilized herbal preparation for migraine headaches is feverfew. It is believed that this preparation may inhibit platelet aggregation and act as a serotonin antagonist, which may help in vascular and migraine headaches. Feverfew may also help with nausea and vomiting. Ginger is another herbal preparation that may help in the treatment of migraine headaches and the associated nausea. Although researched, the mechanism of action is unclear. St. John's wort may be taken for mild depression and anxiety, but it is not effective in treating headaches. St. John's wort has not been shown to be effective in moderate or severe depression; in fact, when combined with an SSRI, there is a higher risk for suicide. The mechanism of action is unknown.

2. Ginger interacts with antiplatelet and anticoagulant drugs. Feverfew also interacts with antiplatelet and anticoagulant drugs. St. John's wort has interactions with many drugs, including central nervous system (CNS) depressants, selective serotonin reuptake inhibitors (SSRIs), and oral contraceptives.

3. As with any herb or drug, the client should be encouraged to keep a list of the drugs and dosages. Although many people believe herbs are automatically "safe" since they are natural, this is not always the case. Herbal preparations do not pass through an FDA approval process as drugs do, so strength, amount of filler, and impurities may vary. Herbal preparations may also vary from one company to another, so the client should be encouraged to continue to obtain the preparation from the same reliable source or company.

CHAPTER 6: PEDIATRIC CONSIDERATIONS

1. fewer; increased
2. age; health status; weight; route of administration
3. 2; 3
4. body fluid composition; tissue composition; protein-binding capability
5. 2 years; higher
6. e
7. d
8. a
9. b
10. c
11. a, b. Absorption depends on the drug formulation (basic [alkalotic] or acidic). A low pH environment favors acidic drug absorption, whereas a high pH favors basic drug formulations.

12. c. The dosage for a water-soluble medication may need to be increased in this age group because their bodies are about 70% water up until age 2 years. Therefore, there is more water in which the drug will be distributed.

13. d. Immature blood-brain barrier allows drugs to pass easily into the central nervous system tissue (brain), increasing the risk of toxicity. As a child matures, the blood-brain barrier becomes more impervious to drugs.

14. a. The drug will absorb faster. One of the factors in which the degree and rate of drug absorption is age. The skin of infants and young children is thinner than that of adults. Furthermore, the ratio of body surface area to body mass is proportionately higher than for adults. Topical drugs are readily absorbed and toxicity can result. Sex of a child does not influence drug absorption.

15. a, b, c, d. Pharmacokinetics include drug absorption, distribution, metabolism, and excretion.

16. a, b, c, e. In early adolescence, renal tubular function decreases, which may lead to impaired excretion and a higher risk for toxicity. Dehydration can also decrease renal function and may lead to toxicity. Because the client is nauseated and vomiting, drugs should not be administered orally. When providing care to any client, developmental levels should be considered.

17. b, c, d, f. If necessary, a child may be lightly restrained but should not be forcibly held down. The child should be praised for taking the drug. At no time should a child be threatened, forced, or made to view the medication as punishment. Depending on the developmental level of the child, explanations should be given to the child about what to expect, but the child should not be given the option of debating whether to take the drug. Herbal preparations are not usually given to children; however, cultural traditions should be respected as much as possible.

Case Study

1. Preschoolers may respond age-appropriate explanations. They may also benefit from a familiar toy or stuffed animal as support. Allow the child to verbalize being scared or upset. Whenever possible, allow the child options and control. Do not argue with the child or tell the child that she is being punished for falling from the tree. Tell the child what will happen before it happens. Do not just surprise the child.

2. A topical anesthetic like a eutectic mixture of local anesthetics or topical lidocaine may be utilized to lessen the pain of establishing an intravenous (IV) site. The downside to using these topical anesthetics is that they must be in place 60 to 90 minutes before the IV can be started for anesthetic effect.

3. Answers can vary. Caregivers may be involved in child care (if they choose to be) by helping to gently restrain the child. They can also provide distraction

("What color sling would you like?" or "What should we have to eat tomorrow morning when we get up?"). Reassuring the preschooler can also be beneficial.

CHAPTER 7: OLDER ADULT CONSIDERATIONS

1. absorption, distribution, metabolism
2. low; gradually; response
3. sensory; physical; aging
4. receptor; affinity
5. sotolol, all NSAIDs, meperidine, glyburide, metformin, exenatide, nitrofurantoin, potassium-sparing diuretics, thiazide diuretics, olmesartan, and new anticoagulants
6. c
7. b
8. d
9. a
10. Angiotensin converting enzyme inhibitor (ACE-I)
11. Beta blockers
12. Psychotropics
13. Angiotensin II-receptor blockers (ARBs)
14. False. Risk factors associated with polypharmacy *includes* advanced age in addition to female gender, having multiple health care providers, use of herbal therapies, use of over-the-counter (OTC) drugs, multiple chronic disorders, and frequency of hospitalizations and care transitions.
15. True
16. True
17. False. Risk factors associated with polypharmacy *include* over-the-counter (OTC) drugs, in addition to female gender, having multiple health care providers, use of herbal therapies, advanced age, multiple chronic disorders, and frequency of hospitalizations and care transitions.
18. False. Beers criteria is a document developed by the American Geriatric Society listing drugs to *avoid among older adults and information on renal dosing and drug-drug interactions.*
19. True
20. True
21. a. Creatinine clearance is determined by the glomerular filtration rate (GFR). Normal working kidneys will have a GFR of 100 to 125 mL/min. Aspartate aminotransferase (AST) measures the liver function. Troponin is a type of protein found in skeletal and heart muscles. Urea is a waste product.
22. b. Renal function is decreased in older adults, which can cause electrolyte imbalance. Also, decreased renal function can lead to prolonged half-life and elevated drug levels. Certain antihypertensives like ACE-I, potassium-sparing diuretics, and thiazide diuretics can worsen electrolyte imbalance.
23. a. There is no reason that the client cannot work outside while taking digoxin, and the client's symptoms are not related to the digoxin. Diphenhydramine can be very sedating among older

adults, and there are substitutes that are equally effective with fewer side effects. Fluoxetine, an SSRI, is prescribed for depression. Clients of all ages should be advised not to take each other's medications.

24. c. Drugs with a shorter half-life will be eliminated from the body faster than drugs with longer half-life without interfering with its therapeutic effect. Quicker elimination will decrease the risk of adverse/toxic drug effects. More protein binding the drug has, the less active drug is available to exert its therapeutic effect. Fat-soluble drugs have greater volume of distribution and a prolonged period of action. This can also increase the risk for toxicity.

25. a, b. BUN (blood urea nitrogen) and creatinine clearance are assessed to determine renal function. The ability for the kidneys to excrete drugs decrease with age. CBC (complete blood count) is a test that evaluates red blood cells, white blood cells, and platelets. Lipase is a pancreatic enzyme. Triglycerides are a type of fat.

26. d. Dizziness when going from a supine to a standing position is referred to as *orthostatic hypotension*. Although bradycardia may cause dizziness, this is not the most likely cause.

27. a. Changing positions slowly should assist in decreasing the dizziness associated with hypotension related to changes in position. Taking a deep breath and checking heart rate will not affect dizziness. Having a chair close to the bed may be beneficial if the client feels dizzy but may also pose a safety risk; the client may strike the chair with fainting.

28. c. When a person has been hospitalized, a drug reconciliation has been completed. Depending on the client's response, drugs may be added to or subtracted from the regimen and dose adjustments may be made. The client should take only those drugs that have been prescribed at discharge.

29. a. Although a family member could assist with the daily drug regimen, the client will be able to maintain more independence using a non-childproof cap. Using a non-childproof cap should make the container easier for the older adult client to grasp and open.

30. b. Maintaining independence for as long as possible is crucial for an older adult client. A client who has visual challenges can, with assistance, fill a drug-dispensing container for the upcoming week. The client must have assistance in the setup to assure that the correct drugs are in each separate compartment. Leaving the drug bottles on the counter could lead to a mix-up if they are displaced. Writing down which drugs need to be taken is not beneficial if the patient has visual challenges.

31. a, c, d, e. Of the listed factors, only height does not have a role in dosage adjustment. Older adults have more adipose tissue, so a greater amount of lipid-soluble drug would be absorbed. Protein is required for binding of some drugs, so if a patient is malnourished, there would be less protein available, leading to more free drug; this can lead to drug toxicity. Laboratory results, specifically those that assess renal and hepatic function, are important to trend, as well as those drug levels (digoxin, INR) needed to measure toxicity. As with any population, it is important to evaluate the client for responsiveness to the drug.

32. a, b, d, e. Older adults have less protein available for binding, so it is important to know if a drug is highly protein bound. Drugs with a short half-life are less likely to cause problems for the client. Certain drugs (some antibiotics, digoxin, warfarin) have very narrow therapeutic ranges, so they must be monitored closely. Vital signs may vary as a client ages; therefore, it is important to obtain baseline vital signs to know the client's norm.

Case Study

1. Because both renal function and hepatic function are important in drug metabolism and excretion, and both decrease with aging, the nurse would anticipate that measurement of liver enzymes, BUN, creatinine, and creatinine clearance would be ordered. Because this client also has diabetes, the client's blood glucose level will be evaluated.

2. There are a variety of sleep aids besides triazolam that could be utilized. Because M.Z. is also taking a diuretic, it would be important to suggest the client to take the diuretic in the morning to prevent frequent awakenings during the night to go to the bathroom. Some nonpharmacologic measures include taking warm baths, decreasing stimulation in the evening, and eliminating caffeine intake late in the day. The client also likes chamomile tea, which may help induce sleep. A light bedtime snack will help maintain blood sugar levels throughout the night.

3. The nurse should recognize and support the client's desire to adhere with the drug regimen; however, the client does need further education about "doubling up" on drugs. A variety of methods can be used to help M.Z. remember to take the prescribed drug. These can include using commercial pill dispensers, making a list, keeping a calendar, or setting an alarm.

CHAPTER 8: DRUGS IN SUBSTANCE USE DISORDER

1. b
2. c
3. a
4. dopamine, neurotransmitters
5. reward circuit
6. epigenetics
7. inhibits
8. methadone or buprenorphine, or naltrexone
9. GHB (gamma-hydroxybutyrate)
10. euphoria, tranquility, blocks
11. CAGE

12. personality, behavior, job performance, job attendance
13. False. Electronic cigarettes are *not* safer than tobacco products.
14. False. DHEA is found in many dietary supplements, and there is *no* evidence that DHEA slows aging, increases energy levels, or increases muscle strength.
15. True
16. b
17. a
18. d
19. c
20. a. Cocaine can cause dilated pupils (not pinpoint pupils) and restlessness. It can also cause hypertension (not hypotension), tachycardia, insomnia, erratic behaviors (not fine tremors), and tachypnea (not respiratory depression).
21. c. Methadone is a long-acting opioid that is effective in treating persons addicted to opioids by blocking the sensation of euphoria and tranquility produced by opioids, and it prevents opioid withdrawal and craving. Dronabinol is a synthetic cannabis, lorazepam is a benzodiazepine to decrease anxiety, and naloxone is a reversal agent for opioid-induced respiratory depression.
22. a, c, e. A client must be ready and motivated to quit any addictive substance, or the likelihood of success is decreased. This is a difficult process that will require the client's commitment. Certain triggers, like places where a person smokes or times that trigger the craving for a cigarette, should be identified and alternatives determined. There are a variety of aids, both pharmacologic and nonpharmacologic, that can be utilized to help a client quit smoking. Ideally, a quit date of 1 to 2 weeks should be set so the client stays motivated. Tobacco in any form is still addictive, so chewing tobacco or smoking tobacco in a pipe instead of a cigarette is still abusing tobacco. Although it is difficult, some clients prefer to quit smoking "cold turkey" or without the use of aids.
23. d. It is estimated that 10–15% of nurses have a substance use disorder, including cannabis, cocaine, narcotics, opiates, alcohol, and nicotine.
24. d. Bath salts are synthetic cathinones that have amphetamine-like stimulant effects.

Case Study
1. Even though the client appears to be intoxicated, other causes of his unresponsiveness need to be evaluated. There is no antidote for alcohol intoxication other than supportive care. The client's respiratory rate is insufficient, and his respirations must be assisted. Treatment should be aimed toward airway management and supplemental oxygenation, supportive care, and IV hydration.
2. A person with alcohol toxicity can aspirate on vomitus and asphyxiate and develop severe dehydration, seizures, hypothermia, and eventually brain damage and death.

3. Disulfiram inhibits acet aldehyde dehydrogenase, the enzyme needed to metabolize alcohol. Disulfiram keeps clients from ingesting alcohol because of its side effects. It is slowly metabolized by the liver. The side effects can occur up to 2 weeks after cessation of drug therapy. Side effects can occur within 10 minutes of ingesting alcohol (including mouthwash, cough medicine, or foods containing or cooked in alcohol). Side effects include nausea, headache, vomiting, chest pains, dyspnea (difficulty breathing), rash, drowsiness, impotence, acne, and a metallic aftertaste.
4. Metronidazole, an antimicrobial, and paraldehyde, a sedative, when taken concomitantly with disulfiram can produce the same side effects as if the person had been ingesting alcohol.

CHAPTER 9: SAFETY AND QUALITY

1. Safety
2. Client-family-centered care
3. Collaboration and teamwork
4. Quality improvement
5. Informatics
6. Evidence-based care
7. c
8. f
9. j
10. g
11. a
12. h
13. b
14. d
15. e
16. i
17. a
18. a
19. b
20. a
21. b
22. a
23. a. intradermal, yes; b. morphine sulfate or multiple sclerosis, no; c. every other day, no; d, drops, yes; e. kilograms, yes; f. 1 milligram, no; whole numbers should not contain trailing zeros; g. milligram, yes; h. every day or daily, no; i. keep vein open, yes; j. intravenous piggyback, yes; k. with, no; l. before, no; m. twice daily, yes
24.

Abbreviation	Meaning
CR	controlled release
ER	extended release
IM	immediate release
XR	extended release
XT	extended release

25. c. Antibiotics must be taken at regularly spaced intervals to maintain therapeutic blood levels. All antibiotics should be completed even if the client feels better. The dosage of antibiotics should not be increased, even if the client does not feel better.
26. b. ac is before meals and hs is at bedtime. However, it is best not use these abbreviations.
27. c. "Tall man" letters promote safety between drugs with similar names by calling attention to differences in spelling, such as quiNIDine and quiNINE.
28. c. A nurse must never administer a dose that seems large or out of range without rechecking the calculations. If there continues to be a question, another nurse should double-check the dose as well.
29. a, b, d
30. a. The nurse's first action is to document the refusal immediately. It is important to remember that the refusal to take a medication is the client's right. The nurse should determine the client's reasoning behind refusing to take a medication and stress the importance of the medication regimen. The health care provider should be notified of the refusal.
31. b, c, d, e. The "Do Not Use List" of abbreviations include q.d., U, IU, and MS. q.d. should be written as "daily" or "every day"; U is to be written as "unit"; and IU as "International Unit." MS can be confused for morphine sulfate or magnesium sulfate; instead, write out the drugs.
32. d. Unused drugs should not be disposed in a manner that is connected to the sewage. Instead, it is best to dispose of them by taking the drug to a facility that has a "take-back" program. If this is not available, then drugs should be mixed whole in an unpalatable nonfood substance, such as kitty litter or dirt prior to placing them in the regular trash. It should not be crushed prior to mixing it.

Case Study

1. The "six rights" are 1) the right client, 2) the right drug, 3) the right dose, 4) the right route, 5) the right time, and 6) right documentation.
2. Ask the client to state their full name and birth date and compare these with the client's identification (ID) band and the medication administration record (MAR).

   Many facilities have electronic health records (EHRs) that allow the nurse to directly scan the bar code from the client's ID band. Once the band is scanned, the nurse can see the client's medication record.

   If the client is an adult with a cognitive disorder or a child, verify the client's name with a family member. In the event a family member is unavailable and the client is unable to self-identify, follow the facility's policy. Many facilities have policies that include a photo ID on the band with the client's name and birth date affixed to the band.

   Distinguish between two clients with the same first or last name by placing "name-alert" stickers as warnings on the medical records.

3. The nurse should check the drug with the medication administration record and physician's order to ensure they are the correct drugs. If the drugs are dispensed in a unit dose method, the drugs should be taken out of its package at the client's bedside. Show the package to the client. Many facilities dispense drugs using unit dose method to reduce drug errors.

CHAPTER 10: DRUG ADMINISTRATION

1. Enteric-coated; timed-release
2. fine particle
3. semi-Fowler's or high Fowler's
4. 30
5. 30
6. c
7. a
8. b
9. ventrogluteal
10. vastus lateralis
11. deltoid
12. ventrogluteal
13.

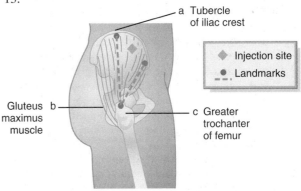

Ventrogluteal injection site

14. c. The oral route is contraindicated in a client who is vomiting. Parenteral routes are preferred.
15. a. In children younger than 3 years old, straighten the external ear canal by pulling the auricle down and back. In older children and adults, straighten the canal by pulling the auricle upward and outward.
16. d. The ventrogluteal muscle is the preferred site for many IM injections because it is a deep muscle, situated away from major nerves and blood vessels.
17. c. Vastus lateralis is the preferred site because of easy access; however, ventrogluteal can also be used. Dorsogluteal muscle is no longer used. Deltoid muscle is not developed.

18. a. Over-the-counter drugs and herbal preparations may interact with prescription drugs. Clients must be encouraged to discuss the use of these preparations with their pharmacist or health care provider.

19. a, b, e. Nurses have the responsibility of teaching clients about their drugs. Teaching includes expected therapeutic effects, dietary considerations, and instructions should be written. Other aspects of teaching include possible side and adverse drug effects, possible laboratory tests that may be required, and ensuring continuous supply of the drug, among others. c is incorrect because not all drugs are stored in the refrigerator. d is incorrect because clients do not need to know how the drug was tested and developed.

20. b. The client should rinse out the mouth after administering a dose from a metered-dose inhaler. This will help prevent secondary infection and irritation. a is incorrect because the MDI must be used as prescribed. Overuse can increase side effects and tolerance can result. c is incorrect because the mouth is not placed tightly over the end. It is closed around the MDI with the opening toward the back of the throat or it can be positioned 1-2 inches from the mouth if a spacer is not used. d is incorrect; subsequent doses should be spaced 1-2 minutes apart.

Case Study Answers

1. 18-25 gauge needle that is 5/8 – 1 ½ inches long and 1-3 mL syringe. The size of the syringe depends on the mL drawn for the correct dose.

2. The potential sites for IM injections include deltoid, ventrogluteal, or the vastus lateralis. The preferred site for anyone at any age is the ventrogluteal. Ventrogluteal muscle is a deep muscle that is away from major nerves and blood vessels. The deltoid is easier to access, but not all clients have developed deltoids. These are reserved for small volume of drug. Vastus lateralis would be appropriate, but it is usually hard to access.

3. Promethazine is irritating to tissue. It should be given deep IM. The best method would be to use the Z-track. The ventrogluteal is the preferred site for Z-track IM administration. Z-track seals the drug in the muscle which can minimize local skin irritation.

CHAPTER 11: DRUG CALCULATIONS

Metric and Household Systems

1. b
2. f
3. g
4. c
5. i
6. j
7. o
8. e
9. n
10. m
11. d
12. l
13. a
14. k
15. h
16. A. 1000 mg; B. 1000 mL; C. 1000 mcg
17. 3000 mg
18. 1500 mL
19. 100 mg
20. 2.5 L
21. 0.25 L
22. 0.5 g
23. 4 pt
24. 32 fl oz
25. 48 fl oz
26. 2 pt
27. 3 mg
28. 15 mL
29. 1 fl oz
30. 3 tsp
31. 1000 mg
32. 0.5 g
33. 100 mg
34. 1 L; 1 qt
35. 8 fl oz
36. 1 fl oz; 2 T; 6 t
37. 1 t
38. 1 ½ fl oz; 9 t
39. 150 mL; 10 T

Drug Calculations for Enteral and Parenteral Drugs

1. d. When calculating drug dosages, it is most helpful to convert to the system used on the drug label.

2. b, c, d, e. Parenteral routes are any routes that do not involve the gastrointestinal (GI) system and generally bypass the hepatic system. These routes include subcutaneous, intramuscular, intradermal, and intravenous.

3. c, d. All insulins and heparinized products can be given subcutaneously. Regular insulin and fractionated heparin can be given intravenously.

4. self-sealing rubber tops; reusable if properly stored

5. a, b. Once a drug in a multi-dose vial has been reconstituted, the nurse should label the vial with the date and time the drug was reconstituted or when to discard the vial and also with the nurse's initials.

6. c. The body's habitus must be considered when administering IM injection. 19, 20, and 21 gauges with 1, 1½, and 2 inches in length are appropriate for the average adult.

7. b. Any parts of the syringe that can touch or be injected must remain sterile, which includes the needle, plunger, and inside of the barrel.

8. b. Subcutaneous injections can be administered at 45-, 60-, or 90-degree angles, depending on the person's body habitus.

9. c. Because the volume to be administered is less than 1 mL, a tuberculin (TB) syringe should be

selected. A TB syringe is a 1-mL syringe. An insulin syringe is measured in units and not in mL. The 3-mL and 5-mL syringes can be used; however, they are too big and the amount drawn in these syringes may not be as accurate.

10. d. A 5-mL syringe should be used to measure 3 mL of saline solution to mix the powdered drug. The solution of saline and drug will be more than 3-mL; therefore a 3-mL syringe would be too small.

11. c. Since the drugs are compatible, use one syringe to draw up the correct amount of volume from each drug and attach the syringe to a syringe pump for infusion. Total volume of drug is 13 mL; one 20-mL syringe will suffice.

Interpreting Drug Labels

12. A. Viread;
    B. a generic name is not available;
    C. 300 mg/tab;
    D. tab

13. A. hydrocodone bitartrate and acetaminophen;
    B. 5 mg/300 mg per tab;
    C. yes; it is a schedule II drug
    D.

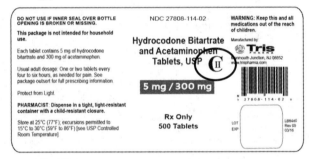

    E. Tab;
    F. controlled room temperature between 59° F and 86° F;
    G. Tris Pharma

14. A. phenytoin sodium;
    B. no;
    C. cap;
    D. 100 mg;
    E.

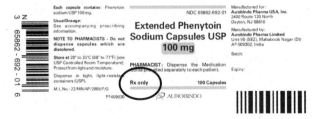

    F. in its original container at controlled room temperature and protect from light and moisture

15. A. dextromethorphan polistirex;
    B. Robitussin;
    C. no;
    D. liquid;
    E. 30 mg/5 mL;
    F. 89 mL;

    G. 10 mL q12h;
    H. approximately 9 doses

16. A. influenza A (H1N1)
    B. liquid;
    C. multi-dose;
    D. in an environment that is 35° to 46° F;
    E. IM

17. A. interferon gamma-1b;
    B. Actimmune;
    C. refrigerated

18. A. d;
    B. d; solution:

$$x \, tab = \frac{1\,tab}{100 \, \cancel{mg}} \times \frac{1000 \, \cancel{mg}}{1 \, \cancel{g}} \times \frac{0.5 \, \cancel{g}}{X}$$
$$= 5 \, tab$$

19. A. a; B. b

20. A. d; B. b

21. d

22. A. b; concentration is 350 mg/mL after reconstitution. The amount 1 g does not need to be factored into the equation since the resulting concentration is given in mg.
    B. 3 mL syringe

23. A. b

24. A. losartan potassium;
    B. Cozaar;
    C. 30 tab;
    D. b

25. A. a; since both tab are scored, then 10 mg can be divided into ½ tab for the ordered dose;
    B. b

26. A. furosemide;
    B. Lasix;
    C. room temperature;
    D. c

27. A. Extended Release tablet; oral liquid is not extended release, and the bioavailability will be decreased;
    B. c; The nurse cannot switch the formulation of a drug without an order from a prescriber.
    C. a; liquid solution; drugs in ER cannot be crushed; liquid solution can be given via NGT; b. 7.5 mL.

28. A. a; B. a

29. A. 1 tab; B. 2 tab

30. A. 5.7 mL; B. d

31. A. subcut;
    B. 40 mg/0.8 mL;
    C. 0.8 mL;
    D. a, c; tuberculin syringe is a 1-mL syringe. Insulin syringe is measured in units. Less accurate dosing can occur with 3-mL syringe.

32. A. c; B. c

33. A. a and b or just a or just b;
    B. 1 tab from 2.5 mg and 5 mg; 3 tab from 2.5 mg; or 1.5 tab from the 5-mg tab.

34. d. This lithium level is too high, and adjustments need to be made. Withhold the dose and contact the health care provider.

35. A. b; B. a
36. A.

B. d;
C. d
37. b
38. d
39. c
40. c. The nurse should acknowledge the client's concerns and provide an appropriate answer. The first two responses negate the client's concerns, while the last response is incorrect.
41. a
42. d
43. A. No, Duramorph is morphine and is much weaker in strength than hydromorphone;
B. d
44. d
45. c
46.

47. A. Topamax;
B. topiramate;
C. sprinkle capsules;
D. 1 cap/dose

Drug Calculations using Body Weight
48. A. b;
B. d; *solution:*

$$mL = \frac{5\ mL}{400\ 000\ units} \times \frac{200\ 000\ units}{x}$$

$$= \frac{1000\ mL}{400} = 2.5\ mL$$

49. A. b, *solution:*

$$min = \frac{10\ mg}{1\ kg} \times \frac{1\ kg}{2.2\ lbs} \times \frac{75\ lbs}{24\ h} \times 12\ h = 170\ mg;$$

$$max = \frac{15\ mg}{1\ kg} \times \frac{1\ kg}{2.2\ lbs} \times \frac{75\ lbs}{24\ h} \times 12\ h = 256\ mg;$$

the dose of 200 mg is between the recommended dose; the question is asking if 200 mg is appropri-

ate; therefore, do not include the ordered dose of 200 mg into the equation.
B. d
50. A. a; the dose is too low; child should receive 133–150 mg/dose;
B. a; 225 mg/d
51. c
52. A. 2.1 mL;
B. 350 mg/mL;
C. b; *solution:*

$$mL = \frac{1\ mL}{350\ mg} \times \frac{50\ mg}{kg} \times 8\ kg = 1.1\ mL$$

53. A. b; no, the dose is too low; B. d
54. A.

$$\frac{(20\ mg/1\ kg \times 1\ kg/2.2\ lb \times 22\ lb)}{3}$$
$$= 66.7\ mg\ and$$
$$\frac{(50\ mg/1\ kg \times 1\ kg/2.2\ lb \times 22\ lb)}{3}$$
$$= 133.3\ mg;$$

B. Yes, the dose ordered is between the minimum and maximum dosage range;
C. b
55. A. b;
B. b;
C. a
56. A. 11.4 kg;
B. 114 mg - 171 mg; Range provided by using weight 11 kg (after rounding)
Dimensional Analysis:

$$X\ mg = \frac{10\text{-}15\ mg}{1\ kg} \times \frac{1\ kg}{2.2\ lbs} \times \frac{25\ lbs}{?}$$
$$= 113.6 - 170.5\ mg = 114 - 171\ mg\ per\ rounding\ rule$$

Notice with Dimensional Analysis, all conversion factors were included in the equation. Only the final answer had to be rounded.
C. Yes, it is within the recommended dose

57. 523 mg; *solution:*

$$mg = \frac{50\ mg}{1\ kg} \times \frac{1\ kg}{2.2\ lb} \times 23\ lb$$
$$= 523\ mg\ per\ rounding\ rule$$

58. A. 2954.5 mg; *solution:*

$$mg = \frac{100\ mg}{1\ kg} \times \frac{1\ kg}{2.2\ lb} \times 65\ lb = 2955\ mg$$

B. 1477 mg; *solution:*

$$mg = \frac{2955\ mg}{2\ doses}$$

Drug Calculations using Body Surface Area

59. All answers are approximates.
    A. 0.17–0.18 m²;
    B. 0.52 m²;
    C. 0.9–0.95 m²
60. All answers are approximates.
    A. 0.88 m²;
    B. 0.9 m²;
    C. 0.56 m²
61. A. 0.51 m²; *solution:*

$$\sqrt{\frac{25\times32}{3131}}=\sqrt{0.256}=0.51\text{ m}^2$$

    B. 0.66 m²; *solution:*

$$\sqrt{\frac{58\times48}{3131}}=0.94\text{ m}^2$$

    C. 0.66 m²

$$\sqrt{\frac{40\times34}{3131}}=0.66\text{ m}^2$$

62. A. 0.25 m²; *solution:*

$$\sqrt{\frac{8\times28.2}{3600}}=0.25\text{ m}^2$$

    B. 1.02 m²; *solution:*

$$\sqrt{\frac{28.1\times133.4}{3600}}=1.02\text{ m}^2$$

    C. 0.77 m²; *solution:*

$$\sqrt{\frac{85.5\times25}{3600}}=0.77\text{ m}^2$$

63. A. 1.06 m²;
    B. 1.01 m²; *solution:*

$$\sqrt{\frac{80\times40}{3131}}=1.01\text{ m}^2$$

    C. 101 mg; *solution:* 100 mg × 1.01 m² = 101 mg
64. A. 1.10 m²; B. 55 mg
65. A. 0.85 m²; B. 30 mg
66. A. 1.31 m²; B. 176 mg
67. A. 1.17 m²; B. 263 mg
68. A. 1.46 m²; B. 5 mg
69. A. 0.78 m²; B. 273 mg
70. A. 1.45 m²; B. 247 mg

Drug Calculations for Drugs Requiring Reconstitution

71. A. 5.4 mL; 250 mg/1.5 mL; B. c
72. A. 3.4; 250 mg/mL; B. b
73. b
74. c
75. d

Drug Calculations for Intravenous Drugs and Fluids

76. c; the question was asking for dosage for infusion. mL/h would be flow rate for infusion. gtt/min is the flow rate when calculating the rate for infusion using gravity and the drop factor is known.
77. d. Any method of drug calculation can be used, however dimensional analysis is the best method when conversion factors are needed. Rounding is conducted at the end.
78. d
79. a
80. c
81. a
82. b
83. d
84. 10–20 gtt/mL; 60 gtt/mL
85. keep vein open; 250-mL IV bag
86. calibrated cylinder with tubing
87. volumetric
88. uniform concentration of the drug, client control and ownership of the pain
89. 28 gtt/min; solution:

$$\frac{\text{gtt}}{\text{min}}=\frac{10\text{ gtt}}{1\text{ mL}}\times\frac{1000\text{ mL}}{6\text{ h}}\times\frac{1\text{ h}}{60\text{ min}}=28\text{ gtt / min}$$

90. 31 gtt/min
91. 50 gtt/min; *solution:*

$$\frac{\text{gtt}}{\text{min}}=\frac{15\text{ gtt}}{1\text{ mL}}\times\frac{100\text{ mL}}{30\text{ min}}=\frac{50\text{ gtt}}{\text{min}}$$

92. A. 1000 mL;
    B. 2500 mL;
    C. 104.2 mL/h; *solution:*

$$\frac{\text{mL}}{\text{h}}=\frac{2500\text{ mL}}{24\text{ h}}=104.2\text{ mL / h}$$

93. A. e;
    B. 28 gtt/min; *solution:*

$$\frac{\text{gtt}}{\text{min}}=\frac{10\text{ gtt}}{1\text{ mL}}\times\frac{500\text{ mL}}{3\text{ h}}\times\frac{1\text{ h}}{60\text{ min}}=\frac{28\text{ gtt}}{\text{min}}$$

94. A. c;
    B. d
95. d; partial drops cannot be administered; therefore, round 12.5 gtt up to 13 gtt/min
96. A. 3.4 mL;
    B. 250 mg/mL;
    C. b
97. 25 gtt/min; see problem 18B for example solution.
98. 67 gtt/min
99. A. 614 mcg;
    B. 307 mcg;
    C. 127.5 mL/h; flow rate is based on 255 mL = 250 mL fluid + 5 mL of drug

D. 42 gtt/min; *solution:*

$$\frac{127.5 \text{ mL}}{1 \text{ h}} \times \frac{1 \text{ h}}{60 \text{ min}} \times 20 \text{ min} = 42.5 \text{ mL infused;}$$

therefore,

$$\frac{20 \text{ gtt}}{\text{mL}} \times \frac{255\text{-}42.5 \text{ mL}}{100 \text{ min}} = \frac{43 \text{ gtt}}{\text{min}} \text{ per rounding rule}$$

100. 200 mL/h
101. A. 1.6 mL;
   B. 203.2 mL/h; add 1.6 diluent to the total fluid amount to equal 101.6 mL
102. 84.2 mL/h
103. 100 gtt/min
104. 50 gtt/min
105. A. 1250 units/h; *solution:*

$$\frac{\text{units}}{\text{h}} = \frac{30000 \text{ units}}{1 \text{ day}} \times \frac{1 \text{ day}}{24 \text{ h}} = 1250 \text{ units / h}$$

   B. 25 mL/h; *solution:*

$$\frac{\text{mL}}{\text{h}} = \frac{250 \text{ mL}}{12500 \text{ units}} \times \frac{1250 \text{ units}}{\text{h}}$$

106. A. 81.8 kg;
   B. 6544 units;
   C. 14.7 mL/h; *solution:*

$$\frac{\text{mL}}{\text{h}} = \frac{250 \text{ mL}}{25000 \text{ units}} \times \frac{18 \text{ units}}{1 \text{ kg}} \times \frac{81.8 \text{ kg}}{\text{h}}$$

$$= 14.7 \text{ mL / h}$$

107. A. 10.1 mL/h; *solution:*

$$\frac{\text{mL}}{\text{h}} = \frac{1 \text{ mL}}{100 \text{ unit}} \times \frac{18 \text{ unit}}{1 \text{ kg}} \times \frac{1 \text{ kg}}{2.2 \text{ lb}} \times \frac{123 \text{ lb}}{\text{h}}$$

$$= 10.1 \text{ mL / h}$$

   B. 2236.4 units; 11.2 mL/h
108. A. 11.3 mL/h;
   B. 2520 units; 12.6 mL/h
109. A. 25.2 mL/h;
   B. 21 mL/h
110. A. 39 mg; *solution:* (0.25 mg × 65 kg) + (0.35 mg × 65 kg) = 39 mg
   B. 10 mL/h
111. 7.6 mL/h (NOTE: both mcg and mg measurements are provided. Use the mcg measurement when calculating dosage.); *solution:*

$$\frac{\text{mL}}{\text{h}} = \frac{1 \text{ mL}}{1000 \text{ mcg}} \times \frac{2 \text{ mcg}}{1 \text{ kg}} \times \frac{63 \text{ kg}}{1 \text{ min}}$$

$$\times \frac{60 \text{ min}}{1 \text{ h}} = 7.6 \text{ mL / h}$$

112. A. 23.4 mL/h (NOTE: both mcg and mg measurements are provided. Use the mcg measurement when calculating dosage.)
   B. 32.8 mL/h
113. 16.7 mL/h (NOTE: no conversion factors are needed.)
114. 75 mL/h
115. 33 mL/h
116. 10.4 mL/h; *solution:*

$$\frac{\text{mL}}{\text{h}} = \frac{250 \text{ mL}}{500 \text{ mg}} \times \frac{1 \text{ mg}}{1000 \text{ mcg}} \times \frac{5 \text{ mcg}}{1 \text{ kg}} \times \frac{1 \text{ kg}}{2.2 \text{ lb}}$$

$$\times \frac{152 \text{ lb}}{1 \text{ min}} \times \frac{60 \text{ min}}{\text{h}} = 10.4 \text{ mL / h}$$

117. 14.3 mL/h
118. 11.1 mL/h
119. 11.3 mL/h
120. 8 mL/h
121. A. 4 mg/min; *solution:*

$$\frac{\text{mg}}{\text{min}} = \frac{1000 \text{ mg}}{1 \text{ g}} \times \frac{2 \text{ g}}{250 \text{ mL}} \times \frac{30 \text{ mL}}{1 \text{ h}} \times \frac{1 \text{ h}}{60 \text{ min}}$$

$$= \frac{4 \text{ mg}}{\text{min}}$$

   B. 30 mL/h. (NOTE: The flow rate is already provided in the question.)
122. A. 3 mcg/kg/min per rounding rule; *solution:*

$$\frac{\text{mcg}}{\text{kg / min}} = \frac{1000 \text{ mcg}}{1 \text{ mg}} \times \frac{100 \text{ mg}}{250 \text{ mL}} \times \frac{29 \text{ mL}}{1 \text{ h}}$$

$$\times \frac{1 \text{ h}}{60 \text{ min}} \times \frac{2.2 \text{ lb}}{1 \text{ kg}} \times \frac{1}{143 \text{ lb}}$$

(NOTE: calculate for mcg/kg/min)
   B. 29 mL/h

CHAPTER 12: FLUID VOLUME AND ELECTROLYTES

1. d
2. f
3. b
4. e
5. a
6. c
7. b
8. a
9. c
10. d
11. a. Oral potassium supplements can be irritating to the stomach and should be taken with at least 8 ounces of fluid and/or with a meal. The client is correct in that the tablet should not be chewed.
12. d. IV potassium must be given using a rate-controlling device and cannot be allowed to run freely. In many hospitals, the nurse does not prepare this medication, and it is either mixed in

the pharmacy or comes prepackaged from the manufacturer. IV potassium is never given as a bolus (IVP).

13. d. Potassium is very irritating to the vein. If the site has become reddened and swollen, the IV should be discontinued immediately and another IV site should be started. The rest of the potassium is then infused. If another peripheral IV access is not possible, the health care provider should be contacted for possible central venous access.

14. b, c. Hyperkalemia can cause cardiac dysrhythmia, such as tachycardia. Other clinical manifestations of hyperkalemia include paresthesia to the face, tongue, and extremities; gastrointestinal hyperactivity (nausea, vomiting, and abdominal cramps), and acidosis may be present. Client with hyperkalemia will most likely have hyperglycemia, not hypoglycemia.

15. d. Administering sodium bicarbonate intravenously (IV) (50 mEq/L) as a one-time dose may help temporarily by driving potassium back into the cell. A client with hyperkalemia will most likely have hypermagnesemia. Saline will not help move the potassium back into the cell. $D_{10}W$ is high in glucose, and glucose pulls the potassium out of the cell which will worsen hyperkalemia.

16. a, b, d, e. A client who is taking a potassium supplement orally should be taught the signs and symptoms of both hypo- and hyperkalemia and when to notify the health care provider. Since there is a narrow range for potassium level, the client should anticipate routine blood work to evaluate if the potassium level is in the expected range. Because potassium is irritating, the supplement should be taken with a meal or a full glass of liquid and the client should remain upright for a minimum of 30 minutes to prevent esophagitis.

17. b. Normal serum osmolality (isoosmolar) is 275 to 295 mOsm/kg. Levels below 275 mOsm/kg is considered hypoosmolar. Levels greater than 295 mOsm/kg is considered hyperosmolar.

18. c. 285 mOsm/kg is normal (isoosmolar). Levels below 275 mOsm/kg is considered hypoosmolar. Levels greater than 295 mOsm/kg is considered hyperosmolar. There is no such thing as neoosmolar.

19. b. 3% saline is considered hypertonic solution. Any solution that is greater than 0.9% sodium chloride is considered hypertonic. Hypotonic fluid has less than 0.9% saline, such as 0.45% sodium chloride.

20. b. Around 80-90% of potassium is excreted in the urine. 8% is excreted in feces.

21. a, c. A client with pancreatitis will most likely have hypocalcemia due to calcium shifting into cells and hypomagnesemia.

22. b. Vitamin D helps the absorption of calcium from the small intestine, primarily in the ileum. Products in the large intestine are waste. Kidneys do help with resorbing calcium, but not with the help of vitamin D. Liver does not absorb calcium.

23. b. The majority of calcium is located in bones and teeth. Of the remaining calcium, 50% is bound to protein. The other 50% is circulating free (ionized calcium) to assist with cellular functions.

24. b. D_5W and $D_51/2NS$ are considered crystalloids. Crystalloids help maintain and/or temporarily correct hydration; they cause early plasma expansion. They do not contain proteins. Colloids contain protein, lipids, and/or carbohydrates and are given to increase serum osmolality; they are also called plasma expanders. Examples of colloids are albumin, and dextran. Lipids are fats and are considered colloids. Parenteral nutrition is intravenous nutrition containing protein, fats, and many minerals and electrolytes and are considered colloids.

25. b. $D_51/2NS$ is considered to be hypertonic solution. But, once it is in the body, it becomes hypotonic since the body metabolizes the glucose rather quickly, leaving free water and 0.45% saline.

26. a. Dextran is a colloid (volume expander) made from glucose. It is given to persons with major burns to temporarily restore circulating volume. No other drugs, including blood, should be infused in the same line as dextran.

27. a. Plasma has similar electrolyte content as lactated ringers.

28. c, d, e. This client is hypokalemic. Early signs of hypokalemia usually do not occur until serum K^+ level falls below 3.0 mEq/L and may include muscle weakness, anorexia, nausea, and vomiting. Untreated hypokalemia can lead to cardiac arrest and death.

29. a. Decreased magnesium (hypomagnesemia) is associated with hypocalcemia. Other electrolyte imbalance associated with low magnesium is hypokalemia.

30. a. A potassium level of 3.2 mEq/L is considered hypokalemia and may require a supplement. Potassium supplements are taken over an extended period and not just a few days. Hypokalemia is rarely caused by inadequate intake. This response is also accusatory and is not therapeutic. Gastrointestinal (GI) losses attributable to vomiting and diarrhea may lead to hypokalemia; constipation will not.

31. c. A sodium level of 150 mEq/L is considered hypernatremia. The normal range for serum sodium is 125–135 mEq/L. All other electrolytes are in normal range.

32. a, d, e. gastrointestinal (GI) disturbances, such as abdominal cramps; paresthesias of the face, hands,

and feet; and arrhythmias are commonly seen with hyperkalemia.

33. c, d, e. Insulin moves the potassium back into the cells while exogenous glucose maintains serum glucose level. Sodium polystyrene sulfonate binds with potassium, then it is excreted in feces while sorbitol maintains serum glucose level. Sodium bicarbonate shifts potassium intracellularly while calcium gluconate decreases myocardial irritability.

34. a, b, e. This client is hypocalcemic. Signs of hypocalcemia include anxiety, irritability, tetany, seizures, hyperactive deep tendon reflexes, and carpopedal spasms.

Case Study

1. D.M. is in hemorrhagic shock from massive blood loss as indicated by the vital signs. Stab wounds to the chest and abdomen can penetrate vital organs, causing large blood loss and risk of death. The priority assessment for this client is homeostasis, which includes circulation and airway. Circulation and airway are always a priority. During a systematic assessment of the client, two large-bore IVs (14 or 16 gauge) should be established in large veins to replace fluids rapidly. Another option is to assist the health care provider in placing a central line for rapid fluid resuscitation with colloids and crystalloids.

2. The client needs to be resuscitated with blood and blood products (colloids) and crystalloids.

3. Whole blood may be more beneficial for this client because it contains all the components (plasma, platelets, and RBCs); however, uncrossmatched packed red blood cells (PRBCs) may be easier to obtain in the emergent setting of trauma. Volume can be expanded using volume expanders.

CHAPTER 13: VITAMIN AND MINERAL REPLACEMENT

1. a
2. b
3. b
4. a
5. a
6. a
7. a
8. a
9. b
10. b
11. a
12. d
13. c
14. e
15. a
16. b

17.

ChooseMyPlate.gov

18. d. Vitamin D is needed to regulate calcium and phosphorous. It is also necessary for calcium absorption from the small intestines. Vitamin A is essential for bone growth and maintenance of epithelial cells. Vitamin B_{12} is essential for DNA synthesis, conversion of folic acid to its active form, and maintenance of the integrity of the nervous system, among others. Vitamin C is absorbed in the small intestine and aids in the absorption of iron and conversion of folic acid.

19. c. Vitamin K is needed to help the blood to clot. Newborns are vitamin K–deficient at birth, and it is a common practice in the United States to administer a one-time dose of vitamin K to prevent hemorrhagic disease of the newborn, which can present up to 6 months after birth.

20. c. Vitamin E has antioxidant properties to protect red blood cells from hemolysis and cellular components from being oxidized. Vitamin A is aids in the formation of the visual pigment needed for night vision, bone growth/development, and promoting integrity of the epithelial cells. Vitamin D is needed to regulate calcium and phosphorous. It is also necessary for calcium absorption from the small intestines. Vitamin K is needed for synthesis of prothrombin and various clotting factors.

21. a. Folic acid is very important during the first trimester of pregnancy to prevent neural tube defects such as anencephaly or spina bifida. All women who may become pregnant should be encouraged to take folate 400 mcg/day, since frequently a woman does not know she is pregnant until well into the first trimester. Multivitamin with iron should be taken *during* pregnancy according to the RDA recommendations.

22. c. Iron is essential for hemoglobin (Hgb) regeneration. Bleeding decreases the number of Hgb and vitamin A can assist in increasing Hgb. Chromium

is needed for proper metabolism for carbohydrate, lipid, and other essential nutrients. Copper is needed for formation of red blood cells (RBCs), not hemoglobin regeneration. Selenium is needed for protection from oxidative damage and infection, among other functions.

23. b. Vitamin B_1 is also known as *thiamine*. Thiamine deficiency is evident in Wernicke encephalopathy, which, if left untreated, leads to Wernicke-Korsakoff syndrome and irreversible brain damage. Thiamine should be administered before dextrose. Vitamin B_6 deficiency can also be seen in alcohol abusers but does not necessarily create the above symptoms.

24. a. Vitamin C is a water-soluble vitamin that is needed for collagen synthesis, aiding in absorption of iron, and assisting in converting folic acid to its active form. Vitamin D, a fat-soluble vitamin, helps in absorption of calcium. Iron, a mineral, is needed for hemoglobin regeneration. Zinc, a mineral, is important for growth, appetite, and skin integrity, among others.

25. c. Antacids will decrease the absorption of iron from the intestines. It do not help each other do its job. Iron must be taken daily, not every other day. Iron does not decrease the effectiveness of the antacids; instead, antacids decrease the absorption of iron.

26. d. Liquid iron can discolor teeth; therefore, taking liquid iron through a straw can decrease the discoloration.

27. b. Vitamin A deficiency can be seen in clients with biliary and pancreatic disorders. Celiac disease damages the lining of the intestine and impairs absorption of vitamin A.

28. b. Vitamin A, a fat-soluble vitamin, is excreted in urine and feces.

29. a, b, c, d. Vitamin A is a fat-soluble vitamin and is stored in the liver. Toxicity can occur. Any dose changes should be discussed with the health care provider before changes are made. Symptoms of hypervitaminosis A include nausea, vomiting, anorexia, lethargy, peeling skin, hair loss, and abdominal pain. Alcohol ingestion will decrease the absorption of vitamin A.

30. b. Pyridoxine or vitamin B_6 might be considered beneficial for a client with neuritis from INH therapy. Signs and symptoms of neuritis include numbness, tingling, "pins and needles" feeling, and difficulty gripping an object. Niacin can be used to alleviate Pellagra and elevated cholesterol. Riboflavin can be used for dermatologic disorders. Thiamine for persons with Wernicke-Korsakoff syndrome with central nervous system disorder. Wernicke-Korsakoff syndrome is usually associated with alcoholism, not due to drug therapy.

31. d. Clients who are receiving parenteral nutrition (PN) are at risk for zinc deficiency. Zinc will also be crucial for this client for wound repair and tissue healing. With continued PN, deficiencies of copper and iron can also occur.

32. c. Chromium is needed for metabolizing carbohydrate, fats, and nucleic acid. It might help normalize glucose in those with type 2 diabetes. Vitamin E has been used for Alzheimer disease. Vitamin C has been used to treat the "common cold." Vitamin B3, niacin, might be useful for Raynaud's phenomenon.

33. d. Shellfish is rich in copper. Other foods with rich copper include liver, nuts, seeds, legumes, and cocoa. Broccoli is rich in vitamin K. Grapefruit would be high in vitamin C. Lamb is rich in zinc.

34. d. Vitamin K is needed for synthesis of prothrombin and the clotting factors VII, IX, and X. Vitamin K_1 (phytonadione) is the only form that is available to treat an overdose of an oral anticoagulant.

Case Study

1. Vitamin A is a fat-soluble vitamin necessary for bone growth and for maintenance of epithelial tissues, eyes, and hair and has antioxidant properties. Excessive dosages can be toxic, causing alopecia, anorexia, abdominal pain, lethargy, nausea, and vomiting. Vitamin C is a water-soluble vitamin absorbed from the small intestine. Vitamin C helps absorb iron, assists in carbohydrate metabolism, and is involved in collagen, protein, and lipid syntheses. Toxicity from vitamin C is rare since excess dosages are excreted unchanged by the kidneys. Too much vitamin C can cause GI upset. Vitamin E is a fat-soluble vitamin with antioxidant properties, protecting the red blood cells from hemolysis. Excessive amounts of vitamin E may include fatigue, weakness, nausea, GI upset, headache, bleeding, and breast tenderness. Vitamin E may prolong the prothrombin time (PT). Clients on warfarin and vitamin E should have their PT monitored closely.

2. Vitamins C and D and certain foods can affect warfarin. Vitamin C has an antagonistic effect to oral anticoagulants; on the other hand, vitamin D has a synergistic effect. Vitamin K increases the synthesis of prothrombin, which is necessary for clotting. Vitamin K promotes clotting and is used as an antidote for warfarin. Foods high in vitamin K include dark green leafy vegetables, liver, cheese, egg yolk, and tomatoes. If consumed, the therapeutic effects of warfarin will decrease.

3. Advise client to consult with the health care provider if the client wants to continue taking vitamins and eating fresh fruits and vegetables. The dose of anticoagulant may need adjustment. Explain the potential effects of the vitamins to the anticoagulant; complications of the atrial fibrillation can occur. Explain to the client that a well-balanced diet usually negates the need for vitamin supplements. Educate on the signs and symptoms of hypervitaminosis. Also educate how certain vitamins and minerals can affect the therapeutic effects of warfarin.

1. metabolic processes
2. 50%
3. hydration; electrolyte
4. multidisciplinary team approach
5. PEG; surgically; endoscopically; radiologically
6. True
7. True
8. False. Parenteral nutrition is delivered IV and enteral nutrition is delivered into the GI system.
9. True
10.

Nasogastric   Nasoduodenal/nasojejunal   Gastrostomy   Jejunostomy

11. d. It is best used for ambulatory patients so that they are not connected to tubings.
12. a
13. b
14. c
15. a. The enteral nutrition of choice for a diabetic client is specialty formula for diabetes. It has modified macronutrient to promote glycemic control. Polymeric formula mimics macronutrients with fiber and used as supplements for persons without mal-absorptive disorders. Immune modulating formula is a specialty formula that contains pharmacologically active substances aimed at modulating the immune response for improved outcome. Modular formula contains single macronutrient (carbohydrates, protein, or lipids).
16. d. Enteral tube feeding is best if the client has a functioning GI system. However, a client who is at risk for aspiration needs enteral feeding that will deliver the food below the pyloric sphincter or below the stomach; enteral via jejunostomy is the best answer. Nasogastric tube is placed in the stomach which is above the pyloric sphincter. Parenteral nutrition is reserved for those whose GI system is not functioning.
17. d. Intermittent enteral feeding occurs over short time every 3-6 hours. It mimics when person usu-

ally eats. Bolus feeding is given usually in less than 15 minutes with a syringe. Enteral feedings can occur by gravity or by infusion pump.

18. b. Clients with burns have a higher calorie requirement than most other types of clients. In the acute phase, this is due to a hypermetabolic state. The client requires nutritional support to assist in wound healing. Total parenteral nutrition (TPN) would be an option; however, there is an increased risk of infection. The best response is cyclic tube feeding in which the nutrition is administered over 8–16 hours, allowing the client to be ambulatory and active during that time.

19. d. Because of the irritation to the veins from the high glucose content, TPN must be administered through a central venous line. Central lines are usually accessed through the subclavian vein or internal jugular vein. The brachiocephalic vein is used for peripherally inserted central catheter (PICC) for parenteral nutrition for short-term therapy (less than 4 weeks).
20. d. TPN provides 60-70% of carbohydrates. TPN provides 3.5-20% of protein and about 30% of fat.
21. b. Continuous enteral feedings occur over 24 hours. Enteral feedings over 30-60 minutes are considered intermittent feedings. Enteral feedings to be administered over 15 minutes are considered bolus feedings. Enteral feedings over 8-16 hours are considered cyclic feedings.
22. a, b. Diarrhea and constipation are a common side effect associated with enteral tube feedings due to multiple reasons. Other complications include dehydration and aspiration.
23. c. If a client is receiving continuous enteral nutrition, residuals should be checked every 2–4 hours. A residual greater than 150 mL indicates potential delay in gastric emptying. If the residual is more than 150 mL, stop the infusion for 30 minutes to 1 hour and then recheck. If the residual continues to be high, stop the feeding and contact the health

care provider. Some studies suggest withholding if greater than 500 mL. However, it is always prudent for the nurse to assess the client regarding the tolerance of enteral tube feeding.

24. a, c, d. Enteral nutrition is the preferred method if there is a functioning GI tract. It tends to be much less expensive than TPN and has a lower risk of infection, since TPN must be administered through central access. There is no risk of central line–associated bloodstream infection (CLABSI) from enteral feeding, because it is administered into the gastrointestinal tract. Enteral tube feeding has a risk of aspiration. Both enteral and parenteral can promote healing.

25. a, c, d. Complications associated with TPN include air embolism, hyperglycemia, and pneumothorax. Air embolism can occur when air enters the central line catheter. TPN consists of hypertonic dextrose solution which can increase serum glucose. Pneumothorax is air or gas in the pleural space causing the lungs to collapse. This can occur due to punctured lung during the procedure in inserting the central line. Aspiration can occur with enteral tube feeding, not because of TPN.

Case Study

1. Transitioning a client from TPN to enteral nutrition is common when a client has a long-term need for nutritional support. Certain steps must be followed for a successful and safe transition. The first step is to see if a client is ready for enteral feeding and how much the client will tolerate. This is accomplished by giving small amounts of feeding at a slow rate while the TPN rate is gradually reduced. TPN can be discontinued when the client is able to tolerate taking approximately 75% to 80% of of caloric needs by the enteral method. It is important to remember that a critically ill client may require between 3000 and 5000 calories/day.

2. A client who will require long-term enteral nutrition will likely require a gastrostomy tube. Before that time, the client may have received nutrition via a nasogastric or orogastric tube. Aspiration is a serious risk for those clients receiving tube feedings and may lead to aspiration pneumonia. Elevating the head of the bed between 30 and 45 degrees when possible may be beneficial. This is not an option if there is a question of spinal cord injury. The nurse should aspirate to check for residual before administering the next feeding and every 4 hours between feedings.

CHAPTER 15: ADRENERGIC AGONISTS AND ANTAGONISTS

1. c. Alpha$_1$ blocker causes vasodilation. Alpha$_2$ blocker causes vasoconstriction.
2. d. Beta blockers can decrease heart rate. Beta$_1$ affects the heart; whereas, Beta$_2$ affects bronchioles, uterus and glycogenolysis.
3. b. Has greater affinity for certain receptors

4. e. The sympatho*mimetic mimics* the sympathetic nervous system.
5. a. Blocks action of sympathetic nervous system
6. effector
7. adrenergic
8. do
9. sympatholytics
10. phentolamine mesylate
11. propanolol
12. Beta blocker; many drugs can cause depression. Beta blockers should not be abruptly discontinued.
13. nonselective
14. asthma; chronic obstructive pulmonary disease (COPD)
15. The adrenergic blocker will be an antagonist which would negate the therapeutic actions of the adrenergic agonist.
16. d
17. a, c
18. a
19. a
20. b
21. d
22. c
23. d
24. b
25. b. Although albuterol will increase the client's heart rate, this may cause a feeling of nervousness and not an ease of breathing. It has no effect on urinary output. Albuterol causes smooth muscle dilation, not constriction or contraction. Bronchodilation and relaxation of smooth muscles will improve air flow into the lungs.
26. a. Ensuring a patent airway is the first step in providing care to any client. There is no indication currently for an electrocardiogram. Although epinephrine is beneficial in allergic reactions, 1 mg of 1:1000 exceeds the subcutaneous dosage. Establishing an IV would not be the first action to take.
27. d. Although all pieces of information are important, the nurse should ask the client how many puffs of the inhaler were taken to determine that the client did not overdose on the drug. Other side effects of albuterol, besides shaking and trembling, include sweating, nausea, headaches, blurred vision, and flushing.
28. b, c, e. Albuterol is a beta agonist and amphetamine is a sympathomimetic.
29. c. Dopamine is a vasopressor (adrenergic agonist) that acts on alpha$_1$- and beta$_1$-receptor sites. Dopamine can cause tissue necrosis. Phentolamine mesylate is an adrenergic antagonist and is an antidote to stop further tissue necrosis. Dobutamine and epinephrine are also adrenergic agonists that can cause tissue necrosis. Although reserpine is an adrenergic neuron antagonist, it is used to treat hypertension.
30. a, b, c. Carvedilol is an adrenergic blocker. The other three drugs are adrenergic agonists. Adrenergic agonists are contraindicated in narrow-angle glaucoma.
31. b. Many OTC drugs, such as nasal decongestion, contain pseudoephedrine, which is a sympathomimetic; they can worsen hypertension.

32. b. Dopamine acts primarily on dopaminergic receptors and are located in renal, mesenteric, coronary, and cerebral arteries. These dopaminergic receptors can only be activated by dopamine. When these receptors are stimulated, vasodilation and increased blood flow occur, which can increase renal flow.

33. c, e. Beta$_1$ receptors are primarily located in the heart and in the kidney.

34. a. St John's wort can decrease the hypotensive effects of reserpine.

35. b. The proper dosage for timolol is initially 10 mg b.i.d., with a maximum dose of 60 mg/day. The above-ordered dose is 10 times the initial starting dose.

36. a. Catecholamines are substances that can produce a sympathomimetic response. Endogenous catecholamines include epinephrine, norepinephrine, and dopamine. Exogenous catecholamines are isoproterenol and dobutamine.

Case Study

1. An epinephrine auto-injector contains epinephrine, which is a naturally occurring catecholamine useful in the treatment of allergic reactions and anaphylaxis. It acts on both alpha and beta receptors and promotes CNS and cardiac stimulation and bronchodilation. It also decreases mucous congestion by inhibiting histamine release. Although epinephrine can be used for a variety of processes, including cardiac arrest and hypotension, an epinephrine auto-injector is used specifically for allergic and anaphylactic reactions and must be used at the first indication of difficulty breathing, hoarseness, hives, itching, or swelling of the lips and tongue.

2. The epinephrine auto-injector must be stored in a cool, dark place, and the solution must be clear and without particles. It is crucial that the client appreciate and understand that the drug must always be available.

3. Proper use of an epinephrine auto-injector includes pressing the device firmly against the outer thigh and holding the device in place for 5–10 seconds. The injection must be delivered into the subcutaneous tissue. Massage the area for 10 seconds to promote absorption and decrease vasoconstriction.

CHAPTER 16: CHOLINERGIC AGONISTS AND ANTAGONISTS

1. c
2. e
3. g. Also known as acetycholinesterase inhibitors
4. d
5. h
6. a
7. b
8. f. Direct-acting acts like cholinergic agonists. Indirect-acting acts like cholinesterase inhibitors.
9.

b Eye (constrict pupil)

c Lungs (constrict bronchioles and increase secretions)

d Heart (decrease heart rate)

e Blood vessel (dilates)

PARASYMPATHETIC

a.2. Ganglion

a.1. Spinal cord

f Gastrointestinal tract (increase peristalsis and secretions)

g Bladder (contract)

h Salivary gland (increase salivation)

10. d. Pralidoxime chloride is an anticholinergic that inhibits the actions of acetylcholine. It is given for cholinesterase inhibitor toxicity and oragnophosphate pesticide toxicity. Bethanechol is a direct-acting cholinergic agonist and is used to treat urinary retention. Metoclopramide, a direct-acting cholinergic agonist, is used to treat gastrointestinal (GI) symptoms.

11. a. Bethanechol, a direct-acting cholinergic agonist, is used to treat urinary retention. Metoclopramide, a direct-acting cholinergic agonist, is used to treat gastrointestinal (GI) symptoms. Neostigmine bromide is used to treat myasthenia gravis.

12. b. Anticholinergics inhibit the acetylcholine receptors and include muscarinic and nicotinic receptors. Anticholinergic eyedrops causes dilated pupils (mydriasis). Cholinergic agonists will constrict pupils. Direct-acting cholinergic agonists will decrease intraocular pressure.

13. c. Anticholinergic drugs are contraindicated in a client with glaucoma because they increase the intraocular pressure. Therefore, the nurse should hold the drug and contact the prescriber.

14. b. Bethanechol is a direct-acting cholinergic agonist. Agonists promote tissue response.

15. c. Bethanechol, a direct-acting cholinergic agonist, works on the muscarinic receptor. Nicotinic receptors work on skeletal muscles. Anticholinergics inhibits muscarinic and nicotinic receptor.

16. c. Bethanechol, a direct-acting cholinergic agonists stimulates the muscarinic receptors to contract bladder which increases urination.

17. a, c. Cholinergic drugs are parasympathomimetics in that they mimic the parasympathetic responses. One response is the dilation of blood vessels, which decreases blood pressure. Other responses include pupillary constriction (miosis), bronchoconstriction and increased bronchial secretions, decreased heart rate, increased gastrointestinal peristalsis and secretions, bladder contraction, and increased salivation.

18. d. Bethanechol is used to treat urinary retention but will not be effective and should not be used in the case of a mechanical obstruction. If this client was prescribed bethanechol for urinary retention and the urine output is decreasing, the health care provider should be notified to investigate another cause.

19. d. Bethanechol is a cholinergic agonist. The client is experiencing an adverse response, and the treatment of choice is atropine. The nurse should obtain an order to administer atropine, the antidote for cholinergic overdose. The nurse should document the client's experiences, but it is not the best action by the nurse. Abdominal cramps is due the action on the muscarinic receptors, not due to constipation. Increasing fluid intake will not relieve the side effects of bethanechol.

20. c. Neostigmine bromide is used to *treat* myasthenia gravis (MG). Bethanechol is used to treat urinary retention. Pilocarpine is used to treat glaucoma.

21. a, b. Atropine would be beneficial as a preoperative drug to help control oral secretions. It is also used for clients who are symptomatic with a heart rate less than 50 beats per minute and is symptomatic of decreased cardiac output. Bethanechol is for urinary retention. Benztropine is for paralytic ileus. Propantheline bromide is used for gastric ulcers.

22. d. Atropine-like drugs should not be administered to clients with narrow-angle glaucoma because they will increase the intraocular pressure.

23. c. Because of the decrease in gastrointestinal motility that can be associated with propantheline, the client should be encouraged to eat foods that are high in fiber and drink adequate amounts of liquid to prevent constipation.

24. a, b, c, e. Hyoscyamine is an anticholinergic drug that will have similar side effects to the prototype drug atropine. Adequate fluid intake will help prevent constipation. Vision may be blurry, and the client should be advised not to drive until the effects of the drug on the vision are known. Sucking on hard candy or sugar-free ice pops, as well as increased fluid intake, may help with dry mouth. The client should be educated as to baseline heart rate and advised to report tachycardia (rates above 100 beats/minute) to the health care provider. Increased sweating is not a common side effect.

25. a, c, d. Anticholinergic drugs block the normal parasympathetic responses of the pupils, lungs, heart, blood vessels, gastrointestinal tract, bladder, and salivary glands. Therefore, anticholinergic drugs are contraindicated in clients with any heart disease and diabetes mellitus.

26. d. Anticholinergics, such as biperiden and benztropine, are used to treat early Parkinson. Anticholinest*erase,* not anticholinergics, are used to treat myasthenia gravis.

27. b, c, d, e. Common side effects of anticholinergic drugs, like benztropine, may include dry mouth, constipation, and urinary retention. Dizziness and hallucinations should be reported to the health care provider because these may become dangerous to the client. Because there is a decreased ability to perspire, life-threatening hyperthermia may develop. Palpitations may be due to tachycardia.

Case Study

1. Tolterodine tartrate blocks cholinergic receptors selectively in the bladder to decrease the incidence of incontinence.

2. The common side effects are those associated with other cholinergic drugs and may include dizziness, vertigo, dry mouth, nausea, vomiting, weight gain, and urinary retention. Adverse drug effects include angioedema, chest pain, and dementia.

3. Tolterodine is contraindicated in clients with glaucoma, gastric paresis, urinary retention, and in women who are breastfeeding.

4. Besides discussing side effects and adverse reactions with the client, H.H. should be encouraged to take the drug on an empty stomach since absorption is delayed with food. Grapefruit juice should also be avoided because it decreases drug levels. Before taking any other drugs, the health care provider should be consulted because this drug interacts with several other classes of drugs such as phenothiazines, macrolides, and antifungals.

CHAPTER 17: STIMULANTS

1. brain; spinal cord
2. dysregulation
3. norepinephrine; dopamine
4. stimulant; suppress appetite
5. analeptics
6. a, c, d. CNS stimulants, such as amphetamines, analeptics, and anorexiants, are approved to treat ADHD, narcolepsy, and PTSD.
7. a, b, c, d. Methylphenidate is a stimulant to treat ADHD and narcolepsy. Clients taking methylphenidate should not operate hazardous equipment when they experience tremors, nervousness, or increased heart rate; avoid other stimulants, such as caffeine; and that nervousness or tremors can occur. The drug should be taken before meals. Weight loss can occur, not weight gain.
8. b. Analeptics stimulate the brainstem and medulla to stimulate respiration. Anorexiants stimulate the satiety center in the hypothalamic and limbic areas of the brain. Amphetamines stimulate the cerebral cortex.
9. a, b, c, d, f. Methylphenidate can cause euphoria, headache, hypertension, irritability, and vomiting. Hypotension is an adverse effect, not a common side effect.
10. b. An immediate-release drug can be taken in 2 or 3 divided doses. An extended-release drug should be taken once daily.
11. a. Phentermine hydrochloride should not be taken within 14 days of monoamine oxidase inhibitors (MAOIs) such as selegiline. Combinations of the two drugs intensify the stimulation and vasopressor effects of phentermine that can cause severe cardiovascular and cerebrovascular responses. Therefore, the nurse should contact the health care provider to verify the prescription.
12. d. Phentermine-topiramate is used for short-term weight management.
13. b. The nurse should include that counseling should be obtained while on methylphenidate. Diarrhea, not constipation, is a common side effect. Methylphenidate is usually prescribed long term and should not be stopped abruptly. Weight loss, not gain, can occur.

14. a, b, e. Methylphenidate and MAOIs taken together can increase hypertensive crisis. Methylphenidate can increase the effects of anticoagulants. The effects of methylphenidate can be increased by caffeine.
15. c. Hemorrhagic stroke is the most likely diagnosis of those listed. There is a high risk for hemorrhagic stroke attributable to hypertensive crisis in clients taking appetite suppressants or anorexiants. Pregnancy-induced hypertension is a possibility, but the client has been trying to lose weight, not become pregnant. However, a pregnancy test should be obtained; anorexiants are contraindicated in pregnancy.
16. a, d, e. CNS stimulants are absolutely contraindicated in clients with coronary artery disease, hypertension, and liver failure. Cautious use is recommended for clients with any amount of liver disease.
17. a. Caffeine can stimulate the respiratory system to help the neonate breathe better. It will not cause the baby to gain weight and increase body's temperature.

Case Study

1. Methylphenidate is absorbed from the GI tract and is taken before breakfast and lunch. It should be given at least 6 hours before sleep since it can cause insomnia. Methylphenidates decrease hyperactivity and improve attention span.

2. The drug is a CNS stimulant that is used in conjunction with appropriate counseling for treatment of ADHD. The best time to give the drug is 30–45 minutes before meals, so the nurse will need to review the lunch schedules of the students and plan accordingly on how best to administer the drugs.

   Baseline height, weight, and vital signs should be obtained and monitored throughout the course of treatment. A record of the students' complete blood count, including a white blood cell count with differential and platelet count, should be on file. Routine vital signs should be assessed since these drugs can cause an elevation in heart rate and blood pressure, especially if taken in conjunction with caffeine. Clients should also be monitored for an increase in hyperactivity.

   Health teaching is important not only for the student but also for the family and the teachers on staff. The goals of these drugs are to increase focus and attention and decrease impulsiveness and hyperactivity. The student and family should be encouraged to eat three nutritious meals per day along with healthy snacks because anorexia may be a side effect. Dry mouth may also occur, and if possible within school policy, the student should be allowed to chew gum or suck on hard candy. The importance of avoiding caffeinated beverages and foods, including chocolate, sodas, and energy drinks, must be stressed because high plasma levels of caffeine can be fatal.

Drug administration at school must be handled with tact and ease. If possible, the school nurse's office should not be open and in the main hall where all other students can observe the comings and goings of the students requiring drug or care. Privacy is crucial.

CHAPTER 18: DEPRESSANTS

1. rapid
2. rapid
3. slow
4. rapid
5. rapid
6. rapid
7. sedative-hypnotics; general anesthetics; analgesics; opioid and nonopioid analgesics; anticonvulsants; antipsychotics; antidepressants
8. rapid eye movement; nonrapid eye movement
9. sedation
10. may
11. short
12. central nervous; pain; consciousness
13. surgical; analgesia; excitement or delirium; medullary paralysis
14. spinal
15. respiratory distress or failure
16. saddle block
17. are
18. short
19. zolpidem tartrate (also eszopiclone, zaleplon, and ramelteon)
20. flumazenil
21. esters; amides
22. d
23. f
24. e
25. a
26. b
27. c
28. c. Sedative-hypnotics are commonly prescribed to treat sleep disorders. Analeptics are CNS stimulants. Anesthetics are CNS depressants and are not prescribed for sleep. Triptans help with migraines.
29. b. Long-acting barbiturates, such as phenobarbital, are used to control seizures. Intermediate-acting barbiturates, such as butabarbital, use useful to sustain sleep. Short-acting, such as secobarbital, may be used for sedation. Ultra-short-acting barbiturates, such as methohexital sodium, are used for anesthesia induction.
30. c, d. Postdural-puncture headache can occur because of a decrease in pressure due to fluid leakage from the cerebrospinal space. Maintaining the client flat in bed for 24 to 48 hours and encouraging adequate oral fluid intake as tolerated may help prevent a spinal headache. The client may also require IV fluids to supplement oral intake.

31. c. By explaining the reason for positioning (either seated with an arched back or fetal position), the client will feel more control. The nurse can reassure the client that assistance in her maintaining the proper position will be provided.
32. d. Zolpidem may be ordered. It is a nonbenzodiazepine for short-term treatment of insomnia. Flumazenil is an antidote for benzodiazepine overdose. Phenobarbital, a long-acting barbiturate, is used to treat seizures. Triazolam is a benzodiazepine. While this class of drug can help with insomnia, a nonbenzodiazepine is a better choice.
33. d, e. Lidocaine is used for local and spinal anesthesia that has a rapid onset with its effects long-lasting.
34. a. Antihistamines, such as diphenhydramine, are the primary ingredient in over-the-counter sleep aids.
35. a, b, c, e. Older clients may have more problems with Stage 3 and Stage 4 nonrapid eye movement (NREM) sleep and awaken frequently. Establishing a bedtime routine, maintaining a schedule of going to bed and arising in the morning, and avoiding caffeine and alcohol at bedtime may help. Although it sounds intuitive to take naps, they may hinder a client from obtaining a good night's sleep if the naps last longer than 20–30 minutes. Diuretics should be taken in the morning and fluids should be limited at bedtime to prevent frequent trips to the bathroom, which may interrupt sleep.

Case Study

1. Benzodiazepines are frequently prescribed before surgery. They increase the action of the inhibitory neurotransmitter gamma-aminobutyric acid (GABA) to the GABA receptors and reduce the excitability of the neurons. Drugs such as alprazolam or lorazepam might be prescribed for anxiety.
2. Balanced anesthesia includes many parts leading up to surgery. By using a variety of agents, less general anesthetic is needed, fewer cardiovascular side effects occur, less nausea and vomiting occur, pain is decreased, and a quicker recovery is promoted. This is also true if utilizing a laparoscopic approach instead of an "open" approach to this surgery.

   The night before the surgery, a medication such as zolpidem might be prescribed to ensure a good night's sleep. After the client has arrived in the preoperative area and approximately 1 hour before surgery, a combination of an opioid or anxiolytic and an anticholinergic such as atropine might be given. The purpose of the anticholinergic is to decrease secretions, and therefore the risk of aspiration. Once the client is transferred to the operating room, a short-acting sedative such as pentothal, propofol, or etomidate may be given and the client will be given inhaled anesthetics. This procedure will require general anesthesia, so the client will also receive a muscle relaxant to facilitate endotracheal intubation and maintain neuromuscular blockade.

CHAPTER 19: ANTISEIZURE DRUGS

1. d
2. a
3. e
4. b
5. c
6. electroencephalogram (EEG)
7. idiopathic
8. generalized; partial
9. preventing; do not
10. are not
11. phenytoin
12. over-the-counter
13. intramuscular
14. a, b. Carbamazepine and diazepam are given for tonic-clonic seizures. Ethosuximide and acetazolamide are indicated for absence seizures.
15. b. Although it is important to know the client's medical history regarding seizures, the best response is asking about the drugs that have been prescribed. Most antiseizure drugs have teratogenic properties. Women with seizure history are at increased risk for seizures during pregnancy. The risk versus the benefits need to be discussed. Abruptly stopping antiseizure drugs can also increase the risk of seizures.
16. a, c, d. Hydantoins, such as fosphenytoin, barbiturates, such as phenobarbital, and benzodiazepines, such as diazepam or lorazepam are used for status epilepticus. Diazepam is the drug of choice. Carbamazepine and topiramate are indicated for tonic-clonic and partial seizures.
17. b. Phenytoin prevents sodium from entering the cells. This reduces the activities of cells. Antiseizure drugs inhibit neurotransmitters; they do not destroy them. Antiseizure drugs suppress entry of calcium; they do not increase the influx.
18. a, b, d. Valproic acid is taken in divided doses. Doses start at 10–15 mg/kg/day and increase to a maximum of 60/mg/kg/day until seizures are controlled. Frequent labs are needed to monitor serum levels and liver functions. Antiseizure drugs control the frequency and severity of seizures, it does not cure.
19. b, c, d. An absolute contraindication is heart block and bradycardia. Cautious use is recommended for clients with hypoglycemia and hypotension. Dilantin is excreted in small amounts in the urine. Urine output should be monitored afterward, but not hourly.
20. d. Intravenous phenytoin is irritating to the tissue, and the nurse should discontinue the IV and restart

the infusion at a different site. It is recommended that a central line or peripherally inserted central catheter (PICC) line be utilized when possible. The health care provider does not need to be notified immediately to change the medication to oral form. Continuing the infusion, even with a saline flush, may cause sloughing of the tissue.

21. a. Although a variety of antiseizures may be utilized over a client's lifetime, at this time, there is no cure for seizure disorders. The client will most likely need to take an antiseizure for one's lifetime.
22. b. 18 mcg/mL is within the therapeutic range of 10 to 20 mcg/mL for bound phenytoin and 1 to 2 mcg/mL for unbound/free drugs. 8 mcg/mL is below the therapeutic range and the client may be at risk for seizure. 28 and 38 mcg/mL are too high, drug toxicity can occur.
23. a, b, d, e. Documenting the types of movements (tonic/clonic), the duration of seizure activity, and the locations where the movements started and progressed are important pieces of gathering the history of the seizure event. It is important to know, if possible, what the client had been doing before the event and if the client reported any warning before the seizure. The client is unable to stop true seizure activity voluntarily.
24. c. Nosebleeds and sore throats may be a sign of blood dyscrasias and should be reported to the health care provider. A reddish pink discoloration of the urine may be expected. To prevent injury to the gums, a soft toothbrush should be utilized. Orthostatic hypotension is not associated with phenytoin use.
25. a. Gingival hyperplasia is a common side effect of phenytoin. Excessive thirst and weight gain are not common with phenytoin.
26. a. The first-line drug of choice for status epilepticus is diazepam. Midazolam, propofol, and high-dose phenobarbital are administered for continued seizures.
27. a, b, c. Up to 33% of women with history of seizures can have increased seizure activity during pregnancy. Many antiseizure drugs have teratogenic properties. Antiseizure drugs increase the excretion of folic acid; therefore, pregnant individuals should take daily folate supplement. Antiseizure drugs inhibit vitamin K, contributing to bleeding.
28. c. Valproic acid and topiramate are indicated for migraine. Diazepam can be used additionally to those with spasms, anxiety, and alcohol withdrawal. Clorazepate can be used for anxiety and alcohol withdrawal.

Case Study

1. Oxcarbazepine is taken by mouth with an initial dose of 300 mg twice daily. One of the benefits of this drug is that there are fewer adverse effects than

with carbamazepine and drug level monitoring is usually not necessary, which may be more convenient in the client's role of elementary school teacher. Client teaching is required for safe handling of the drug. As with other antiseizure medications in the iminostilbene family, dizziness, drowsiness, and ataxia can occur. The client needs to be instructed to closely monitor for any seizure activities since oxcarbazepine is indicated for partial seizures.

2. The nurse should tell the client that many antiseizure drugs have teratogenic properties that increase the risk for fetal malformations. Carbazepines have been known to cause fetal anomalies; whereas there is a decreased risk with oxcarbazepine. However, as with any drug, caution is advised in taking drugs while pregnant. If the client is contemplating pregnancy, then the client should consult with the health care provider to determine risk versus benefit.

CHAPTER 20: DRUGS FOR PARKINSON'S AND ALZHEIMER DISEASE

1. c
2. a
3. d
4. e
5. b
6. dopamine; acetylcholine
7. dopamine
8. levodopa
9. carbidopa
10. donepezil or rivastigmine
11. enhance
12. selegiline
13. carbidopa, levodopa, entacapone
14. trihexyphenidyl (also benztropine)
15. a. Dizziness is a common side effect of carbidopa-levodopa. Constipation is a side effect, not diarrhea. Anxiety and nasal stuffiness are not a side effect of carbidopa-levodopa.
16. b, c, d, e. Carbidopa-levodopa may make the client's movements smoother, although at high doses, dyskinesia may be noted. Jaundice will not result from missing doses. Extended release drugs should not be crushed or cut; if the client is unable to swallow tablets, then other preparations, such as liquid or oral disintegrating tablets, are available. Nausea and vomiting are side effects, so taking the drug with meals may be beneficial. There is no indication that carbidopa-levodopa affects glucose levels.
17. a, b, e. Tyramine rich foods should be avoided, such as, aged cheeses, chocolate, and yogurt. These foods should be avoided when taking selegiline to prevent a hypertensive crisis from occurring. Peanut butter and wheat bread are not high in tyramine.

18. d. An order for tricyclic antidepressant should be questioned. Tricyclic antidepressants decrease the effect of rivastigmine.
19. c. The nurse understand that levodopa only will be decreased. When taken with levodopa, COMT inhibitors like entacapone will increase the levodopa combination in the brain.
20. a. Anticholinergic drugs are contraindicated in persons with glaucoma. Extreme caution is warranted for persons with heart problems and those with urinary retention, not urinary frequency. Shingles and diabetes are not contraindications.
21. a, c. Even though most drugs for Parkinson disease can cause hallucinations, they are more common with bromocriptine and pramipexole.
22. c. Memantine is prescribed for the treatment of mild to severe Alzheimer disease. Increased wandering and hostility can indicate that the disease is progressing and an increase in the dose may be beneficial. The maximum dose for memantine is 20 mg per day.
23. a. Sucking on hard candy or chewing sugarless gum may help with dry mouth associated with anticholinergic drugs such as benztropine mesylate. This drug is initially taken at bedtime and twice per day in divided doses as a maintenance dose. The nurse should remind the client that all drug adjustments need to be made by the health care provider. Urinary retention is a side effect of anticholinergic drugs; however, the nurse should encourage the client to urinate when the urge is felt and not on a set schedule.

Case Study

1. Alzheimer disease is a progressive disease of cognitive decline, and the progression may occur over many years or decades. During the early stages of Alzheimer disease, symptoms are usually considered mild, and the client may start to show some signs of decreased ability to function in work or social settings and have problems with recall and memory. Anxiety may also be a component. As the disease progresses, J.T. may require more assistance with performing complex tasks, leading to the need for a higher level of assistance as the client needs reminders to bathe, lock doors, and turn off stoves, for example. Disorientation becomes more noticeable and the client may become tearful; this marks the beginning of early dementia. Later in the disease, the client needs assistance with activities of daily living and may have incontinence of urine and feces. Psychological disturbances such as paranoia, agitation, delusions, and violent behavior become more prominent. In late dementia, the client is unable to care for self and may make only sounds or speak a few words. Clients will eventually become comatose.

2. Rivastigmine is an acetylcholinesterase inhibitor (AChE) that is used in the treatment of mild to moderate Alzheimer disease. Rivastigmine in-

creases cognitive function by preventing the breakdown of acetylcholinesterase, which allows for more acetylcholine to be available as a transmitter.

3. Safety is a primary concern as J.T. moves into a new home with the family. As Alzheimer disease progresses, the client may begin to wander more and is at higher risk for falling. Removing obstacles from the J.T.'s path may help prevent falls, as will eliminating loose rugs and quickly cleaning up spills. Assuring adequate locks on outside doors may prevent the client from wandering outside unattended; however, the client should be able to have an escape route from the house as needed. Door alarms are also available. Covers may be placed over dials for the burners on a stove. These are like those utilized for preventing young children from adjusting the burners. The family will need additional resources and support, as caring for a someone with Alzheimer disease is a full-time job. Organizations such as the Alzheimer's Association can provide direction.

CHAPTER 21: DRUGS FOR NEUROMUSCULAR DISORDERS AND MUSCLE SPASMS

1. b
2. d
3. a
4. c
5. traumatic; debilitating disorders
6. hyperactive; antiinflammatory
7. decrease; increase
8. Myasthenia gravis is an autoimmune disorder that involves an antibody response against acetylcholine receptor (AChR) sites, eventually destroying the receptor sites for acetylcholine (Ach). Drugs used to treat myasthenia gravis (MG) are the acetylcholinesterase (AChE) inhibitors (cholinesterase inhibitors and anticholinesterase), such as neostigmine or pyridostigmine. They inhibit the action of AChE, which allows more activation of the cholinergic receptors.
9. Multiple sclerosis (MS) is an autoimmune disorder that attacks the myelin sheath of the nerve fibers of the central nervous system, resulting in plaques. Drugs used to treat MS include corticosteroids and immunomodulators, such as teriflunomide, alemtuzumab, and glatiramer acetate.
10. b. Pyridostigmine increases muscle strength in clients with myasthenia gravis. Increased salivation and miosis are signs and symptoms of overdose. Bradycardia, not tachycardia can be an adverse drug effect.
11. b. Drooling, excessive tearing, sweating, and miosis are signs of a cholinergic crisis, an overdose of AChE inhibitors.
12. a. Atropine is the antidote for AChE inhibitor.

13. c. Multiple sclerosis is difficult to diagnose. MRI, assessing brain's electrical activity, or analysis of cerebrospinal fluid can aide in confirming the diagnosis.
14. d. There is an increased toxicity when taken with tetracycline.
15. c. Azathioprine is an immunosuppressant and interferon-β is an immunomodulators. Both decrease the inflammatory process of the nerve fibers. Interferon-β delays neurological deterioration. Decreased inflammation and delaying of deterioration will decrease spasticity and hopefully muscular movement will improve. They do not form new neurons and axons nor will they stop the progression of the disease, but they can delay the deterioration.
16. b. Centrally acting muscle relaxant, such as baclofen, has actions to the neuronal activities in the brain and spinal cord. They suppress hyperreflexia and muscle spasms that do not respond to other forms of therapy. By suppressing the spasms, pain is decreased, which allows increased movement.
17. a, c. Centrally acting muscle relaxants, such as methocarbamol, can cause drowsiness and change the color of the urine. Other side effects include dizziness, lightheadedness, headaches, altered taste, and anorexia, not increased appetite.
18. b. Diazepam can increase intraocular pressure and is contraindicated in narrow-angle glaucoma.

Case Study

1. Clients with spinal cord injuries may have spasticity attributable to hyperexcitability of neurons caused by increased stimulation from the cerebral neurons or lack of inhibition in the spinal cord or at the skeletal muscles.
2. Carisoprodol is a centrally acting muscle relaxant and is utilized for muscle spasms. Baclofen is used specifically for muscle spasticity, either caused by trauma or resulting from multiple sclerosis.
3. Side effects of these drugs include drowsiness, dizziness, nausea, and hypotension. They should not be taken with other central nervous system depressants or alcohol. Baclofen can be used for an extended period without developing tolerance. It does not have abuse potential. Carisoprodol is now a Schedule IV drug and has the potential for abuse.

CHAPTER 22: ANTIPSYCHOTICS AND ANXIOLYTICS

1. e
2. d
3. f
4. g
5. a
6. h
7. b

8. c
9. thought processes; behaviors; dopamine
10. dihydroindolones; thioxanthenes; butyrophenones; dibenzoxazepines
11. drowsiness
12. pruritus; photosensitivity
13. decrease
14. are not
15. tolerance
16. sedative-hypnotics
17. c
18. a
19. a
20. b
21. b
22. c
23. c. Neuroleptics are considered antipsychotics that modify psychotic behaviors and exert antipsychotic effects. Anxiolytics treat anxiety and insomnia. Antidepressives treat depressive disorders; antipsychotics worsen depression.
24. b. The nurse should inform the client that antipsychotic drugs can take 3 to 6 weeks before full therapeutic effects occur. While psychotherapy may help, it is not required for antipsychotics to have therapeutic effects. While the onset may be minutes to hours, its full therapeutic effect does occur until weeks later.
25. b. Orthostatic hypotension may occur with phenothiazines and nonphenothiazine drugs within this class. The client should be encouraged to change positions slowly to prevent orthostatic hypotension. Clients should abstain from alcohol while on antipsychotics, it can worsen drowsiness, dizziness, and hypotension. Any antipsychotics should not be abruptly stopped.
26. d. Pseudoparkinsonism, major side effect of typical antipsychotics, are symptoms similar to Parkinson disease. Shuffling gait is one example of EPS. Other EPS include masklike facies, rigidity, tremors at rest (not intentional tremors), pill-rolling, motions of the hands, and bradykinesia.
27. a. Benztropine, an anticholinergic antiparkinson drug. Bethanechol is an antispasmodic for urinary retention. Buspirone is an anxiolytic. Doxepin is an antidepressant.
28. b. Fluphenazine belongs to the piperazine subclass of phenothiazines. Chlorpromazine is an aliphatic phenothiazine. Thioridazine is a piperidine. Thioxanthene is a nonphenothiazine.
29. c, d, e. There are numerous side effects associated with fluphenazine, including dizziness, headache, and nausea; the client should be encouraged to notify the prescriber if any of these symptoms occur. The drug is to be taken daily. Alcohol should not be consumed while on any antipsychotics. Either hypo- or hypertension may be an indication of an adverse reaction. Although it may be safe to take some herbal medications while taking fluphenazine, taking kava kava can increase dystonic reactions.
30. c. Because of less effective hepatic and renal function, doses of antipsychotics should be decreased by 25% to 50% in older clients.
31. d. Overdose on phenothiazines can cause respiratory compromise. Maintaining a patent airway is a priority. Once airway is patent, then establishing an IV, administering activated charcoal and anticholinergics may be necessary.
32. a. Haloperidol has a sedative effect on clients. Haloperidol is contraindicated in clients with liver dysfunction. In older adults, the dosage may need to be decreased. Like other neuroleptics, it can cause extrapyramidal syndrome.
33. c. Atypical antipsychotics, such as risperidone and clozapine block serotonin and dopaminergic receptors. Butyrophenones, phenothiazines, and thioxanthenes are typical antipsychotic drugs.
34. c. D_2 antagonists can cause EPS. Atypical antipsychotics have a weak affinity to these receptors, thus decreasing the amount and severity of EPS.
35. d. Atypical antipsychotics have a strong affinity for D_4 and they block serotonin receptors.
36. b. Hyperglycemia is a side effect of taking risperidone. Blood glucose levels should be obtained at baseline and monitored carefully.
37. b. Alprazolam is a benzodiazepine. Benzodiazepines are used for severe or prolonged anxiety.
38. a, b, c, d. Clients with glaucoma, liver damage, subcortical brain damage, and any continued blood dyscrasia should not take fluphenazine.
39. a, b, d, e. Lorazepam is a frequently prescribed anxiolytic and is also indicated for clients with alcohol withdrawal, anxiety with depression, preoperative induction (lessen anxiety), and status epilepticus.

Case Study

1. Clonazepam is a benzodiazepine that is in the same family as diazepam and alprazolam. It is used for anxiety associated with depression and seizures.
2. Benzodiazepines enhance the action of gamma-aminobutyric acid (GABA), an inhibitory neurotransmitter. It has a rapid mechanism of action and is readily absorbed from the gastrointestinal tract.
3. Side effects include drowsiness, dizziness, and coma if taken in large doses. The action of benzodiazepines is potentiated when taken with alcohol.
4. H.K. may have taken an overdose. A respiratory rate of 8 breaths/minute and an O_2 saturation of 78% require immediate action by the nurse. Maintaining an airway is the priority intervention. Oxygen should be administered, and an airway adjunct should be inserted. Her ventilations should be assisted with a bag-mask and high-flow oxygen until her airway can be secured. An IV will need to be established and flumazenil, a benzodiazepine

antagonist, administered. Flumazenil acts very quickly but is only effective for benzodiazepine overdoses. An emetic is not an option for this client because she is unresponsive. Gastric lavage is the intervention of choice. Blood pressure may need to be supported with IV vasopressors.

CHAPTER 23: ANTIDEPRESSANTS AND MOOD STABILIZERS

1. False. Herbal supplements, such as St. John's wort decrease reuptake of the neurotransmitters, such as serotonin, norepinephrine, and dopamine.
2. True
3. False. Serotonin modulators, such as selective serotonin reuptake inhibitors (SSRIs) and serotonin norepinephrine reuptake inhibitors (SNRIs) are considered first-line therapy for depression. MAOIs are used for clients who do not respond to tricyclic antidepressants.
4. False. Amitriptyline is a tricyclic antidepressant (TCA).
5. True
6. 2 to 4 weeks
7. increase; increase; decrease
8. St. John's wort
9. second-generation antidepressants; dopamine, norepinephrine, serotonin
10. stimulate; central nervous system
11. Lithium; bipolar affective
12. narrow; 0.8 to 1 mEq/L
13. increase; caffeine; loop; decrease
14. generalized anxiety disorder, and social anxiety disorder
15. grapefruit juice; toxicity
16. b, c
17. c
18. b, c
19. b, c
20. c
21. b, c
22. a, b, c
23. a
24. a
25. b
26. d
27. c
28. b
29. c. Imipramine, a tricyclic antidepressant (TCA) is also indicated for enuresis, involuntary urination while sleeping.
30. d. The maximum daily dose of phenelzine is 90 mg. The initial dose is 15 mg/day in three divided doses.
31. b. Orthostatic hypotension is a frequent side effect of tricyclic antidepressants (TCAs). The client should be encouraged to change positions slowly to avoid this side effect. Amitriptyline can cause

tachycardia, not bradycardia. The onset of amitriptyline is 1-3 weeks, not 12 hours. Since amitriptyline has an anticholinergic action, it should be taken at night, not during the day.
32. a, b, e. Foods high in tyramine, such as bananas, chocolate, and wine are contraindicated in a client who is taking a monoamine oxidase inhibitor (MAOI), such as isocarboxazid. Other foods that are high in tyramine include aged cheeses, processed meats, and soybeans or soy products. These foods have sympathomimetic-like effects and can cause hypertensive crisis.
33. d. St. John's wort is a common herbal remedy for depression. St. John's wort, when taken in combination with selective serotonin reuptake inhibitor (SSRI) drugs, such as fluoxetine, can precipitate serotonin syndrome, which presents as headache, sweating, and agitation. Ephedra and ginseng can cause palpitations, heart attack, and hypertensive crisis when taken with MAOIs, not SSRIs.
34. c. SSRIs has less sedative effect. They also do not cause hypotension, anticholinergic effects, or cardiotoxicity. However, SSRIs can cause sexual dysfunction.
35. c. Monitoring the client is one of the most important roles of the nurse. Trending vital signs, weight, and lab work will be important to the client's ongoing care. The client needs to maintain a fluid intake of 2–3 L of fluid/day initially and must be especially vigilant to maintain an adequate intake in hot weather. Clients during manic phase frequently stop taking their drug when they feel better. They must be advised to continue taking the drug even if they feel better.
36. a. Monitoring hepatic and renal function in a client taking lithium should be completed with weekly blood work, which includes BUN and creatinine level measurements.
37. b. The client's lithium level is still subtherapeutic, and he remains in a manic phase. Therapeutic range for lithium is 0.8 to 1.2 mEq/L.
38. a. The client needs further education requiring the purpose of the drug. Lithium may be used in bipolar disorder as a mood stabilizer, but its effect is on the manic phase. The drug should be taken with food. Tyramine rich foods, such as caffeine should be avoided.
39. d. Venlafaxine is a serotonin-norepinephrine reuptake inhibitor (SNRI). Side effects of venlafaxine may include drowsiness, insomnia, photosensitivity, and ejaculatory dysfunction, among others. Taking St. John's wort while taking venlafaxine increases the risk of serotonin syndrome or neuroleptic malignant syndrome.
40. a, d. Some studies have linked lithium to a congenital anomaly involving the tricuspid valve of the heart if taken during the first trimester of pregnancy.

Case Study

1. SSRIs block the reuptake of the neurotransmitter serotonin at the nerve terminal. One of the possible causes of depression is a lack of circulating serotonin. By preventing the reuptake, more serotonin is available and depression is lessened. SSRIs may be effective in the treatment of depression in cases where the client was nonresponsive to a TCA. Additional benefits of SSRIs are prevention of migraine headaches.

2. In the initial interview, the nurse should inquire about medical history, prescription and OTC drugs, allergies, and past coping behavior. The nurse should directly ask the client about suicidal thoughts. The use of herbal products should also be investigated. A thorough psychiatric history should be obtained with a specific focus on past episodes of depression and treatments. Vital signs should be obtained as well as weight. Baseline laboratory work should be reviewed, since fluoxetine should be used with caution in clients with a history of renal or liver problems.

3. Discharge teaching should include recommendations for counseling, since studies have shown that drug and counseling together are more successful than either modality alone. Support groups have also shown benefit. The nurse should teach the client to take fluoxetine as prescribed and inform the client that it may take 2–4 weeks for the onset of action. Alcohol should be avoided while taking SSRIs. Fluoxetine should be taken with food. Dry mouth may be a side effect that can be relieved somewhat with sucking on hard candy or chewing gum. If the client feels suicidal at any time, she should contact the health care provider or suicide hotline or go to the emergency department immediately. Even though SSRIs can have additional benefits in the prevention of migraine headache, it can precipitate headache. F.K. is postmenopausal. She needs to be taught that sexual dysfunction can increase.

CHAPTER 24: ANTIINFLAMMATORIES

1. d
2. c
3. e
4. h
5. b
6. a
7. f
8. g
9. i
10. injury; infection
11. redness (erythema); swelling (edema); heat; pain; loss of function
12. delayed
13. does
14. higher (or increased)
15. arthritic
16. d. The vascular phase of the inflammation is associated with vasodilation and increased vascular permeability. This allows leukocyte and other substances to filter into the inflamed tissue.

17. a, c, d, e. Heartburn can be a side effect of NSAIDs. Taking NSAIDs with food may help decrease heartburn. Dark, tarry, or bloody bowel movements are an indication of GI bleeding, which is an adverse effect of NSAID use. The dosage range for NSAIDs varies from drug to drug, but large doses may cause erosive esophagitis, which would cause indigestion-type pain. There are many types of heartburn, including those associated with acute myocardial infarction. Not all heartburn is of GI origin attributable to a drug effect.

18. b. NSAIDs inhibit the production of prostaglandin, thereby, decreasing inflammation and pain. Ibuprofen is not a COX-2 inhibitor. Ibuprofen does not bind to opiate receptor sites and it does not promote vasodilation.

19. a. Warfarin is an anticoagulant that may be taken by clients with atrial fibrillation. Aspirin displaces warfarin from its protein-binding site. This increases the anticoagulant effect and may lead to excessive bleeding, which may initially be indicated by bruising. Although the other drugs may have drug-drug interactions, they do not cause increased anticoagulant effects, as evidenced by the bruising.

20. d. Aspirin should not be given to young children due to the risk of Reye syndrome, which can be fatal. Hypersensitivity reactions, such as ringing in the ears can occur in any person, but it is not the most concerning. Side effects, such as GI distress can occur in anyone taking NSAIDs, but it is not the most concerning.

21. c. Sulfasalazine, a salicylate derivative, can cause bronchospasms in a client with asthma; therefore, its use is contraindicated to those with known sensitivity.

22. a. Ibuprofen is a propionic acid derivative, which has a decreased risk of GI disturbances. Ibuprofen should be taken with food. It has a short half-life and is highly protein bound. There are many drug-drug interactions. Ibuprofen can increase bleed time when taken with warfarin. When taken with aspirin, the effects of the ibuprofen are decreased.

23. b. Since ibuprofen is excreted in the urine, adequate fluid intake and urine output should be maintained. Ibuprofen can have negative consequences during early pregnancy and is contraindicated during third trimester. It can cause GI upset and diarrhea.

24. c. Piroxicam has a long half-life (50 hours). Because of its long half-life, it is taken once daily. Like other NSAIDs, it can cause GI irritation. It

has many drug-drug interactions, and its onset is delayed.

25. a. Colchicine inhibits the migration of leukocytes to the inflamed area; thereby decreasing inflammation. Colchicine does not inhibit the synthesis of uric acid nor does it block the reabsorption or remove uric acid. Colchicine does not block the release of prostaglandins.

26. b. Probenecid is used for the inhibition of the reabsorption of uric acid in the kidneys; thereby, increasing the excretion. Its primary action is not the retention of urate crystals. Ureters are tubes for the pathway of urine; it is not the primary action of probenecid.

27. a. Etanercept neutralizes tumor necrosis factor (TNF). This neutralizing alters the inflammatory process. Anakinra, not etanercept, inhibits IL-1 from binding to interleukin receptors found in bones and cartilages. Celecoxib inhibits COX-2 receptors to alter the inflammatory process. Uricosurics, such as probenecid, blocks the reabsorption of uric acid.

28. c. Steroids should be tapered over 5-10 days.

29. a, c, d. Corticosteroids may be used for a variety of disease processes including flare-ups of arthritic conditions. They have a long half-life and are usually taken once a day in a large prescribed dose and then the dose is tapered for 5–10 days. Lengthy corticosteroid therapy is never stopped abruptly. They may be given in combination with other drugs including prostaglandin inhibitors.

30. b, c, d, e. Fluid intake should be increased to promote uric acid excretion. Avoiding alcohol is important because alcohol causes an overproduction, as well as an underexcretion, of uric acid. Purine is required to synthesize uric acid. Taking the drug with food will help avoid GI upset. Some studies have shown that vitamin C may help increase uric acid elimination; however, large doses of supplemental vitamin C are not recommended, and since vitamin C is an acid, there is a higher risk of kidney stone formation.

31. d. Although side effects of infliximab may include headache, dizziness, cough, nausea, and vomiting, an adverse reaction to the drug is severe infection attributable to immunosuppression. A fever of 101.9° F in an adult who is taking infliximab needs to be evaluated.

Case Study

1. The normal therapeutic dosage is 325–650 mg q4h as needed, up to a maximum of 4 g/day. If the client takes 975 mg every 4 hours as stated, this client will be taking 5850 mg/day, which exceeds the maximum daily dose.

2. Side effects may include anorexia, nausea, vomiting, dizziness, abdominal pain, and heartburn.

3. Signs of overdose or adverse reactions include tinnitus, GI bleeding, blood dyscrasias including thrombocytopenia and leukopenia, and liver failure.

4. The client appears to be hypotensive, tachycardic, and tachypneic. These vital signs could be indicative of a hypovolemic state, potentially attributable to a GI bleed. Interpretation of the vital signs is compounded because of the use of caffeine with the aspirin. Metabolic acidosis due to aspirin overdose can also cause tachypnea.

CHAPTER 25: ANALGESICS

1. gate, nociceptors
2. endorphins
3. peripheral, prostaglandins
4. increased
5. c
6. f
7. e
8. a
9. b
10. d
11. central nervous system; peripheral nervous system
12. respiration; coughing
13. antitussive; antidiarrheal
14. head injury; respiratory depression (shock and hypotension are also acceptable answers)
15. side effect; health care provider
16. IV
17. c
18. b
19. e
20. a
21. f
22. g
23. d
24. a. A major side effect of meperidine is decreased blood pressure (hypotension). All opioids have the potential to decrease (not increase) pulse rate, respiratory rate, and urine output.
25. c. Opioid toxicity will cause pinpoint pupils, not dilation. Respiratory depression, nausea, vomiting, constipation, and urinary retention can also occur with opioid overdose.
26. b. Monitoring fluid intake is the least important. The nurse should monitor bowel sounds to identify constipation, a common side effect of opioids. The client's pain should be frequently assessed using a pain scale. The nurse should assess vital signs, noting rate and depth of respirations for future comparisons; opioids commonly decrease respirations and systolic blood pressure.
27. b, c, d, e. There are no dietary restrictions associated with the use of opioids. The client should not exceed the recommended dosage. Adequate fluid intake and inclusion of fiber in the diet will assist with constipation. Clients should always be taught the side effects to report.

28. d. Drugs with long duration of action (long half-life) are more beneficial to clients dealing with chronic pain. If chronic pain needs treatment, nonopioid drugs are preferred over opioids. If opioids are used, in addition to long duration of action, they should be oral or transdermal formulation, not injectable.

29. b. An opioid antagonist is naloxone. Flumazenil is an antagonist to benzodiazepines. Butorphanol and pentazocine are opioid agonist-antagonists.

30. b. Opioid agonist-antagonists may be used to decrease substance use disorder. Opioid agonist-antagonist can cause renal failure and respiratory depression. There is still a potential to cause dependence. They are indicated for acute moderate to severe pain.

31. b. Withdrawal symptoms attributable to physical dependence can result 24 to 48 hours after the last opioid dose and include irritability, diaphoresis, restlessness, muscle twitching, tachycardia, and hypertension.

32. c. Controlled-released morphine has 8-12 hours of pain relief. Other types of morphine have a duration of action of 3-6 hours.

33. b, d, e. The best people to assess how a child is acting are those who are with the child the most. Ask the parents or other caregivers how the child usually acts due to pain. Utilizing developmentally appropriate communication skills and pain scales should yield the best result for the nurse treating a child's pain. Opioids are appropriate to utilize if nonopioid methods are ineffective.

34. b. Cholestyramine will decrease the effectiveness of acetaminophen. An alternative nonopioid would be an option for the client instead of stopping the cholestyramine.

35. d. A priority assessment for a client taking opioid agonist-antagonist is respiratory depression. While opioids can cause constipation and dysuria, they are not a priority over respiratory system. A client effectively managed on opioids will have hypotension, not hypertension.

36. b. The best action by the nurse is to administer the dose and contact the health care provider. Dose should be withheld for respiratory rate 10 and below, not 12. Since the client is not in respiratory distress, the dose should not be withheld due to inadequate pain relief. The dose should be given, then contact the health care provider.

37. c. The dose may be too high for the client. Older adults should use a lower dose fentanyl transdermal patch to avoid severe side effects. Side effects from the use of opioids are more pronounced in older adults. The rates of metabolism and excretion of drugs are decreased; thereby, drug accumulation may occur.

38. c. Alcohol must be avoided while taking opioid pain medications. Alcohol can intensify the CNS effect of the opioid. The client should take the drug as prescribed and should avoid other drugs, including over the counters, that contain NSAIDs. Opioids can cause constipation and laxatives may be warranted.

39. c. Ketorolac is used for short-term pain management and should not be taken for more than 5 days.

40. a, b, d. Nonopioid pain drugs, such as acetaminophen, ibuprofen, and aspirin are appropriate for minor injuries such as abrasions and minor aches and pains. Some nonopioids, such as aspirin and ibuprofen, have antiinflammatory effects that can further lessen pain and swelling. But, aspirin also has an antiplatelet effect and should not be taken concomitantly with other antiplatelets or anticoagulants. Hydrocodone and morphine are opioids and should not be taken for mild pain.

Case Study

1. Migraines are caused by neurovascular events in the brain causing neuronal hyperexcitability in the cerebral cortex. The exact cause is unknown, but specific factors that trigger a migraine headache include foods with monosodium glutamate and aspartame, fatigue, stress, missed meals, odors, light, and hormone changes, among others.

2. Two types of migraines include migraine with an aura and migraine without an aura. Migraine headaches, with or without an aura, are characterized by a unilateral throbbing headache accompanied with nausea, vomiting, and photophobia. Migraines are more common in women. Cluster headaches are also unilateral, but nonthrobbing pain behind the eyes and they are not associated with an aura. Cluster headaches are more common in men.

3. Treatment may include analgesics, beta-adrenergic blockers, anticonvulsants, and tricyclic antidepressants. Other treatments include ergot alkaloids and selective serotonin$_1$ receptor agonists (triptans). The triptans, 5-HT receptor agonists (i.e., sumatriptan, naratriptan, zolmitriptan), should be taken as early as possible during a migraine to be effective. All triptans are contraindicated if the client has coronary artery disease, uncontrolled hypertension, cerebrovascular disease, and peripheral vascular disease.

CHAPTER 26: ANTIBACTERIALS

Penicillins and Cephalosporins

1. f
2. b
3. g
4. e
5. a
6. h
7. c
8. d
9. i
10. d. Superinfection is a secondary infection caused by the disturbance of the normal microbial flora

during antibiotic therapy. Common signs and symptoms of superinfection include vaginal itching and discharge due to fungal overgrowth. While poor hygiene can cause infection, the client has been taking antibiotics. It is less likely the infection is due to poor hygiene. Hypersensitivity reactions usually include rash and difficulty breathing, not infection. Kidney infection is usually exhibited with dysuria and hematuria, not vaginal itching.

11. a. The nurse will teach the client that ceftriaxone is given via IM or IV. It is not given orally. About 10% of population who has hypersensitivity to penicillin has cross-reaction to cephalosporin, such as ceftriaxone. Ceftriaxone, when taken concomitantly with anticoagulants, increases risk of bleeding. Ceftriaxone can increase liver enzymes and international normalized ratio (INR).

12. b. Cefprozil monohydrate is given for skin infections. The usual dosage range for adults is 250 to 500 mg/d, with a maximum dose of 1 g/d. Clients with CrCl <30 mL/min, adjust dose by half; therefore, the maximum dose would be 500 mg/d.

13. c. The appropriate dose for aztreonam would be 1500 mg q8h. The range for an adult dose is 1 to 2 g q8h to q12h, with a maximum dose of 8 g/d. The amount and frequency of drugs should be considered to obtain therapeutic response and a steady state. 500 mg q8h is too low of a dose to achieve therapeutic response. 500 mg q6h is too low of a dose. 2000 mg daily will result in low serum level.

14. c. Loop diuretics, such as furosemide, can cause nephrotoxicity when taken concomitantly with ceftriaxone. Other class of drugs that can cause nephrotoxicity include intravenous calcium salts. ACE-I, antidysrhythmics, and NSAIDs are not implicated in causing nephrotoxicity when taken with ceftriaxone.

15. a. Loss of appetite, diarrhea, nausea, and vomiting are common side effects of cephalosporins, such as ceftriaxone. These side effects could cause weight loss. The nurse should encourage the client that when the antibiotic is completed, appetite will resume, and weight loss will stop. It is possible that GI bleeding can occur, but the client is concerned about weight loss, not bleeding. Ceftriaxone is administered IM or IV, not orally; therefore absorption problem is not a concern. It is possible the client will begin to eat more and regain weight as her illness is cured; however, the antibiotic is what is causing the side effects, not the illness.

16. b. Acidic fruits or juices, such as orange juice, may make dicloxacillin less effective. Abdominal pain is a possible side effect. The entire course of antibiotics must be completed to prevent the development of resistance. Rashes can be associated with dicloxacillin but may also be an indication of an allergic reaction. The client would need to be evaluated for other indications of an allergic reaction, such as difficulty breathing or hives.

17. d. Uricosurics, such as probenecid, compete for renal tubular clearance which can decrease the excretion of cefotetan. Intravenous calcium salts are contraindicated when taking some cephalosporin; they can deposit crystals in the lungs and kidneys. They do not increase serum levels of cefotetan. Laxatives do not increase levels of cephalosporins. Opioid solutions that contain alcohol can have a disulfiram-like reactions if coadministered with cefotetan; it does not increase the serum levels of cefotetan.

18. b. Penicillin's beta-lactam ring structure inhibits bacterial cell-wall synthesis. Penicillins, including penicillin V, can be both bacteriostatic and bactericidal. Amphotericin B and polymyxin alter membrane permeability. Aminoglycosides and tetracyclines are some drugs that inhibit protein synthesis. Sulfonamides and trimethoprim are some antibiotics that interferes with cellular metabolism.

19. c. Antibiotics, especially penicillins, may make oral contraceptives less effective, so an alternate method of birth control should be utilized. The client does not need to increase dietary calcium or stop fexofenadine. While some antibiotics can increase photosensitivity, wearing sunscreen at all times is not necessary. Sunscreens should be worn when being exposed to sun is likely.

20. a, c, d. Ideally, culture and sensitivity should be obtained before starting antibiotics. Allergic reactions are a possibility with any antibiotic. Because cephalosporins are eliminated in the urine, monitoring for adequate urine output is important. Ceftazidime is administered q8-12h, not daily. Fluid intake is encouraged since the drug is excreted in urine.

21. c. Caution is advised in administering amoxicillin to clients with asthma. Use in pediatric clients and diabetic clients are not contraindicated. Amoxicillin is generally safe during pregnancy.

22. c. A dose of IR 750 mg every 8 hours would be too much. The standard dose for adults is 250–500 mg q8h for immediate release or 500 mg q12h for extended release.

Macrolides, Oxazolidinones, Lincosamides, Glycopeptides, Ketolides, Tetracyclines, and Glycylcyclines

1. b
2. e
3. a
4. c
5. a
6. d
7. a
8. a. Common side effect of doxycycline is gastrointestinal distress, which includes nausea, vomiting, and diarrhea. These side effects could cause a decrease in serum potassium due to potassium loss. Serum calcium, platelets, and hemoglobin/hematocrit are not commonly affected.

9. c, d, e. Doxycycline should be taken with meals or milk for improved absorption. There are no restrictions regarding eggs.

10. a, b, c, e. Outdated drugs of any kind should be discarded; however, tetracycline will break down into toxic by-products so it must be assured it is discarded. Superinfections, which occur when normal bacteria are destroyed, are common with the use of antibiotics. Tetracycline should not be taken during the first and third trimesters of pregnancy because of possible teratogenic effects. Tetracycline increases photosensitivity and sunscreen should be used when exposed to sun or limit sun exposure. Tetracycline does not cause urinary urgency.

11. a, b, c, e. Iron, which is found in prenatal vitamins and antacids prevent absorption of doxycycline. Studies have shown that the effects of warfarin may be increased by taking doxycycline, placing the client at higher risk for bleeding. Cautious use should be exercised in a client taking doxycycline and a proton pump inhibitor like omeprazole. There are no known interactions with doxycycline and morphine.

12. b, c, d, e. Drugs in the tetracycline family should be stored away from light to prevent breakdown. Cautious use is recommended in clients with renal and/or liver disease. Baseline levels should be assessed and reevaluated as needed. Because of mutations within the strains of various sexually transmitted infections, a culture and sensitivity should be obtained before starting treatment. It is also possible that various sexually transmitted infections could be present at the same time, and it would be beneficial to the client if the most effective antibiotic is prescribed for each. Tetracyclines may make oral contraceptives less effective, so additional contraceptive use is recommended.

13. c. Aminoglycosides, such as gentamicin, can cause tinnitus, ringing of the ears. Tinnitus is a high-pitch sound due to damage to cranial nerve VIII. Other side effects are pruritus and muscle cramps. Tinnitus is not related to allergy or gender.

14. c. The best action by the nurse is to contact the health care provider. Vancomycin is nephrotoxic, and a decrease in urine output can be an early indication of renal damage. Decreasing renal function is also a part of normal aging, putting an older adult client at higher risk for renal failure. While increasing fluids (orally and intravenously) can improve renal output, it is not the best action. Every assessments, such as decreased urine output, should be documented, but it is not the best answer.

15. c. Conjunctivitis is a possible side effect of azithromycin. If this occurs, the client should not wear contact lenses. Photosensitivity is not a side effect of this drug. Taking azithromycin with food may help prevent nausea. If a headache occurs as a side effect, drugs such as ibuprofen or acetaminophen are not contraindicated.

16. a. Life-threatening infection caused by vancomycin-resistant *Enterococcus faecium* (VREF) is appropriate to use quinupristin-dalfopristin, a combination drug containing two streptogramin antibacterials. Other bacteria the drug is appropriate for includes *Staphylococcus aureus* and *Streptococcus pyogenes*.

Aminoglycosides, Fluoroquinolones, and Lipopeptides

1. aminoglycoside
2. children
3. loop diuretics or methoxyflurane
4. DNA gyrase; DNA
5. increase
6. a
7. b
8. a
9. b
10. c
11. a
12. a. Levofloxacin dosing is daily, not twice daily. All other fluoroquinolone dosings are appropriate.

13. b, e. Ototoxicity is a serious adverse effect of gentamicin. Elevated renal function tests may indicate a decrease in renal function, which increases the risk of nephrotoxicity. Nausea, headache, and photosensitivity may be side effects; however, they are usually not considered serious.

14. b. Peak blood levels are drawn 45–60 minutes after a drug has been administered. Gentamicin is administered intravenously over 30 to 60 minutes. Therefore, peak drug level should be checked at 10:00 am or 10:00 pm. Gentamicin will still be infusing at 9:15 am and 9:15 pm. 10:30 pm is over 60 minutes after drug has completed infusing.

15. b. The correct trough level for gentamicin is less than 1 to 2 mcg/mL. The health care provider should be contacted before administering the dose because it is elevated, which can cause an adverse reaction such as nephrotoxicity. The drug should not be administered because of high trough level. Diphenhydramine can decrease risk of reaction, but the client is not having a reaction; instead the trough level indicates toxicity.

16. c. Superinfection or secondary infection, such as vaginitis, can occur resulting from antibacterial therapy. The client could have been exposed to other infectious agents, but since the client has been on antibiotics, a superinfection is most likely. An allergic reaction is a hypersensitivity and would most likely manifest itself as rash, swelling, or respiratory difficulty. A drug-drug interaction is not able to be determined since the client is on one drug.

17. a, b, c. Because gentamicin can cause hepatotoxicity, liver enzymes (AST and ALT) need to be monitored for signs of liver failure. Gentamicin can also be nephrotoxic; therefore measurement of

the characteristics of urine is necessary. Ototoxicity can occur with gentamicin, causing hearing loss. Gentamicin usually does not affect vision.

18. b. A trough of 5.9 mcg/mL is usually achieved by the third dose. The units are in mcg/mL, not mg/mL.

Sulfonamides and Nitroimidazoles

1. folic acid
2. penicillin
3. trimethoprim
4. are not
5. is not
6. liver; kidneys
7. bacteriostatic
8. increases
9. b
10. b
11. a
12. d. Silver sulfadiazine and mafenide are sulfonamides that are available in cream form to treat burns. Sulfadiazine is used for prophylactic treatment in clients with rheumatic fever. Sulfasalazine is used to treat irritable bowel disease, such as ulcerative colitis. Sulfacetamide sodium is for ophthalmic disorders.
13. b, c, d, e. TMP-SMZ is contraindicated while breastfeeding. It is possible that there is cross-sensitivity between sulfonamides, so it is important to determine if the client is allergic to any other antibiotics. There are a variety of etiologies for kidney stones; however, crystallization of the urine may occur with sulfonamides, which can lead to kidney stone formation. Some clients are more prone to kidney stones than others. TMP-SMZ has a variety of interactions with several drugs, including warfarin, oral hypoglycemic agents, ACE inhibitors, digoxin, phenytoin, and potassium-sparing diuretics.
14. a, b, c, d. To prevent crystallization in the urine, fluids should be encouraged. Urine output should be carefully monitored since this medication is excreted in the urine. Undesired side effects are possible and include abdominal pain, nausea, vomiting, diarrhea, and anorexia. A desired effect of TMP-SMZ will be resolution of the bronchitis as evidenced by decreased coughing and clear lung sounds.
15. b. The usual adult dose of TMP-SMZ is 160 mg TMP/800 mg SMZ every 12 hr. Its half-life is 6 to 12 hrs; thus must be administered twice a day.
16. c. Sulfonamides are not obtained from biological sources. They are bacteriostatic and depending on the dose, can be bacteriostatic. They are effective against bacteria, not viruses and fungi.
17. d. Insomnia is a common side effect from TMP-SMZ. Other side effects include anorexia, nausea, vomiting, diarrhea, depression, and headache, among others. Confusion, constipation, and fever are not common.

18. a. The maintenance dose for sulfasalazine is 500 mg every 6 hours, with a maximum dose of 4 g/day. While 1000 mg every 6 hours are within the maximum dose, it is not the best answer. 1250 mg/d and 1500 mg/d are too small of a dose.

Case Study

1. TMP-SMZ is a sulfonamide that is bacteriostatic. Trimethoprim and sulfamethoxazole inhibit the bacterial synthesis of folic acid, which is required for bacterial growth. The standard oral dosage is 160 mg of TMP/800 mg of SMZ q12h.
2. Client and/or caregiver teaching will include the need for adequate fluid intake to maintain a urine output of more than 600 mL/d to prevent crystalluria. The drug should be taken on an empty stomach. The nurse will educate on the potential side effects of anorexia, nausea, vomiting, diarrhea, and abdominal pain. Other side effects include headache, fatigue, vertigo, and insomnia. The client should be advised to ask for help when getting out of bed or ambulating because of the potential for vertigo and risk of falling. Other plan of care instructions includes teaching to monitor for any rash or bruises, and if observed to notify the provider. TMP-SMZ can increase the effects of warfarin. The blood glucose level should be monitored more closely because of increased risk for hypoglycemia.
3. The nurse will need to be aware of the potential for increased effects of anticoagulation, such as bruising and bleeding, because of the interaction between warfarin and TMP-SMZ. There is also a potential for increased hypoglycemic effects of glyburide. The nurse will need to carefully monitor lab work, including BUN and creatinine levels for renal function as well as liver panel (AST, ALT, ALP). The nurse will also need to monitor for life-threatening adverse effects, including electrolyte imbalances (hyperkalemia, hyponatremia, hypoglycemia), seizures, angioedema, anemias, leukopenia, pseudomembranous colitis, and Stevens-Johnson syndrome (erythema multiforme major). Stevens-Johnson syndrome is characterized by fever, malaise, joint pain, and skin lesions. Severe cases can be life-threatening and may require intensive care hospitalization and the use of immunoglobulins.

CHAPTER 27: ANTITUBERCULARS, ANTIFUNGALS, AND ANTIVIRALS

1. acid-fast, tuberculosis
2. do not
3. speak, sneeze, cough; inhale
4. latent tuberculosis infection
5. kidney, liver; renal or hepatic disorders, alcoholism, diabetic retinopathy, severe hypersensitivity

to pyrazinamide or ethionamide, concurrent MAOI therapy

6. is not (Psychotic behavior is an adverse effect and isoniazid should be discontinued should it occur.)
7. Combination
8. vitamin B_6 (pyridoxine)
9. isoniazid (INH), 9
10. a
11. a
12. a
13. b
14. a
15. b
16. b
17. b
18. a
19. opportunistic
20. histamine-mediated
21. cold sores, genital herpes
22. shingles, dermatome
23. A, B
24. does not
25. B, C
26. b. Other life-threatening effects include blood dyscrasias, seizures, and exfoliative dermatitis.
27. b. Alcoholism is a contraindication for treating tuberculosis with isoniazid. Alcohol ingestion with this drug can increase the incidence of peripheral neuropathy and hepatotoxicity.
28. c. Rifapentine has a long half-life. To minimize drug toxicity but maintain therapeutic level, the drug must be taken twice per week with a minimum interval between doses of 72 hours.
29. a, b, d. Side effects can occur 1 to 3 hours after starting amphotericin B infusion. Side effects include chills, flushing, fever, nausea, vomiting, headache, dyspnea, and tachypnea. To alleviate side effects, diphenhydramine, acetaminophen, and hydrocortisone can be administered 30 to 60 minutes before administering amphotericin B.
30. d. Ribavirin is labeled to treat hepatitis C virus. Acyclovir is given for herpes virus, amphotericin B is an antifungal, and zanamivir is for influenza.
31. b, c, d. It will be important to obtain a history of drugs taken and drug allergies before starting treatment. A history of tuberculosis (TB) exposure and the results and dates of most recent purified protein derivative (PPD) and chest x-rays will also be important information. Blood glucose level is not pertinent in this client; important baseline laboratory values include monitoring liver and renal functions.
32. b. The initial dose is 5 mg/kg/d or over 5 days/week. Other regimen is 15 mg/kg given up to 3 days/week. Maximum dose is 900 mg/day.
33. c. INH can be hepatotoxic; therefore, liver functions must be monitored on a regular basis. Hepatic disease is a contraindication for INH. Clients on

INH should be taught adverse drug effects, including abdominal pain, yellowing of skin/eyes, and clay colored stool. INH is metabolized, not excreted, by the liver. INH has not been implicated in causing liver cancer.

34. c. Antacids should not be taken at the same time as INH. Antacids decrease the absorption of INH.
35. a, b. Vitamin B_6 supplements or increased intake may be necessary to prevent peripheral neuropathy. Alcohol should be avoided since INH can be hepatotoxic. Rifampin, not INH, may turn body fluids brownish-orange.
36. b. Combination therapy is more effective in eradicating TB infection than any single drug.
37. b. The nurse will administer amphotericin B intravenously since it is not absorbed from the GI tract. Because of its risk of toxicity, close monitoring is needed while administering the drug.
38. b. The standard dose range is 0.25–1.5 mg/kg/day. The drug should be further diluted and infused intravenously slowly via an in-line filter while monitoring for side effects, such as fever, chills, flushing, nausea, and vomiting. The drug must be protected from light.
39. c. Amphotericin B is given only via intravenous, and side effects include flushing, nausea, vomiting, hypotension, and chills. The client does not need to be NPO before receiving a dose of amphotericin B, and it may in fact be beneficial to have a light, nongreasy meal or even some crackers to help decrease the nausea. Amphotericin B is nephrotoxic, so any changes in urination should be reported immediately to the health care provider.
40. a, c, d, e. Client should be instructed to maintain hydration and it can be taken at mealtime. Acyclovir can cause orthostatic hypotension and client should be instructed to change or stand up slowly. Client should report decreased urination, dizziness, or confusion. The client should abstain from sexual intercourse or use a barrier method, such as condoms, correctly and consistently. Use of spermicide does not prevent spread of infection.
41. a, b, c. Peginterferon can cause mild to serious side effects. Mild side effects such as flulike symptoms and myalgia can be treated with antiinflammatories. Other side effects are more serious; peginterferon can cause papilledema (which can lead to vision changes), pancytopenia (placing the client at risk for infection, so fever should be reported), and mood changes (which may indicate depression).
42. b. Each tablet has 100 mg. The dose is 150 mg. Therefore, client should take 1.5 tablets.
43. a, b, c, e. Laboratory values that assess hepatic and renal function should be obtained at baseline and trended. Fluconazole can cause hypokalemia. Prothrombin time (PT) may be altered if the client is taking warfarin.

Case Study

1. The nurse must complete a thorough assessment including questions regarding drugs currently taken, allergies, and vital signs. Specific questions regarding vaginal or anal itching should also be asked because nystatin can cause pruritus, urticaria, and rash.

2. Frequent use of antibiotics can destroy the normal flora in the body and cause an opportunistic infection to occur. This infection is likely thrush, which is caused by *Candida* species.

3. To correctly take nystatin, the client should put 4 to 6 mL in her mouth and swish for several minutes to coat the mucous membranes and the tongue. Nystatin should then be swallowed to treat the throat. If ordered, the client can spit out the nystatin.

CHAPTER 28: ANTIMALARIALS, ANTHELMINTICS, AND PEPTIDES

1. c
2. e
3. a
4. b
5. d
6. g
7. f
8. b. The most common site for helminths is the intestine. Person can be infected from soil containing helminths. Other sites include the vascular system and the liver; but they are not common sites.
9. c. Malaria is caused by multiple species of protozoan parasites that are carried by mosquitos and it remains one of the most prevalent protozoan diseases.
10. b. They are all antimicrobials, but chloroquine is a commonly prescribed drug for protozoans causing malaria. If drug resistance to chloroquine occurs, then other treatments can be used. Acyclovir and delavirdine are antivirals. Tobramycin is an antibacterial.
11. c, d, e, f. With the use of chloroquine, red blood cell count, hemoglobin, and hematocrit levels may be lowered. Liver enzymes such as AST may be elevated. Baseline laboratory values should be obtained and monitored.
12. b. Chloroquine is taken for 2 weeks before and 8 weeks after exposure to potentially infected mosquitoes to prevent growth of the parasites. Abdominal cramping, nausea, and vomiting are among the expected side effects. Ringing in the ears may be an indication of ototoxicity and needs to be reported immediately. Taking either antacids or laxatives may decrease the effectiveness of chloroquine.
13. b. Client has most likely developed resistance to chloroquine. Artemether/lumefantrine is a combination drug that has a high success rate and may be used if other drugs have failed because of resistance. It is especially useful in clients. Administering more chloroquine will not improve the health of the client. Thiabendazole is an anthelminthic. Zidovudine is an antiviral to treat HIV.

14. b, d, e. Proper hygiene for a client who has worms includes frequent handwashing, especially after using the toilet and before eating. Because the worms may live on a variety of materials, all clothing, towels, and bedding should be changed daily and washed in hot water. The client should shower instead of sitting in a bathtub and should not swim in pools or use hot tubs while infected. To prevent trichinosis, caused by *Trichinella spiralis,* all pork and pork-containing products must be thoroughly cooked to destroy the larvae.

15. c, d, e. Taeniasis is a parasitic infestation with tapeworms. Praziquantel is prescribed to treat taeniasis. Possible side effects include dizziness, headache, and weakness. Other side effects can include anorexia, malaise, nausea, vomiting, and abdominal pain. Vision and hearing deficits are not side effects.

16. a, c, d. Antibiotics should be taken as prescribed and the full course should be completed, even if the person feels better.

Case Study

1. Helminths are parasitic worms that have been transmitted from infected soil to the person. Helminths feed on the person's tissue.

2. Groups of helminths that infest humans include tapeworms, flukes, and roundworms. They enter humans when the person eats contaminated food, the person is bitten by carrier insects, or the helminth directly penetrates the skin.

3. Helminths are treated with anthelmintics taken orally. The type of helminth infestation will determine the type(s) of anthelmintic(s) prescribed.

CHAPTER 29: HIV- AND AIDS-RELATED DRUGS

1. a
2. d
3. c
4. f
5. b
6. b
7. e
8. a
9. e
10. a
11. binding, fusion, replication, assembly
12. should
13. 95
14. CYP450
15. Efavirenz

16. dosing frequency, food requirement, fluid requirement, pill burden, drug interaction potential, side effect profile

17. IRIS (immune reconstitution inflammatory syndrome)

18. a, d. HIV is transmitted via contact with blood and body fluids, such as semen, vaginal fluids, and breast milk; this also includes donated sperm from an HIV-infected person. Increased risk occurs in those who have unprotected sex; those who have sex with multiple partners; and IV drug users who share contaminated personal care items, such as razors.

19. b. CD4+ T-cell count can be used to determine when to initiate drug therapy and to monitor the efficacy of therapy. Other laboratory tests include plasma HIV RNA quantitative assay (or viral load) and HIV resistance testing.

20. c. Two laboratory tests used to determine the efficacy of treatment include CD4+ count and HIV viral load. CD4+ count reflects the immune status and should increase in response to ART. HIV viral load is indicative of the virus circulating in the blood, which should decrease in response to ART.

21. a, c, e. It is recommended that all who are HIV positive be treated. Tools to promote drug adherence should be provided, which include using a pill planner and setting alarms. The drugs are selected based on results of genotypic resistance testing; comorbidities; potential drug-drug interactions; pregnancy status; and client's willingness and readiness to start therapy. There are many drugs used in various combinations to increase drug adherence. While client's age and support system are important consideration, it is not a determining factor on initiating ART.

22. b, c. Adherence improved because newer drug formulations decreased dosing frequency or pill burden. Also, some ARTs have been combined into one pill, to further reduce pill burden. Newer ARTs have increased potency and/or have fewer side effects.

23. b. Zidovudine's usual adult dosage is 300 mg every 12 hours. Another dosing schedule is 200 mg every 8 hours.

24. b. The oral dose for neonates at 4 weeks old is 12 mg/kg every 12 hours. 9 mg/kg dosing is for intravenous administration. 120 mg/kg and 300 mg/kg would be overdosing the neonate.

25. a, b, c. Zidovudine can cause hepatotoxicity, lactic acidosis, pancytopenia, and myelosuppression. Therefore, CBC with differentials will be monitored for indications of pancytopenia and myelosuppression. A metabolic panel will be checked for signs of hepatotoxicity (elevated ALT/AST) and lactic acidosis (creatinine).

26. a, b, c, d. Seizures would be an adverse reaction, not a side effect.

27. c. Efavirenz is the only NNRTI that crosses the blood-brain barrier (cerebrospinal fluid); neural tube defects to fetuses can occur. Neuropsychiatric symptoms, such as dizziness, sedation, nightmares, euphoria, and loss of concentration, can occur.

28. d. Efavirenz is scheduled on a daily basis, usually at night to reduce CNS side effects, such as dizziness. However, efavirenz can cause insomnia and euphoria.

29. d. All NNRTIs can cause hepatotoxicity, including hepatic failure; therefore, liver panels should be monitored.

30. a, c, d. Most side effects associated with efavirenz are CNS related such as dizziness, insomnia, agitation, and hallucinations. Gastrointestinal side effects include nausea and diarrhea. Other side effects include rash. Seizures are adverse reactions, not side effects.

31. a, c, d. Efavirenz has effects on the liver and increases the potential for liver failure. Efavirenz crosses the cerebrospinal fluid. Alcohol can increase the risk of hepatotoxicity and neuropsychiatric symptoms and should not be consumed while taking efavirenz. The client should discuss the use of any herbal preparations with the health care provider. St. John's wort should not be taken with efavirenz. Vomiting is one of the common side effects, not an adverse reaction.

32. b, c, d. Tenofovir is a nucleoside/nucleotide reverse transcriptase inhibitor (NNRTI) used to treat certain viral infections, such as HIV. Monitoring of liver enzymes and lipid panels (cholesterol and triglycerides) are important while taking tenofovir.

33. a, b, d. St. John's wort should not be taken with any antiretrovirals, as it may change the levels in the blood. A benefit of tenofovir is that it may be taken with or without food. This is important because nausea, vomiting, diarrhea, and flatulence are potential GI side effects.

34. a. Combination therapy is the standard of care for both treatment of maternal HIV infection and prophylaxis to reduce the risk of transmitting HIV to the fetus. During intrapartum, zidovudine IV should be given if the viral load is greater than or equal to 400 copies/mL, regardless of current ART.

35. a, b, c, e. Atazanavir has few side effects. They include rash, cough, diarrhea, vomiting, and nausea.

36. a, b, d, e. Anything that will help the client keep track of timing on drug and increase adherence will be of benefit. This can be in the form of pill organizers, timers to remind the client of dosing schedule, and wall calendars or charts where the drug can be crossed off after it has been taken. Also, taking the drug at the same time each day can increase adherence.

Case Study

1. Although occurring less frequently than in years past, exposure to HIV still occurs to health care

workers. The first step the nurse should take is to completely wash the exposed area with soap and water then report the incident.

2. Postexposure prophylaxis (PEP) should start within 72 hours of exposure and continue for 4 weeks.

3. The common side effects mostly reported include nausea, malaise, and fatigue.

CHAPTER 30: TRANSPLANT DRUGS

1. cadaveric transplantation
2. lymphocytes
3. posttransplant lymphoproliferative disorder, Epstein-Barr virus
4. mTOR, T-cell and B-cell
5. hypokalemia
6. skin, sun
7. Induction therapy includes transplant drugs that provide *immunosuppression.*
8. An example of a living-donor transplantation is when *one kidney* donated by a living person is transplanted into the body with *end-stage kidney disease.* Another example of a living-donor transplantation is when a *portion of a liver* by a living person is transplanted into the body with *severe liver disease.*
9. Transplant recipients receiving immunosuppressive drugs *cannot* receive live vaccines.
10. Sirolimus is primarily excreted in the *feces.*
11. Antithymocyte globulin alters *T-cell* function and prolongs T-cell *deletion.*
12. c
13. e
14. g
15. c
16. f
17. e
18. a
19. d
20. b
21. a, c, e. Cytokine release syndrome is a complex event associated with cytokine release because of an infusion reaction. When cytokines are released into the circulation, systemic symptoms can occur, such as hypotension, tachycardia, dyspnea, and fever (hyperthermia). Other symptoms include chills, nausea, headache, rash, scratchy throat, and asthenia.
22. a. Before receiving immunosuppressive drugs, antipyretics, antihistamines, and/or corticosteroids are administered to reduce the severity of the symptoms associated with cytokine release syndrome.
23. d. Grapefruit and grapefruit juice affect the metabolism of cyclosporine; they increase the blood concentration of cyclosporine.
24. c. Many drugs can interact with cyclosporine, including antibiotics, histamine$_2$-receptor blockers (e.g., cimetidine), antiinflammatories (e.g., ibupro-

fen), and herbal preparations. Fever can indicate an infection, and the client should call the health care provider.

25. a. The dose ordered is incorrect. The maintenance dose for belatacept is 5 mg/kg starting week 17 post renal transplant. The nurse should not give the drug; instead, the nurse should notify the physician for the correct dose. Giving belatacept without an order is not within the scope of nursing practice.

26. d. Mammalian target rapamycin inhibitor (mTOR) is appropriate for persons who had a kidney transplant. Individuals who had other organ transplants are at risk for lymphoma and other malignancies.

27. a, c, d. Mycophenolate mofetil prevents the proliferation of T-lymphocyte cells and formation of antibodies by the B-lymphocytes. It is recommended for recipients of kidney, heart, or liver transplant.

28. c. The adrenal cortex produces and secretes natural glucocorticoids that are necessary for the immune system. High doses of corticosteroids, such as prednisone, suppress adrenal function, more specifically the adrenal cortex. If corticosteroids are discontinued abruptly, the adrenal cortex does not have time to adjust and is not able to produce and secrete its hormones.

29. d. To decrease the incidence and severity of adverse reactions while receiving antithymocyte globulin, a corticosteroid and an antihistamine should be administered. A prophylactic antibiotic is not necessary.

30. a. Infection is a major risk factor for clients on immunosuppressive therapy. Clients and their family and/or caregiver should be taught to wash hands frequently, especially after toileting, and to avoid sick people or crowds. Taking daily blood pressure and temperature is not necessary. Exercise and proper nutrition are encouraged, but cooking all fruits and vegetables is not necessary.

Case Study

1. Cyclosporine modified is a calcineurin inhibitor that inhibits T-lymphocyte proliferation and reduces the synthesis of cytokines. Methylprednisolone sodium succinate is a corticosteroid that decreases the inflammatory response; suppresses neutrophils, the immune system, and adrenal function; and alters vascular permeability.

2. Common side effects for cyclosporine and methylprednisolone sodium succinate include hypertension, edema, acne, hirsutism, nausea and vomiting, headache, and hyperglycemia. Adverse effects include diabetes mellitus, malignancy, infections, and seizures.

3. Immunosuppressive drugs such as cyclosporine and methylprednisolone sodium succinate suppress the immune response and place the client at risk for disseminated infection resulting from the live virus.

1. d
2. f
3. e
4. c
5. b
6. a
7. g
8. 20
9. vaccinations, ages, dosage, route
10. mosquitoes
11. VAERS (Vaccine Adverse Events Reporting System)
12. Herpes, varicella
13. d. Toxoids are inactivated toxins that stimulate the formation of antitoxins but can no longer produce harmful disease. Examples of toxoids are diphtheria and tetanus.
14. b, c, e. Acquired passive immunity is provided through administration of antibodies pooled from another source. Receiving preformed immunoglobulins (Ig) are necessary when exposed persons are at high risk for complications of the disease, when time does not permit active vaccinations, or when persons suffer from an immune deficiency and do not have effective immune response. Fetuses are automatically protected by the maternal immune system. Pregnant women should not receive immunizations, including preformed Ig, with a few exceptions such as the seasonal flu vaccine.
15. c. Passive immunity involves receiving antibodies that are preformed and had short duration of action. On the other hand, active immunity is when the body's own immune response recognizes a pathogen and produces antibodies, which has long duration of protection.
16. d. Seroconversion occurs when a person acquires detectable antibodies after receiving vaccines.
17. d. Vaccines involve the administration of a small amount of antigens, which stimulate an immune response. Not all persons will develop antibodies; thereby immunity. Vaccines are perceived by the body as foreign particles, or antigens. Vaccines rarely cause an allergic reaction and it does not produce a mild form of the disease. Mild reactions, such as swelling and pain at the injection site and low-grade fever, can occur. Persons can develop a hypersensitivity reaction due to vaccine's components.
18. a. A client actively infected stimulates own immune response and acquires natural immunity.
19. a. First vaccine is usually administered at birth. Hepatitis B is the only one vaccine that is recommended at birth.
20. a. Rubella is also known as German measles. Herpes zoster is also known as shingles.
21. a. Adolescents should receive the two doses of varicella zoster vaccine (VZV) 4–8 weeks apart.

22. c. Health care providers must report any vaccine related adverse reactions to the Vaccine Adverse Events Reporting System (VAERS). VAERS is a surveillance system that receives and acts on any reports of adverse events.
23. a. Td is a vaccine that contains inactivated tetanus and diphtheria toxins that stimulate the formation of antitoxins to produce active immunity.
24. c. Attenuated vaccines are composed of live, weakened microbes. Vaccines against MMR and varicella zoster are composed of live, attenuated viruses. Vaccine against hepatitis B is a recombinant subunit vaccine which contains some of the genetic material. Td (tetanus) is a toxoid vaccine.
25. c. Fever, myalgia, and cough are typical signs and symptoms of influenza. Other manifestations include headaches, malaise, and nasal congestion.
26. d. When MMR is not administered on the same day as varicella, then the administration of the two vaccines should be separated by at least 4 weeks.
27. a. The nurse should explain that redness and tenderness are common side effects and prepare to administer the DTaP as scheduled. DTaP should be given intramuscularly, not subcutaneously. Of the routine childhood immunizations, MMR, varicella, and meningococcal are administered subcutaneously.
28. a, b, c, e. Parents should be given a copy of the immunization record as well as an appointment card with a contact phone number for the clinic at the time of discharge. A Vaccine Information Statement (VIS) should be given to any client, not just children, before receiving any immunizations.
29. a. Those traveling abroad should have their immunizations updated based on their age, immunization history, and destination of travel. Current vaccine recommendations for international travels can be obtained from the Center for Disease Control and Prevention (CDC).
30. c. Although diphenhydramine is used for mild allergic reactions, in the case of an anaphylactic reaction, epinephrine should be readily available.

Case Study

1. A concern for a client who has sustained a puncture wound is the potential for tetanus.
2. Signs and symptoms of tetanus include stiffness in the neck ("lockjaw") and abdominal muscles, difficulty swallowing, muscle spasms, and fever. If not treated, tetanus can cause broken bones and difficulty breathing, and can be fatal.
3. The client should receive a Td vaccine. If there are no contraindications, zoster, pneumonia, and, if in contact with infants or young children, pertussis vaccines could also be given.

1. h
2. j
3. a
4. d
5. i
6. c
7. g
8. b
9. f
10. e
11. Acute myelogeous leukemia
12. Skin cancer
13. Non-Hodgkin lymphoma or Hodgkin disease, or nasopharyngeal cancers
14. Cancer of the colon, rectum, breast, uterus, prostate, and ovary
15. Cancer of mouth, throat, esophagus, liver, and breast
16. a. Combination chemotherapy is used as a treatment across all (or most) phases of cell life; therefore, it tends to be more effective and has better response rate than single-drug treatment. Also, combination therapy decreases drug resistance. However, combination therapy results in increased side and adverse drug effects.
17. d. Viruses, such as human papillomavirus (HPV) and Epstein-Barr virus (EBV), have been implicated in cancer. HPV is associated with cervical cancer and EBV Burkitt lymphoma and nasopharyngeal cancer. Benzene can cause acute myelogenous leukemia. Hepatocellular cancer is caused by aflatoxin.
18. c. General side effects and adverse drug reactions are due to the actions on rapidly growing normal cells, such as skin and hair. Anticancer drugs affect all phases of the cell cycle and are not cell specific. Many of the side effects of anticancer drugs are temporary.
19. a. The goal of palliative chemotherapy is not to cure but to help improve the client's quality of life by treating symptoms such as pain or shortness of breath that may be associated with advanced disease.
20. a. White blood cells are used to fight infection. If the white blood cell count is decreased (leukopenia), the client is at higher risk for an infection. Temperature changes, even if slight, may be an indication of a developing illness.
21. a. Chemotherapy causes myelosuppression, involving red cells, white cells, and platelets. Platelets are involved with clotting and healing injured tissue. If the platelet count is low (thrombocytopenia), the client is more prone to occult bleeding (from the GI tract, for example) and may be unable to effectively develop clots to prevent bleeding.
22. d. Caffeine may have a laxative effect, so it should be limited in clients with diarrhea. Fresh fruit and vegetables and high-fiber foods will increase the number of stools. Foods with extreme temperature are not a concern.
23. b. When digoxin and cyclophosphamide are given orally, cyclophosphamide decreases digoxin levels by impairing GI absorption. This can decrease serum digoxin level and have a subtherapeutic effect; thereby increasing the risk of atrial fibrillation. Digoxin dose may need to be altered.
24. d. Metronidazole may increase the toxicity of 5-FU by inhibiting elimination. The dose of 5-FU may need to be decreased. An increase in toxicity will increase the risk of adverse drug effects.
25. c. Doxorubicin may cause cardiac toxicity, including congestive heart failure. Shortness of breath and crackles could be an indication of early heart failure. Methotrexate can cause hematologic and GI toxicities. Although cyclophosphamide can cause hematologic, pulmonary, and cardiac toxicity, CHF is more prevalent in clients taking doxorubicin.
26. c. Antiemetics decrease the severity of nausea and vomiting and should be administered 30-60 minutes prior to administering 5-FU.
27. c. Hemorrhagic cystitis is a result of severe bladder inflammation, which may occur with cyclophosphamide. Adequate hydration before and while giving this drug is important to potentially prevent this complication.
28. a. Hemorrhagic cystitis can occur with cyclophosphamide. Signs of cystitis include hematuria, urinary frequency, or dysuria. Client needs to remain hydrated. Hydration should be started before treatment and maintained throughout. Antiemetics should be given 30–60 minutes before beginning treatment prophylactically.
29. a. Doxorubicin is a vesicant and tissue necrosis can occur 2-4 days after administration. Dexrazoxane is a parenteral chemoprotectant drug used to treat anthracycline extravasation.
30. d. Two pairs of disposable gloves, preferably powder-free gloves (nitrile, polyurethane, Neoprene), should be worn when preparing chemotherapy and changed every 30 minutes or if they become punctured or contaminated.
31. b. The client and his family will need to be alert for signs of infection attributable to the effects of chemotherapy. Assessing the temperature will need to become a part of his routine.
32. a. Aromatases are enzymes that convert other hormones into estrogens that can increase the risk of breast cancer. Aromatase inhibitors block the conversion of androgens to estrogens and slow tumor growth.
33. d. Vincristine lowers the effects of phenytoin, so the client must be carefully observed for an increase in seizure activity.
34. c. An alcohol-based mouthwash will be very uncomfortable for a client with stomatitis. Also, if the skin barrier is broken, using an alcohol-based mouthwash will potentially cause further irritation.

Case Study

1. Cyclophosphamide is an alkylating drug. It works by causing the DNA strand to cross-link, strands to break, and abnormal base pairing to occur. This prevents the cancer cells from dividing. Cyclophosphamide is also a CCNS (cell cycle–nonspecific) drug that kills cells across the life span.

2. Some major side effects of cyclophosphamide include nausea and vomiting, anemia, risk for infection, and bleeding. Some side effects specific to this medication include the potential for hemorrhagic cystitis, discoloration of the nails, cardiomyopathy, and syndrome of inappropriate antidiuretic hormone (SIADH) secretion.

3. A thorough nursing history and physical assessment are crucial for this client throughout the course of therapy. A baseline assessment of laboratory values, x-rays, and vital signs is very important. A psychosocial assessment should also be completed. Careful monitoring of the client's temperature daily is crucial to watch for early signs of infection.

4. The client should be taught that adequate fluid intake (both oral and IV) will be very important to prevent hemorrhagic cystitis. Even if the client is nauseated, small sips of water at frequent intervals may be beneficial. The goal for fluid intake is 2–3 L/day. The client should be advised not to become pregnant while undergoing treatment. Also, before using any OTC drugs or herbal preparations, the client should confer with her health care provider since there are several herbs (ginseng, garlic, kava kava, echinacea, ginkgo, St. John's wort) that may have interactions with chemotherapy. If the client has a desire for complementary therapy, it should be respected as much as possible.

CHAPTER 33: TARGETED THERAPIES TO TREAT CANCER

1. growth factor
2. Proteasomes
3. growth, spread
4. EGFR (epidermal growth factor receptor)
5. Kinases
6. d
7. b
8. a
9. e
10. c
11. d. Shortness of breath could be an indication of an anaphylactic reaction. The infusion must be stopped immediately, and the reaction treated.
12. c. Bevacizumab blocks the VEGF which inhibits tumor angiogenesis. This prevents the tumor from receiving blood and nutrients; thereby, inhibiting tumor's microvascular growth.

13. b. Diarrhea is a common side effect for gefitinib. Other side effects include skin reactions, anorexia, vomiting, and elevated liver enzymes.

14. a, b, e. MAbs are antibodies that are specific to tumor cells that express the target antigen. MAbs include fully human antibodies, murine antibodies, chimeric antibodies, and humanized antibodies.

15. a. Gefitinib is extensively metabolized by the liver, and it can increase the levels of other drugs, such as warfarin, which can increase the international normalized ratio (INR).

16. b. Other drugs, such as ketoconazole, that are CYP3A4 enzyme inhibitors can increase the plasma concentration of sunitinib, leading to toxicity.

17. c. Erlotinib can cause interstitial lung disease. Assessing lung sounds for adventitious sounds is the most important action by the nurse in a client beginning to receive erlotinib. Clients who have preexisting respiratory problems are cautioned in receiving erlotinib because pulmonary fibrosis may occur.

18. a. Imatinib may cause thrombocytopenia and increase the risk for bleeding. This may be initially apparent with bleeding gums, bruising, and petechiae.

19. c. Ziv-aflibercept is an angiogenesis inhibitor. Its primary action is to prevent the development of new blood vessels.

20. b. Notify the health care provider. Rituximab can worsen hypotension when given with antihypertensive drugs. The dose may need to be decreased or the nurse may need to give a bolus of IV fluids; but the nurse must first notify the provider for the order.

Case Study

1. For metastatic ovarian cancer, bevacizumab 10 mg/kg is administered intravenously every 2 weeks in combination with paclitaxel.

2. Bevacizumab binds to vascular endothelial growth factor (VEGF) and prevents the binding of VEGF with its receptors. It blocks angiogenesis, and the goal is to slow the disease progression.

3. Side effects include hypertension, headache, rhinitis, asthenia, dry skin, and back pain. Adverse effects of bevacizumab are GI perforations, encephalopathy, renal toxicity, thromboembolic events, and congestive heart failure. Although there are many side effects and/or adverse effects, bevacizumab is used for those clients with metastatic disease where the benefits outweigh the risks.

4. Because of the many potential side and adverse effects, the client should be informed of when to notify the health care provider. S.M. should notify her provider if she develops any GI symptoms, such as nausea, vomiting, or diarrhea, because of the risk for GI perforation or formation of fistulas.

Chest pain, abdominal pain, or swelling with redness or pain in the legs should be reported immediately. She should also report any blood in the stools. The client should not take NSAIDs because of the risk for bleeding. The client should avoid dehydration and should wear loose clothing to prevent thrombosis.

CHAPTER 34: BIOLOGIC RESPONSE MODIFIERS

1. biologic response modifiers; restore
2. recombinant DNA; hybridoma technology
3. immunomodulation; metastasizing
4. monocytes
5. red blood cells
6. endothelium; neutrophils
7. capillary leak syndrome
8. b
9. c
10. a
11. d
12. a, b, d. The main function of BRMs is to assist the immune system by the following: enhance the immune system, have cancer cells behave like healthy cells, inhibit normal cells from changing into cancer cells, enhance the body to repair or replace damaged cells, and prevent from metastasizing.
13. d. Granulocytes may become sequestered in the pulmonary system and cause dyspnea. This will cause an additional stress on the already compromised client. Special attention should be paid to complaints of difficulty breathing.
14. b. It is important to assess the hemoglobin level. Risk for complications is higher when EPO is administered to clients with a hemoglobin level >11 g/dL.
15. a, b, c. Interferons should be stopped if clients develop severe depression, hematologic toxicity (severe neutropenia and thrombocytopenia), and hepatic decompensation. Dosages are adjusted for hematologic toxicity other than neutropenia or thrombocytopenia.
16. a. Common side effects of interferons are flu-like symptoms, such as fever, chills, malaise, and myalgia. Other common side effects include neurological symptoms, such as paresthesia; alopecia, xerostomia, and dizziness. These and other side effects will subside after the drug is stopped.
17. a, c, d. Dermatologic effects include alopecia, xerostomia, and rash. Ecchymosis is not a common dermatologic effect from interferons.
18. a, b, d. The client should be educated regarding side effects, adverse effects, and how to administer interferon alpha. The side effects from BRM administration usually disappear 72–96 hours after discontinuation of therapy.
19. b, c. GM-CSF should be administered to both allogeneic and autologous BMT recipients. It is not recommended for Kaposi sarcoma. GM-CSF is used for an ANC <1500/mm^3, and it should not be used within 24 hours of chemotherapy.
20. a, c, e. Conventional high dose aldesleukin is associated with significant adverse effects that can affect essentially every organ. Many of the adverse effects are due to capillary leak syndrome, which results from extravasation of plasma proteins into the extravascular space. The dose should be interrupted or discontinued when the nurse observes new arrhythmia, blood in stool, hypoglycemia, any changes to mentation, new skin eruption, myocardial infarction/myocarditis, sepsis, and hepatic failure, among others.

Case Study

1. G-CSF is not a chemotherapeutic drug but is used in conjunction with myelosuppressive chemotherapy to increase production of neutrophils and enhance phagocytosis to help fight infection. It is an adjunct to chemotherapy.
2. Side effects of G-CSF are like those of other BRMs (nausea, vomiting, fatigue, etc.); however, bone pain is consistently reported with G-CSF because of the action on the bone marrow. Bone pain occurs more frequently in clients receiving higher doses.
3. Priority teaching instructions include the use of nonopioids to help relieve bone pain. Should the client want to become pregnant, the health care provider should be notified immediately, as caution should be used in administering this G-CSF to pregnant clients. The client should also report any abdominal pain, including pain referred to the left shoulder, as well as chest pain or unusual bleeding, such as hematuria or bloody stool.

CHAPTER 35: UPPER RESPIRATORY DISORDERS

1. c
2. a
3. d
4. b
5. H$_1$, smooth
6. first-generation; dry mouth; drowsiness
7. nonsedating; anticholinergic
8. tolerance; rebound nasal congestion; 3 days
9. alpha-adrenergic; vasoconstriction; hypertension
10. a
11. b
12. b
13. a
14. b
15. a
16. b. Antihistamines block H$_1$ receptors found in the extravascular smooth muscles. This antagonist effect can cause dryness of the mouth and decreased

secretions. Antihistamines can also decrease nasal itching.

17. a. Second generation antihistamines have fewer anticholinergic effects than first generation antihistamines. Drowsiness is less with second generation antihistamines.

18. d. Phenylpropanolamine was discontinued in all over-the-counter cold remedies and weight-loss aids because of an increased risk of stroke, hypertension, renal failure, and cardiac dysrhythmias.

19. a. The recommended dose to treat allergies with diphenhydramine is 25-50 mg every 6-8 hours, with a maximum dose of 300 mg per day.

20. d. Diphenhydramine is a H_1 antagonist and is one of the most frequently used over-the-counter antihistamine. Diphenhydramine has antitussive effects, in addition to treating allergic rhinitis, sneezing, pruritus, urticaria, and to treat motion sickness.

21. c. Breastfeeding clients need to be instructed that small amounts of diphenhydramine can pass into breast milk. Since children are more susceptible to the antihistamine effects, it is recommended not to use diphenhydramine while breastfeeding.

22. d. Both nasal and systemic decongestants have different mechanism of actions. Nasal decongestants have sympathomimetic actions which stimulate the alpha-adrenergic receptors that cause vasoconstriction. Frequent use of nasal decongestants can have a rebound effect. Systemic decongestants are alpha-adrenergic agonists primarily used for allergic rhinitis. The advantage of systemic over nasal decongestants is that they last longer. But, nasal decongestants have quicker action.

23. c. Expectorant reduces the viscosity of secretions so that they can be eliminated by coughing. The most common ingredient in cold remedies is guaifenesin. However, the best way to help loosen mucus is by maintaining hydration.

24. a, b, c, d. The class of drugs used to treat cold symptoms include antihistamines (H_1 blockers for vasoconstriction), decongestants (vasoconstriction), antitussives (control cough), and expectorants (to thin secretions).

25. a, b, c, d. Decongestants are not contraindicated in obesity unless the client also has any of the other diagnoses.

26. c, d. Antihistamines may cause drowsiness. Diphenhydramine is a common ingredient in OTC sleeping preparations. Should the client choose to take any OTC drugs, the client should be instructed to read the label carefully to check for interactions. The best option, however, is to check with the health care provider or pharmacist. Decongestants taken at bedtime may cause insomnia or jitteriness. Antibiotics are ineffective against a virus.

Case Study

1. Oxymetazoline is a decongestant nasal spray that is used to help constrict the vessels within the nasal cavity. The nasal mucous membranes shrink, and it is easier for the client to exchange air through the nose.

2. The correct dose for this client would be 2 or 3 sprays in each nostril, morning and night. It should not be used for longer than 3–5 days because of the potential for rebound congestion.

3. Rebound congestion occurs because of irritation of the nasal mucosa leading to vasodilation instead of vasoconstriction. Use of nasal decongestants can also lead to nasal dryness and, if overused, epistaxis. Some brands of oxymetazoline are listed as moisturizing. Another option is to use saline nasal drops, although this will only moisturize and not serve as a decongestant. Oral decongestants such as phenylephrine or pseudoephedrine may also be used. Also important with this client is to determine the cause of the nasal congestion. Allergies may be treated with intranasal glucocorticoids and first- or second-generation antihistamines. A common cold will not be treated with glucocorticoids.

CHAPTER 36: LOWER RESPIRATORY DISORDERS

1. d
2. e
3. b
4. f
5. c
6. a, b
7. b
8. f
9. cyclic adenosine monophosphate (cAMP)
10. epinephrine
11. beta$_2$-adrenergic agonists
12. cAMP
13. increases
14. synergistic
15. shorter
16. methylxanthine (xanthine); asthma
17. glucocorticoids
18. prophylactic; histamine
19. rebound bronchospasm
20. beta$_2$
21. is
22. evening
23. 10 mg/day
24. mucolytics
25. antibiotic
26. c. The inhaler should be shaken well before each use. Inhalers do not require refrigeration. By testing the inhaler each time to see if the spray works, the client is losing a dose of the medication.
27. a, b, d, e. Inhaled doses of drugs for asthma have a more rapid onset and fewer side effects than oral preparations. They are shorter-acting. Some inhaled and oral drugs can be taken together.

28. a. The bronchodilator helps open the airway which increases the effectiveness of the inhaled steroid. Beta agonist can cause tachycardia, but it is not the reason to take the beta agonist before the inhaled steroid.

29. a, c. Long-term use of glucocorticoids can cause impaired immune response, hyperglycemia, fluid retention, electrolyte imbalance, hypertension, thinning of the skin, abnormal subcutaneous fat distribution, and purpura. Insomnia, vomiting, and weight loss can be seen with short-term use.

30. b. Ipratropium is an anticholinergic drug that is administered via meter dose inhaler (MDI). It can also be administered via aerosol nebulizer treatment. Unlike albuterol, ipratropium has few side effects which include headache, blurred vision, tachycardia, urinary retention, and constipation.

31. d. Taking theophylline and ephedra together may increase the risk of theophylline toxicity. Hyperglycemia is a sign of theophylline toxicity.

32. a, b, c, d. It is not necessary to wait 5 minutes between inhalations.

33. a, b, c, e. Beta blockers increase the half-life of theophylline. Theophylline increases the risk of digitalis toxicity and decreases the effects of lithium. Phenytoin decreases theophylline levels.

34. b. Cromolyn sodium is used as a prophylactic medication to prevent asthma attacks by preventing the release of histamine and suppressing inflammation in the bronchioles. It will not stop an attack once it has started and is not a bronchodilator.

35. c. The therapeutic range for theophylline is 10–20 mcg/mL.

Case Study

1. Albuterol is a selective beta₂ agonist. It is considered a "rescue inhaler" and can be used on an as-needed basis during an acute asthma attack. Montelukast sodium is a leukotriene modifier. Fluticasone propionate/salmeterol 100/50 is a glucocorticoid combination drug that contains fluticasone propionate 100 mcg and salmeterol 50 mcg.

2. Albuterol is a fast-acting selective beta₂ agonist and provides bronchodilation. It has fewer side effects than with nonselective beta agonists. Leukotrienes are chemical mediators that cause airway edema and increase mucous production. Leukotriene modifiers, such as montelukast sodium, decrease inflammation. They must be taken daily and are not effective to treat an acute asthma attack. Glucocorticoids, such as fluticasone propionate/salmeterol, have antiinflammatory properties, and they work synergistically with beta₂ agonists.

3. H.K. should be encouraged to keep all appointments as scheduled and to contact the health care provider before taking any over-the-counter drugs. If H.K. smokes, information on smoking cessation programs should be given. Female clients should be advised to notify the health care provider if contemplating pregnancy. Clients with asthma should be encouraged to stay hydrated and report any increased use of "rescue inhalers" like albuterol. A client with asthma should also be encouraged to wear a medical identification bracelet or necklace to indicate the drugs being taken.

CHAPTER 37: CARDIAC GLYCOSIDES, ANTIANGINALS, AND ANTIDYSRHYTHMICS

1. b
2. e
3. c
4. d
5. a
6. weakens; enlarges
7. increase
8. digitalis glycosides; inhibit
9. increase; decrease
10. positive inotropic action (increases heart contraction); negative chronotropic action (decreases heart rate); negative dromotropic action (decreases conduction of the heart cells); and increased stroke volume
11. decrease
12. warfarin (or other anticoagulants)
13. hypokalemia, hypomagnesemia, hypercalcemia
14. dilating; arterioles; renal; decreases
15. extensive first-pass metabolism by the liver
16. smooth muscle of blood vessels
17. 1–3; 3
18. headache
19. beta blockers and calcium channel blockers
20. verapamil; diltiazem
21. reflex tachycardia; pain
22. stressed (or exerted)
23. frequently, unpredictable, and progressive
24. is at rest
25. spasm
26. reduction of venous tone or coronary vasodilation
27. hypoxia; hypercapnia
28. fast sodium channel blockers; beta blockers; calcium channel blockers; also drugs that prolong repolarization
29. alcohol; cigarettes
30. b
31. a
32. a
33. c
34. d
35. c. Phosphodiesterase inhibitors, such as milrinone, promote positive inotropic response and vasodilation, not vasoconstriction. Phosphodiesterase inhibitors do not increase serum sodium and potassium levels. Increasing serum sodium can promote water retention, which will worsen heart failure.
36. d. Quinidine is a fast sodium channel blocker that decreases sodium influx into cardiac cells. The response is slowed conduction speed, suppressed automaticity, and increased repolarization time.

37. a. Amiodarone prolongs repolarization and is given intravenously in emergency treatment for ventricular dysrhythmias when other antidysrhythmics are not effective. Atropine is for symptomatic bradycardia; acebutolol is for premature ventricular contractions and is given orally.

38. d. Lidocaine is used to treat ventricular dysrhythmias. Atrial fibrillation, bradycardia, and complete heart block are atrial dysrhythmias.

39. a, c. Constipation is a side effect of verapamil, which is taken three times per day. Verapamil may cause hypotension, not hypertension.

40. d. Calcium channel blockers can affect kidney and liver function, so baseline liver enzymes and renal function should be obtained and trended.

41. c. ANP and BNP are elevated in persons with HF. Both are secreted from the atrial cells of the heart.

42. d. Normal values are less than 100 pg/mL. Greater than 100 pg/mL is considered elevated. Older women tend to have higher normal BNP levels than older men; however, a level of 630 pg/mL is markedly elevated and is of concern for heart failure.

43. a. Digitalis drugs, such as digoxin, can be used for heart failure or atrial fibrillation. Atrial fibrillation is a cardiac dysrhythmia of the atria.

44. a. The usual maintenance dose of digoxin is 0.125-0.5 mg/d. Answers b and c are too low and answer d is too high of a dose. The therapeutic serum level for digoxin is 0.8 to 2 ng/mL.

45. b. Digoxin has a long half of 30-40 hours and has low protein-binding power of 20-30%. Because of these, drug accumulation can occur causing digoxin toxicity. Serum digoxin levels are drawn to assess for possible toxicity. The therapeutic serum level when taken for dysrhythmias is 0.8 to 2 ng/mL. When it is taken for heart failure, the therapeutic level is 0.5 to 1 ng/mL.

46. b. Digoxin-immune Fab can be given to treat severe digitalis toxicity. This drug binds with digoxin so that it can be excreted in the urine.

47. a, b, c. Cortisone, furosemide, and hydrochlorothiazide all promote loss of potassium, which increases the effect of digitalis and can lead to digitalis toxicity. A person taking a potassium-wasting diuretic or cortisol should avoid hypokalemia by eating potassium-rich foods or taking potassium supplements.

48. c. There are no specific drug-food contraindications for digoxin. The client should be encouraged to eat foods high in potassium such as fruits and vegetables (including potatoes). A client with heart failure should avoid hot dogs because of their high sodium content.

49. a, b. Nitroglycerin tablets should not be chewed but should be placed under the tongue. There are no dietary restrictions when taking nitroglycerin. Tablets must be stored in their original amber glass container and away from light to prevent decomposition. A very dry mouth will hinder absorption, so sips of water may be taken. If chest pain persists or worsens after three tablets, client should go to the nearest emergency room by calling rather than notifying their health care provider.

50. c. The duration of action for NTG patch is 18-24 hours. However, clients should be instructed to remove the patch nightly to allow for an 8-12 hours nitrate-free interval to avoid building tolerance.

51. a. Acebutolol is a beta blocker and should not be abruptly stopped because abrupt discontinuation can lead to reflex tachycardia or dysrhythmias.

52. a, d, e. Aloe, Ma-huang, and ginseng should be avoided while taking digoxin. Aloe and Ma-huang can increase the risk of digoxin toxicity; ginseng can falsely elevate digoxin levels.

53. a, b, e. Electrolyte imbalances, especially potassium, calcium, and magnesium, can lead to cardiac dysrhythmias. Excessive catecholamines may lead to rapid atrial or ventricular rates as well as ectopy. Hypoxia and *hyper*capnia may also cause dysrhythmias.

Case Study

1. The three different types of angina are classic, unstable, and variant. Classic angina is fairly predictable and occurs with stress or exertion. Unstable angina is also known as *preinfarction angina*. It is unpredictable and increases in frequency and severity. Unstable angina may or may not be related to stress. Variant angina is also known as *vasospastic* or *Prinzmetal angina*. It occurs at rest. Clients frequently have a combination of both classic and variant angina. Classic angina is caused by an actual narrowing of the coronary arteries, whereas variant angina is caused by vessel spasms. Unstable angina often indicates an impending myocardial infarction (MI).

2. Vasospastic angina or variant angina occurs at rest. But since stress plays a part in anginal attacks, avoiding strenuous activities, heavy meals, and emotional upset may be beneficial nonpharmacologic methods to treat vasospastic angina. Smoking cessation is very important to overall cardiac health. Preventive measures include adequate rest and relaxation techniques.

   Pharmacologic treatments for angina include nitrates, beta blockers, and calcium channel blockers. Antianginal drugs either increase oxygen supply or decrease oxygen demand by the myocardium. Nitrates reduce venous tone, promote vasodilation, and decrease cardiac workload. Beta and calcium channel blockers decrease oxygen demand by decreasing the workload of the heart. Nitrates and calcium channel blockers are effective for treating vasospastic angina.

3. Beta blockers and calcium channel blockers can be used to treat angina. Beta blockers include atenolol, metoprolol, and nadolol. Calcium chan-

nel blockers include amlodipine, diltiazem, and verapamil hydrochloride. Beta blockers should be used in persons with stable angina. Nitrates and calcium channel blockers can be used for variant angina. Nitrates are also used for unstable angina.

4. Nitrates cause relaxation and dilation of blood vessels, including coronary vasculature, which decreases resistance; hence, blood pressure drops. Nitrates also decrease preload and afterload, reducing myocardial oxygen demand.

CHAPTER 38: DIURETICS

1.
a. Tubules: <u>Proximal tubule</u>
Class of drug: <u>Osmotic and carbonic anhydrase inhibitors</u>
Electrolytes: <u>Na$^+$</u>
b. Tubules: <u>Loop of Henle</u>
Class of drug: <u>Loop diuretics</u>
Electrolytes: <u>Na$^+$ and K$^+$</u>
c. Tubules: <u>Distal tubule</u>
Class of drug: <u>Thiazides</u>
Electrolytes: <u>Na$^+$</u>
d. Tubules: <u>Collecting tubule</u>
Class of drug: <u>Potassium sparing</u>
Electrolytes: <u>K$^+$</u>

Laboratory Test	Normal Levels	Abnormal Results
2. Potassium	3.5–5 mEq/L	hypokalemia
3. Magnesium	1.5–2.5 mg/dL	hypomagnesemia
4. Calcium	8.6–10.2 mEq/L	hypercalcemia
5. Chloride	96–106 mEq/L	hypochloremia
6. Bicarbonate	24–28 mEq/L	minimal bicarbonate loss
7. Uric acid	2.8–8 mg/dL	hyperuricemia
8. Blood sugar	70–99 mg/dL	hyperglycemia
9. Blood lipids	Total chol: <200 mg/dL LDL: <100 mg/dL Trig: <150 mg/dL	hyperlipidemia

10. The two main purposes for diuretics are to decrease fluid and decrease hypertension (lower blood pressure).

11. Most diuretics promote sodium and water loss by blocking sodium and chloride reabsorption from the renal tubules. This causes a decrease in fluid volume in the tissues and circulation, which lowers blood pressure.

12. b, d, e. Diuretics are classified according to their mechanisms of action. Loop diuretics promote the loss of potassium and sodium; potassium-sparing diuretics promote the loss of sodium while retaining potassium; and thiazide diuretics promote the loss of sodium and some potassium. All diuretics promote the loss of water. While osmotic diuretics promote the loss of water and sodium, they are not used to treat hypertension and congestive heart failure; instead, they are used to decrease edema, especially cerebral edema. Carbonic anhydrase inhibitors also promote water and bicarbonate loss with minimal influence on electrolytes. Their use is to decrease intraocular pressure, not hypertension and heart failure.

13. b. Spironolactone is a potassium-sparing diuretic. It promotes potassium retention in the renal tubules.

14. a. Furosemide is a loop diuretic, which promotes excretion of water, sodium, and potassium, primarily in the loop of Henle and some in the distal renal tubules. Other electrolytes that are excreted include magnesium, ammonium, phosphate, and calcium.

15. c. Spironolactone blocks the action of aldosterone and inhibits the sodium-potassium pump, so potassium is retained. This is important in maintaining a regular cardiac rhythm. It is frequently prescribed and is not contraindicated in clients who have had a myocardial infarction. Sodium is excreted with this drug. Clients should be advised not to overindulge in foods rich in potassium such as bananas, because this could cause above-normal levels of potassium (hyperkalemia).

16. d. To prevent hearing loss, furosemide must be administered by slow IV push over at least 1–2 minutes. It does not need to be diluted and does not require a central line for administration. Cardiac monitoring is not essential, because furosemide does not generally cause arrhythmias.

17. a, b, d. Hypokalemia, or low serum potassium level, is a risk for clients taking thiazides. This could be a life-threatening condition. Sodium is also lost, causing hyponatremia. Calcium level is elevated because thiazides block calcium excretion. There is minimal effect on bicarbonate levels. Cautious use in hepatic failure clients is recommended, but trending of AST/ALT levels is not always indicated. Baseline values may be beneficial.

18. a. The normal range for serum potassium level is 3.5–5 mEq/L. A level of 5.8 mEq/L is considered hyperkalemia. The dose of spironolactone may need to be held or decreased, and the client should decrease intake of potassium-rich foods such as bananas, apricots, leafy greens, and salmon.

19. a. Acetazolamide is a carbonic anhydrase inhibitor. It blocks the action of carbonic anhydrase, which is an enzyme that affects hydrogen ion balance. If the action is blocked, more bicarbonate will be excreted, leading to metabolic acidosis.

20.	d. Because the onset of action HCTZ is 2 hours, it may be best to take the drug when the client will be awake for several hours so sleep is not disturbed. Hydrochlorothiazide can be taken with food to prevent GI upset. The drug needs to be taken consistently, even if the client is not having symptoms of heart failure.

21.	a. Furosemide will cause an increased loss of potassium (hypokalemia) when given with amiodarone, which may predispose the client to ventricular arrhythmias.

22.	c. Muscle weakness, abdominal distention, severe leg cramping, and cardiac arrhythmias are indications of hypokalemia (low potassium levels). Low potassium levels may occur with the use of loop diuretics.

23.	a. Loop diuretics are contraindicated in clients with anuria. Giving diuretics to a client without any urine output will not force urine production. Clients allergic to sulfa drugs should not take furosemide or bumetanide; these are derivatives of sulfonamides.

24.	d. Daily weights and vital signs need to be trended at home on a daily basis. The client and family should be educated on how to take these measurements or arrangements should be made for assessment by home health services, at least initially. The onset of action for hydrochlorothiazide is 2 hours. Hyperglycemia is a side effect of hydrochlorothiazide, so blood sugar level should be monitored. This medication can be taken with food to prevent nausea.

Case Study

1.	Mannitol is an osmotic diuretic that is used for clients with increased intracranial pressure and increased intraocular pressure. Osmotic diuretics increase osmolality and sodium reabsorption which will allow fluid to shift from the brain tissue to the vasculature. Sodium, chloride, potassium, and water are then excreted. This shift in fluid will cause, at least temporarily, a decrease in intracranial pressure.

2.	The standard dosage range in adults for increased intracranial pressure (ICP) for mannitol is 0.25-1g/kg, followed by 0.25 mg/kg to 1 g/kg infused over 30–60 minutes. The drug can be repeated every 6-8 hours. While there is no true maximum dose, the nurse must closely monitor client's renal function. Mannitol crystallizes easily, so it must be warmed before administration. It is suggested that it be given through an IV administration set with a filter.

3.	For this client, the correct initial dose and maintenance dose would be 20-80 g over 30–60 minutes.

CHAPTER 39: ANTIHYPERTENSIVES

1.	beta-adrenergic blockers; centrally acting alpha$_2$ agonists; alpha-adrenergic blockers; also adrenergic neuron blockers, alpha$_1$- and beta$_1$-adrenergic blockers

2.	diuretics, direct-acting arteriolar vasodilators; also ACE inhibitors, angiotensin II-receptor blockers, and calcium channel blockers

3.	beta blockers; ACE inhibitors; also angiotensin II–receptor blockers, potassium-sparing diuretics, centrally acting alpha$_2$ agonist

4.	diuretics

5.	diminished; lowered

6.	cardioselective

7.	decreased; increased

8.	c

9.	d

10.	b

11.	a

12.	e

13.	f

14.	g

15.	h

16.	b. Nonselective alpha-adrenergic blockers are used for severe hypertension associated with pheochromocytomas (catecholamine-secreting tumors of the adrenal medulla).

17.	d. Direct-acting vasodilators relax the smooth muscles of the blood vessels, mainly the arteries, resulting in vasodilation. This promotes blood flow to the brain, kidneys, and other vital organs. Vasodilation causes the blood pressure to decrease.

18.	d. Diuretics are frequently given with a variety of antihypertensive to decrease fluid retention and peripheral edema.

19.	a, b, c. Angiotensin II binds to cell receptors to increase blood pressure. Angiotensin II also causes vasoconstriction and increases vascular resistance. ARBs inhibit the binding of angiotensin II at receptor sites; thereby, decreasing blood pressure. Without the binding, vasoconstriction does not occur and the peripheral resistance is not increased. ARBs do not increase sodium retention or decrease heart rate.

20.	b. ARBs inhibit the binding of angiotensin II to receptor sites; thereby blood pressure does not increase. Diuretics, such as thiazides, assist in lowering blood pressure by promoting water and sodium loss.

21.	a. The primary side effect of ACE inhibitors is a constant, irritated cough and may be relieved upon discontinuation of the drug. ARBs do not have the side effect of coughing.

22.	d. African Americans are not as responsive to ACE inhibitors as monotherapy but may respond better if they are combined with a diuretic.

23.	c. Calcium channel blockers and alpha$_1$ blockers may be more effective in African American clients for treating hypertension. They do not respond well to direct renin inhibitors, beta blockers, and ACE inhibitors. ARBs have similar mechanism of actions as ACE inhibitors, affecting the RAAS.

24. a. Ma-huang decreases or counteracts the effects of antihypertensives and can even increase the hypertensive state.

25. b. ACE inhibitors, such as captopril, when taken with nitrates, diuretics, or adrenergic blockers can increase the risk of hypotension. Nitrates cause vasodilation, diuretics cause sodium and water loss, and adrenergic blockers decrease sympathetic tone.

26. b. Aldosterone, a hormone secreted by the adrenal cortex, promotes sodium retention and potassium excretion. Captopril is an ACE inhibitor that inhibits the release of aldosterone. This action can increase serum potassium level, and if captopril is taken with a potassium-sparing diuretic, such as spironolactone, hyperkalemia is more likely.

27. b. Adherence with the medication regimen can be very frustrating to a client who "feels better." Stopping an antihypertensive abruptly can lead to rebound hypertension.

28. a. Amlodipine, a calcium channel blocker, is highly protein-bound (93%).

29. a, b, d. Metoprolol is a cardioselective beta blocker that lowers blood pressure, which can cause dizziness, nausea, vomiting, and headache.

30. b. Ankle edema may occur with calcium channel blockers such as amlodipine because of its vasodilatory effect. There are other options that may be utilized to treat the client's hypertension.

31. d, e. Cardioselective beta blockers will help maintain renal blood flow and have fewer hypoglycemic effects than those associated with noncardioselective beta blockers. Rebound symptoms are a possibility if the medication is stopped abruptly. Cardioselectivity does not confer absolute protection from bronchoconstriction.

32. b. Aliskiren can be used for mild to moderate hypertension, either as a monotherapy or with combination of other antihypertensives or diuretics. Aliskiren is not effective in reducing blood pressure among Black clients. Because aldosterone concentration is decreased, aliskiren can cause hyperkalemia, not hypokalemia.

Case Study

1. Chlorthalidone with clonidine combines a thiazide diuretic with a centrally acting alpha$_2$ agonist. Centrally acting alpha$_2$ agonists decrease the sympathetic response from the brainstem to the peripheral vessels. The result is decreased peripheral vascular resistance and increased vasodilation, thereby reducing blood pressure. Because clonidine can cause fluid retention, a diuretic is frequently prescribed, which accounts for the combination of clonidine with chlorthalidone.

2. *Hypertensive emergencies* are episodes of uncontrolled blood pressure that can cause acute impairment of one or more systems (cardiovascular, renal, neurologic). If left untreated, permanent damage may occur. The blood pressure needs to be lowered, but in a controlled setting, such as with sodium nitroprusside in an intensive care unit. Sodium nitroprusside is a potent vasodilator and is administered intravenously in a critical care unit; it is the drug of choice for hypertensive emergencies. The client must be monitored closely in a critical care unit during administration.

3. Priority teaching instructions at discharge for this client include the importance of taking the medication as prescribed. Determining why the client skips doses is important. Missing doses can cause rebound hypertension, tachycardia, and headache. Priority teaching instructions may need to be directed toward the cause of missing doses. If the client remains on a similar drug that is combined with a diuretic, the nurse should suggest the client take the drug during waking hours so sleep is not interrupted. Decreasing stress, increasing exercise, and evaluating the diet are important aspects of the entire care plan for a client with hypertension.

CHAPTER 40: ANTICOAGULANTS, ANTIPLATELETS, AND THROMBOLYTICS

1. artery; vein
2. clot formation; do not
3. do not have
4. venous thrombus; pulmonary embolus
5. subcutaneously; intravenously
6. standard; bleeding
7. warfarin
8. decrease
9. 3-4
10. plasminogen; plasmin
11. bleeding/hemorrhage
12. fondaparinux
13. Order of heparin activity: d, b, a, c
14. c
15. d
16. a
17. a
18. e
19. d
20. f
21. b
22. f
23. c. Warfarin is an oral anticoagulant used to prevent blood clots. Fibrinolytics, not anticoagulants, dissolve existing clots.
24. a, b, c. Most clients on warfarin therapy are maintained at an international normalized ratio (INR) between 2–3 seconds. Clients with mechanical heart valves or recurrent systemic embolism should have an INR of 2.5–4.5 seconds.
25. b, d. Clopidogrel is an antiplatelet and apixaban is a selective factor Xa inhibitor.

26. a. Abciximab is an antiplatelet drug in the glyco-protein (GP) IIb/IIIa receptor antagonist family. It is used primarily for acute coronary syndromes and for preventing reocclusion of coronary arteries following PTCA. Aminocaproic acid is an antagonist to thrombolytics (antithrombolytic) to stop bleeding by inhibiting thrombolysis. Protamine sulfate is an antidote to stop bleeding attributable to heparin or LMWH. Warfarin is an oral anticoagulant.

27. a. The correct dose for continuous infusion is 0.125 mcg/kg/min. This client weighs 76 kg (168 pounds ÷ 2.2 = 76 kg). 76 kg × 0.125 mcg/kg/min = 9.5 mcg/min.

28. d. Clopidogrel is an antiplatelet drug used frequently after a myocardial infarction. When used together with aspirin, the therapeutic effect is more effective than when used alone.

29. a. Various laboratory values will be monitored while a client is taking warfarin. The most important levels to trend will be PT and INR. The INR and PT are closely related.

30. d. Vitamin K is the antidote for warfarin poisoning or overdose. Protamine sulfate is the antidote for heparin overdose. Anagrelide and ticagrelor is an antiplatelet.

31. b. Warfarin is highly protein bound (over 90%). In drugs that are highly protein-bound, such as fluoxetine, there is the potential for drug displacement of warfarin, leading to higher free drug levels in the blood. This can result in bleeding.

32. a. Fondaparinux is a synthetically manufactured antithrombotic that has a selective inhibits factor Xa. The structure is closely related to heparin and LMWH. Uncontrolled bleeding, such as GI bleed, is considered an adverse reaction to fondaparinux. The drug should be discontinued.

33. b. Aminocaproic acid is an antithrombolytic drug that inhibits plasminogen activation, which inhibits thrombolysis. Reteplase is a thrombolytic. Calcium gluconate treats calcium deficiency. Protamine sulfate is the antidote for heparin overdose.

34. a, c, e. Vital signs should be continually assessed while a client is receiving thrombolytics. Cardiac monitoring should be performed to observe for reperfusion arrhythmias. The nurse should also monitor for signs and symptoms of bleeding. Hemorrhage is a serious complication of thrombolytic therapy. Aminocaproic acid can be given as an antidote. Tenecteplase is given as an IV bolus. Liver enzymes are not usually affected. Type and cross-match blood products is not necessary unless there is significant blood loss requiring blood transfusions.

35. a, b, d, e. Anticoagulants would be beneficial for clients with a history of deep vein thrombosis, cerebrovascular accident (embolic stroke) and for those who have received an artificial heart valve. They are also beneficial in clients who have had major orthopedic surgeries, such as hip or knee replacements, to prevent pulmonary emboli.

Case Study

1. Heparin combines with antithrombin III, which accelerates the anticoagulant cascade of reactions that prevents thrombus formation. By inhibiting the action of thrombin, conversion of fibrinogen to fibrin does not occur, and the formation of a fibrin clot is prevented. Heparin will not dissolve a clot like a thrombolytic, but it prevents the formation of further clots. Before discharge, a client must be transitioned to either a low–molecular-weight heparin (LMWH) like enoxaparin sodium, which is administered subcutaneously, or an oral medication such as warfarin.

2. Warfarin inhibits hepatic synthesis of vitamin K, thus affecting clotting factors II, VII, IX, and X. If the blood cannot clot as well, the likelihood of another pulmonary embolus forming is lower.

3. Priority teaching for this client before discharge includes information regarding compliance with lab testing (INR) and communication with the health care provider before taking any medications, herbals, or OTC preparations. Dietary restrictions include limiting the amount of vitamin K–rich foods, such as green leafy vegetables, in the diet, as well as careful consumption of vitamin C. Herbals such as St. John's wort, ginkgo, kava, and ginseng also decrease the effectiveness of warfarin. The nurse should also advise the client that aspirin and NSAIDs should be avoided; acetaminophen may be used as a substitute for pain relief as needed.

Safety precautions should also be taken to prevent anything that would lead to a risk of bleeding. The client should be advised to use a toothbrush with soft bristles and only shave with an electric razor. If the client does sustain an injury, bleeding should be able to be controlled with direct pressure for 5–10 minutes with a sterile dressing. If this is not effective, the client should notify the health care provider or go to the nearest emergency department. Any indications of bleeding such as epistaxis, hematemesis, or blood in the stool should be reported to the health care provider as well.

CHAPTER 41: ANTIHYPERLIPIDEMICS AND DRUGS TO IMPROVE PERIPHERAL BLOOD FLOW

1. Low density lipoproteins (LDL), very low density lipoproteins (VLDL), high density lipoprotein (HDL), chylomicrons
2. protein; fat
3. atherosclerotic plaques; heart disease
4. apolipoprotein
5. HMG-CoA reductase; HMG-CoA reductase inhibitors
6. homocysteine
7. arteriosclerosis; hyperlipidemia
8. b
9. c

10. a
11. a
12. b
13. e
14. d
15. c. There are two forms of apolipoproteins, apoB-48 and apoB-100. Of the two, apoB-100 is a better indicator for CAD.
16. d. Atorvastatin is a statin drug that inhibits HMG-CoA reductase in synthesizing cholesterol in the liver. Rhabdomyolysis is a severe side effect associated with statin drugs, such as atorvastatin. This occurs when muscle tissue breaks down. Rhabdomyolysis can be fatal. Also, serum liver enzymes should be monitored.
17. b. High levels of homocysteine have been linked to loss of flexibility (elasticity) to the vessel walls. Other effects associated with homocysteine include cardiovascular disease, stroke, blood clotting, damage to the vascular endothelial lining, and thickening of the vasculature.
18. c. Intermittent vascular claudications cause vasospasms, and vasodilators improve blood flow to the extremities. Gingko has been taken to treat intermittent claudication.
19. d. LDL contains 50–60% of cholesterol in circulation and with an elevated level increases the risk for atherosclerotic plaques and heart disease.
20. a. An HDL level of 22 mg/dL is low. The normal value should be greater than 60 mg/dL. Low levels of HDL put the client in the high-risk category for cardiovascular disease. A value less than 35 mg/dL is considered high risk.
21. b. Lifestyle changes, such as eating a low-fat, low-cholesterol diet, generally lower the cholesterol level by only 10–30%. Other activities should be instituted, such as implementation of routine exercises to increase HDL level and cessation of smoking.
22. c. Diet, exercise, weight loss, and medication all play a vital role in decreasing cholesterol level. Diet continues to play a vital role, despite the antihyperlipidemic drug that is taken.
23. b, d, e. Cilostazol should be taken 30 minutes before or 2 hours after meals. Grapefruit juice will increase the levels of cilostazol, so it should be avoided. There is no contraindication for the use of acetaminophen. Headache and abdominal pain are both side effects of cilostazol. Blood pressure should be monitored frequently, and the client should be encouraged to change positions slowly to prevent a precipitous drop in blood pressure.

Case Study

1. Atorvastatin is an HMG-CoA reductase inhibitor, or a "statin" drug. By inhibiting cholesterol synthesis in the liver, atorvastatin decreases LDL ("bad") cholesterol, slightly increases HDL ("good") cholesterol, and decreases triglycerides.

2. Atorvastatin is contraindicated to be used during pregnancy, including labor and delivery, and breastfeeding (lactation). S.S. should use a reliable birth control to prevent pregnancy while on atorvastatin. Another form of treatment, other than statin drugs, may be needed to lower LDL.

3. Monitoring the client for the desired effect is an obvious priority, although it is important for the nurse to advise the client that changes in lipid profiles may take several weeks for lipid levels to decline. Liver enzymes should also be drawn at baseline and monitored throughout therapy. Many statin drugs are contraindicated in acute hepatic disease. Vision should be tested at least yearly, because there have been some studies that indicate an increased risk of cataracts in clients taking statins. This risk is higher in clients with diabetes.

4. The nurse should emphasize that treatment of hyperlipidemia is a lifelong commitment. Making dietary changes, exercising, and using pharmacologic therapy will help decrease LDL levels, and therefore potentially decrease the risk of heart disease. Other important points in the health teaching plan for S.S. include the importance of keeping follow-up appointments with health care providers, taking the medication as scheduled even if she does not feel she is making any progress, and reporting any muscle pain or tenderness immediately. These symptoms can be an indication of the life-threatening adverse effect of rhabdomyolysis. She should report any vision changes. The nurse should also emphasize to not abruptly stop taking atorvastatin because of a serious rebound effect that could lead to a heart attack.

CHAPTER 42: GASTROINTESTINAL TRACT DISORDERS

1. f
2. d
3. e
4. b
5. g
6. c
7. a
8. chemoreceptor trigger zone (CTZ); medulla
9. antihistamines, bismuth subsalicylate, phosphorated carbohydrate
10. anticholinergics
11. glaucoma
12. dopamine antagonists
13. nausea, vomiting; serotonin or 5HT$_3$
14. cannabinoid
15. Laxatives; cathartics
16. sodium; magnesium
17. deficit; electrolyte
18. antihistamines, anticholinergics, dopamine antagonists, benzodiazepines, serotonin antagonists, glucocorticoids, cannabinoids, miscellaneous

19. fecal impaction, chronic laxative use, neurologic disorders, bowel obstruction, immobility, delayed defecation, insufficient fluid intake, poor dietary habits, certain drugs such as opioids and anticholinergics

20. Mix psyllium in 8–10 oz of water, stir, and drink immediately, followed by another glass of water.

21. False. Prescription or nonprescription antiemetics *are not safe* for pregnant women to take. Antiemetics are not recommended for pregnant women to consume because of the risk to the fetus. Instead nonpharmacologic treatment should be tried, such as flat soda or weak tea and crackers.

22. False. A person *can have one or more* per day to be "normal." A "normal" bowel movement varies from one person to another. A "normal" number of bowel movements can range from one per day to three per week.

23. True. Chronic use of laxatives can cause a person to become dependent on the laxative for a bowel movement, especially in older adults.

24. False. Even though castor oil is a natural substance, it is *still not safe* for woman in early pregnancy to use for occasional constipation because it can stimulate uterine contractions.

25. a, b, c, e. All but the opioids can be used as antiemetics. Opioids can cause constipation that can decrease intestinal motility, thereby decreasing peristalsis; opioids can be used as antidiarrheals.

26. b. Promethazine is a phenothiazine that blocks H_1-receptor sites on effector cells, impedes histamine-mediated responses, and inhibits the CTZ.

27. a, b, c, d. Drinking weak tea and sodas that have gone flat may help with nausea. Open a can or bottle of soda and let it sit for several hours to remove its carbonation. Unsweetened gelatin may also be helpful. Crackers and dry toast may provide substance in the stomach. Relaxed breathing may help with the feeling of nausea, but it is usually more beneficial to breathe in through the nose and out through the mouth as is used in relaxation techniques.

28. a. When poison is ingested, vomiting should not be induced because regurgitating these substances can cause esophageal injury. Instead, activated charcoal is administered to absorb the poison.

29. a, b, e. Diphenoxylate with atropine is an antidiarrheal. Usual side effects are caused by atropine, an anticholinergic; these include headache, drowsiness, and urinary retention. It also causes hypotension (not hypertension), nausea, and vomiting. It does not cause hypoglycemia.

30. b, d, e. Laxatives and/or cathartics include bulk-forming, emollients, and stimulants. Adsorbents are considered antidiarrheal, and emetics are used to induce vomiting.

31. a. Bisacodyl is a stimulant laxative used for bowel preparation and for prevention and short-term treatment of constipation. Its action increases peristalsis by directly affecting the smooth muscle of the intestine.

32. b. Mineral oil absorbs the fat-soluble vitamins so the body cannot absorb them. This can lead to vitamin deficiency.

33. d. Clients with any kind of bowel obstruction or severe abdominal pain should not take laxatives.

34. a, c, d, e. Promethazine is an antihistamine given for nausea and/or vomiting. Antihistamines inhibit histamine-mediated responses and have anticholinergic side effects, which include blurred vision, drowsiness, dry mouth, and hypotension.

35. c, d. A client with diarrhea should avoid "heavy" fried foods and milk products. Promoting fluid intake and replacing electrolytes are priority interventions when the client is experiencing diarrhea.

Case Study

1. Constipation has a variety of causes, including decreased fluid intake, poor diet, lack of exercise, and current drugs. Lack of appetite is a frequent complaint among the older adult. Poor dentition may lead to inability to eat raw fruits and vegetables. The opioid L.B. is taking for postoperative hip pain, as well as the potential for decreased mobility and lack of exercise, may also lead to constipation.

2. Bisacodyl is a stimulant laxative that promotes defecation by irritating the smooth muscle of the intestine.

3. Omeprazole and other proton pump inhibitors will decrease the effect of bisacodyl, so dosage adjustments may need to be made. Calcium supplements can decrease the dissolving of bisacodyl. There are no serious interactions with either digoxin or hydrocodone.

4. It will be important for the nurse to encourage L.B. to eat well and exercise as much as possible. Including bran and whole grain in the diet may be beneficial. Bulk-forming laxatives can provide the fiber that L.B. may not be getting in a regular diet. When possible, the client should discontinue use of the opioid pain reliever. The nurse should also advise L.B. that the drug should be taken whole, with a glass of water. Milk should be avoided around the time of administration, because milk also reduces the effectiveness of the laxative. L.B. should be instructed on the side effects of bisacodyl, such as abdominal cramps.

CHAPTER 43: ANTIULCER DRUGS

1. g
2. a, h
3. e
4. b
5. f
6. c

7. i
8. a
9. e
10. d
11. c
12. d
13. a
14. d
15. c
16. e
17. b
18. d
19. b
20. b. Antacids neutralize hydrochloric acid and should be taken 1–3 hours after meals and at bedtime. Chewable and liquid antacids should be followed by 2-4 ounces of water to ensure the drugs reach the stomach. They should not be taken with meals because of the delayed gastric emptying time, which can increase acid production. Some antacids can cause acid rebound (increased acid production). Antacids should not be taken with other oral drugs concomitantly due to multiple drug-drug interactions.
21. b, c, d, f. Antiulcer drugs include anticholinergics, antacids, H_2 blockers/antagonists, and PPIs. Other antiulcer drugs include tranquilizers, pepsin inhibitors, and prostaglandin E_1 analogues.
22. c, e. Commonly used drugs to treat GERD include H_2 blockers/antagonists and PPIs. Anticholinergics and pepsin inhibitors are commonly used to treat ulcers. Antacids are used to decrease acid production, which can prevent ulcers.
23. d. Propantheline is an anticholinergic that inhibits gastric secretions and is used to treat peptic ulcers. Anticholinergics should be taken before meals to decrease acid secretion and at bedtime. It should not be used as a monotherapy.
24. a, b, c. Nizatidine should not be taken with meals, because it will delay absorption. The abdominal pain should have improved within 1–2 weeks, depending on the cause. Healing of the ulcer may take 4–8 weeks.
25. a, b, d, e. Side effects of ranitidine and other H_2 blockers/antagonists include confusion, headache, erectile dysfunction, and nausea. Other side effects include dizziness, constipation, abdominal pain, diarrhea, vomiting, blurred vision, malaise, and weakness.
26. a, b, c. There are no documented interactions between esomeprazole and either lisinopril or propranolol. Esomeprazole interferes with the absorption of ampicillin, digoxin, and ketoconazole.
27. c. Hyperglycemia is an adverse reaction to sucralfate. Although the normal range for blood glucose may vary, a blood glucose level of 185 mg/dL is considered elevated. Another adverse reaction includes hypophosphatemia. Hgb, serum potassium, and INR are all normal.

Case Study

1. There are seven groups of antiulcer drugs: tranquilizers, anticholinergics, histamine$_2$ blockers/antagonists, proton pump inhibitors, pepsin inhibitors, prostaglandin E_1 analogues, and antacids.
2. Aluminum hydroxide is a nonsystemic antacid composed of alkaline salts and aluminum. Antacids, as their name implies, neutralize acids that destroy the gastric mucosal barrier. They may be taken alone or in combination with other medications for ulcers.
3. The usual dose for aluminum hydroxide is 10 mL, 1 to 3 hours after meals and at bedtime, however the dosage is variable and may be more depending on the reason for taking antacids.
4. The priority teaching right now for this client is about the proper dose. The client should be advised to drink 2–4 ounces of water with the aluminum hydroxide and to decrease or eliminate consumption of alcohol and caffeinated beverages. Aluminum hydroxide should not be taken with milk or foods high in vitamin D because of the risk for hypophosphatemia and hypercalcemia. S.S. should also avoid spicy or high-fat foods and caffeinated beverages, which can further irritate the gastric mucosa. There are many predisposing factors for ulcers, including environmental factors such as a high-stress job. Learning to utilize relaxation techniques and decrease stress may help the client's discomfort. The client should also be advised of the potential side effects, including anorexia and constipation.

CHAPTER 44: EYE AND EAR DISORDERS

1. locally
2. artificial eyes
3. NSAIDs; corticosteroids
4. tear
5. intraocular; trabecular
6. angle-closure glaucoma (closed-angle glaucoma)
7. diuretics; glaucoma
8. cycloplegics
9. increase
10. conjunctivitis
11. carbonic anhydrase inhibitors
12. parasympathomimetic
13. h
14. f
15. i
16. a
17. b
18. d
19. c
20. j
21. g
22. e
23. c. Mydriatics dilate pupils for better visualization during a diagnostic procedure. Carbonic anhydrase

inhibitors decrease intraocular pressure by decreasing the production of aqueous humor. Cerumenolytics softens and breaks up the cerumen in the external ear canal.

24. c. Acetazolamide is a systemic carbonic anhydrase inhibitor used to decrease IOP. Acetazolamide is also a diuretic and can cause fluid and electrolyte imbalances.

25. b. Carbamide peroxide is an OTC drug that helps break up cerumen so it can be washed away. Bimatoprost is a prostaglandin inhibitor to treat open-angle glaucoma to decrease IOP. Echothiophate is a cholinergic agonist used to treat open-angle glaucoma. Proparacaine is a topical anesthetic instilled in the eyes to conduct a comprehensive examination.

26. a, c, d, e. Pilocarpine is a cholinergic agonist with minimal systemic effects, but they can occur. The side effects are similar to that of cholinesterase inhibitors, which include blurred vision, eye pain, and headache. Cardiac dysrhythmias and respiratory depression are adverse reactions and are deemed an emergency.

27. e. There are two types of age-related macular degeneration, wet and dry. Dry AMD is more common, with vision being gradually lost. There is no known treatment or drug for dry AMD. Treatment for wet AMD targets vascular endothelial growth factor (VEGF).

28. a, b, c, d. Tetracaine is a topical anesthetic. The other medications listed are decongestants to help with the eye irritation attributable to allergies. Ophthalmic allergy drugs contain antihistamines and/or mast cell stabilizers.

29. b. A cotton wick is placed inside the external auditory canal (EAC) for medication to reach the length of the EAC. When the swelling subsides, the wick will fall out or it can be manually removed.

Case Study

1. Open-angle glaucoma occurs when there is too much aqueous humor that causes pressure and damages the optic nerve, which leads to decreased vision. As aqueous humor is formed, excess fluid drains through the trabecular meshwork structure of the eye. In open-angle glaucoma, the trabecular network is clogged, and the excess fluid cannot drain. Open-angle glaucoma occurs gradually, and the cause is unknown.

2. There are several different classes of medications that are used to treat glaucoma. Timolol is a nonselective beta-adrenergic blocker. Beta blockers are usually the first-line drugs in glaucoma treatment. Beta blockers work by decreasing the production of aqueous humor.

3. The client should wash hands before administration of the drug and be very careful not to touch the tip of the bottle to the eye. The head should be tipped back, and one drop instilled in the conjunctival sac of the lower lid. The client should not rub the eyes after the drug is instilled. A tissue can be used to dab at the extra drug. Eyedrops should be instilled before any eye ointment.

4. No. This dose is too high. The standard dose is 1 gtt of 0.25–0.5% solution bid initially; then it can be decreased to 1 gtt/day as the condition stabilizes. The client must be carefully observed for bradycardia, bronchospasm, and indications of developing or worsening heart failure, since this drug may cause systemic effects.

CHAPTER 45: DERMATOLOGIC DISORDERS

1. c
2. d
3. b
4. a
5. f, h
6. h
7. b, c, d, e
8. a
9. b, c, d
10. athlete's foot, ringworm
11. Comedones; whiteheads; blackheads
12. teratogen; iPLEDGE
13. multisystem; skin; joints
14. rebound
15. T-cell
16. desquamation
17. thinning; atrophy
18. a, c, d. Acne vulgaris is a common skin disorder treated nonpharmacologically or with pharmacotherapy. Drugs used to treat acne include antibiotics, corticosteroids, and keratolytics. Antifungals can be used for skin disorders caused by tineas. Nonsteroidal antiinflammatories are not effective for skin inflammation. A T-cell antagonist, such as methotrexate, is a folate antimetabolite for systemic treatment of psoriasis.

19. a. Calcipotriene is a synthetic vitamin D analogue that enhances keratinocyte differentiation while inhibiting their proliferation. There is no cure for psoriasis, but there are periods of remissions and exacerbations.

20. b. Infliximab is a biologic response modifier; specifically, it inhibits tumor necrosis factor and is given in a controlled environment via IV injection at prescribed intervals.

21. b, c, e. Contact dermatitis, a common form of eczema, can cause local manifestations, such as rash, swelling, and stinging at the affected skin site. Common skin irritants include cosmetics, dyes, and plants. Anesthetics and peanuts can also cause an allergic response, but usually the manifestations are systemic, such as anaphylaxis.

22. a. The standard initial dose for tetracycline is 125–250 mg q6h for 1–2 weeks; then the dose can be decreased to 125–500 mg daily or every other day.

23. a, b, d. The client should be encouraged to report to the health care provider if she is pregnant or plans on becoming pregnant because tetracycline has possible teratogenic effects. Harsh cleansers may be irritating to skin that may already be sensitive. Tetracycline taken in combination with isotretinoin will increase the potential for adverse effects. Sunscreens with SPF15 and higher are recommended for all adults. Also, tetracycline can cause tooth discoloration to developing teeth.

24. c. Hair loss or alopecia can be treated with minoxidil solution to stimulate hair growth. Acitretin and methotrexate are for psoriasis. Tretinoin can be used for acne and warts.

25. a, b, c. Contact dermatitis attributable to skin irritants can be treated with antiinflammatories or topical corticosteroids, such as triamcinolone and dexamethasone, and/or antihistamines, such as diphenhydramine. Fluconazole is an antifungal. Salicylic acid is used to treat acne, psoriasis, or verruca vulgaris.

Case Study

1. Full-thickness burns extend down and include the epidermis, the dermis, and the subcutaneous tissue. They have also been referred to as *third-degree burns*. Full-thickness burns may appear red, black, or white and are not painful because the nerve endings have been destroyed. Partial-thickness burns do not extend as deep; there may be blistering. Partial-thickness burns are very painful. Frequently partial-thickness (second-degree) burns surround a full-thickness burn.

2. Mafenide acetate is a broad-spectrum antibiotic that is applied topically (1.6 mm thick once or twice daily) to the burned area. Mafenide is a sulfonamide derivative, and it interferes with bacterial cell-wall synthesis and metabolism.

3. Another treatment option is silver sulfadiazine. It is also applied topically to the burned surface. Silver sulfadiazine acts on the cell membrane and cell wall. It is less likely to cause metabolic acidosis than mafenide.

4. Priority nursing interventions for this client are adequate fluid resuscitation, pain control, and prevention of infection by providing sterile dressing changes. It will be easier for this client to receive skin grafting when appropriate with minimal to no infections.

CHAPTER 46: PITUITARY, THYROID, PARATHYROID, AND ADRENAL DISORDERS

1. f
2. h
3. i
4. a
5. m
6. b
7. l
8. n
9. c
10. g
11. d
12. j
13. k
14. e
15. Addison Disease: Adrenal hyposecretion (hypocortisolism): anemia, hyponatremia, hyperkalemia, hypoglycemia, weight loss, fatigue, hypotension, tachycardia, diarrhea, hyperpigmentation. Cushing Syndrome: Adrenal hypersecretion (hypercortisolism): weight gain, hyperglycemia, buffalo hump, edema, delayed wound healing, hyperlipidemia, peptic ulcers, hirsutism, hypertension, hypernatremia, hypokalemia.
16. a
17. d
18. e
19. g
20. c
21. b
22. f
23. c. The normal dose is 25–50 mcg/day initially, with a maintenance dose of 50–200 mcg/day.
24. d. Manifestations from hypothyroidism are usually alleviated within 2 to 4 weeks without having symptoms of adverse reactions. Activity level is usually improved within 4 weeks of thyroid treatment.
25. a, c, d. Symptoms of hyperthyroidism include palpitations, excessive perspiration, and tachycardia. Constipation is a symptom of hypothyroidism, not hyperthyroidism.
26. a. Levothyroxine should be taken on an empty stomach at least 30 to 60 min before breakfast.
27. a, e. Over-the-counter drugs are generally contraindicated in clients with hypothyroidism. Clients with thyroid disorders should be encouraged to wear a medical alert identification. Drugs for hypothyroidism should be taken on an empty stomach. Numbness and tingling of the hands occurs with hypoparathyroidism, not hypothyroidism. Hypothyroidism causes weight gain; it is not a priority to teach clients to increase food and fluid intake.
28. d. Prednisone is a glucocorticoid steroid. Long-term use can cause sodium and fluid retention.
29. b. Prednisone is a corticosteroid and should be taken with food to prevent irritation of gastric mucosa.
30. b, c, d, e. Concurrent use with NSAIDs including aspirin can increase the risk of GI bleed; phenytoin can decrease the effect of glucocorticoids; digitalis toxicity can occur and may cause dysrhythmias; and diuretics can increase potassium loss, increasing the risk of hypokalemia.
31. c, d, e. Obtaining a drug history is important before starting a client on prednisone, because there are

many drug interactions possible with glucocorticoids. Vital signs and daily weights should be monitored. Hypernatremia, not hyponatremia, can occur with prednison. Weight gain is a side effect of prednisone.

32. b. Glucocorticoids can lead to fluid retention. Adequate fluid intake should be ensured but not forced.

33. b. Corticosteroids can decrease serum potassium and cause hypokalemia. Herbal laxatives or diuretics taken concurrently with corticosteroids can worsen hypokalemia.

34. b. Corticosteroids increase metabolism and can cause insomnia; these effects can worsen when taken with herbal stimulants, such as ginseng.

35. a, b, e. Levothyroxine has many drug-drug interactions. Levothyroxine can increase the effects of an anticoagulant, such as warfarin. Levothyroxine can decrease the effects of digoxin and oral antidiabetic drugs. There are no strong interactions with diuretics and NSAIDs.

Case Study

1. Signs and symptoms of adrenal insufficiency include muscle wasting, apathy, nausea, vomiting, electrolyte imbalances, hypovolemia, anemia, and cardiovascular collapse.

2. Hydrocortisone 20–240 mg/d in 2–4 divided doses can be given orally. Hydrocortisone, depending on its formulation, can be administered IV, IM, or subcut; the dose and frequency may be different.

3. Priority teaching for this client is to recognize and report symptoms of Cushing syndrome, which includes puffy eyelids, edematous feet, increased bruising, dizziness, and bleeding. Also, the client should be advised against abruptly stopping the drug for adrenal insufficiency. Laboratory values will be monitored closely to watch for hypoglycemia, anemia, and electrolyte imbalances. The client should be encouraged to carry a medical alert identification and a current list of drugs. Herbal preparations should be avoided unless discussed with the health care provider. Teach client to weigh daily.

CHAPTER 47: ANTIDIABETICS

1. d
2. f
3. h
4. c
5. g
6. e
7. a
8. b
9. 120 days; 3
10. obesity, stress, insulin resistance
11. abdomen
12. gastrointestinal secretions
13. lipodystrophy; rotating
14. insulin resistance; allergy
15. c
16. a
17. f
18. b
19. e
20. d
21. regular
22. Somogyi effect
23. Hyperglycemia; dawn
24. hypoglycemia
25. biguanide; glucose; absorption; receptor; peripheral
26. 48 hours; lactic acidosis
27. type 2
28. a, b, e. Three major symptoms of diabetes are characterized by the three *p*'s that include polydipsia (increased thirst), polyphagia (increased hunger), and polyuria (increased urination).
29. a, b, d. Certain drugs increase serum glucose level (hyperglycemia), including cortisone, hydrochlorothiazide, and epinephrine. Doxepin is a tricyclic antidepressant that can lower blood glucose level. Thiazolidinediones are a class of oral antidiabetic drugs that lower blood glucose level.
30. b, c, d, e. The client experiencing hypoglycemia can have headache, sweating, nervousness, and tremor. Abdominal pain and vomiting can occur because of a reaction to oral antidiabetic drugs.
31. b, c, d, e, f. Signs and symptoms of ketoacidosis include dry mucous membrane, fruity breath odor, Kussmaul respirations, polyuria, and thirst. The client can also develop tachycardia, not bradycardia.
32. d. Tolazamide is a first-generation intermediate-acting oral antidiabetic drug. Oral drugs in this class should not be used by clients with type 1 diabetes; instead, insulin is used.
33. a, b, c, d. Oral antidiabetic medications should be taken on a regular, prescribed basis and not adjusted by glucose testing results.
34. a. Unopened insulin vials should be kept in the refrigerator, and an opened vial can be kept in the refrigerator or kept at room temperature. They should not be stored in the freezer, exposed to direct sunlight, or left in a high-temperature area.
35. c. Cloudy insulin is mixed by rolling the vial. Shaking the vial can cause bubbles, which can lead to an inaccurate dose.
36. a, c, e. The client needs to develop a rotation pattern to prevent lipodystrophy and promote insulin absorption. Insulin is not administered IM. The ADA's suggested actions do not include injection into a different area of the body every day.
37. a. Regular insulin is short-acting, with an onset of 30 minutes to 1 hour.
38. b, d, e. Insulin glargine is a long-acting insulin that is evenly distributed over a 24-hour duration of action and is usually administered in the evening

(bedtime). It is available in a prefilled cartridge, and some clients have complained of pain at the injection site. Hypoglycemia can still occur, but it is not as common as with other insulins. Some clients may need coverage with rapid-acting or short-acting insulins.

39. c. Insulin pumps are used for type 1 diabetics and they reduce the number of hypoglycemic reactions. An insulin pump is not used with intermediate insulin, such as NPH, because of unpredictable glucose control. Insulin pumps use a needle to insert a cannula under the skin; the needle does not stay inserted.

40. a. Depending on the class of oral antidiabetic drugs, they can increase the insulin cell receptor sensitivity, increase insulin release from the pancreas, decrease hepatic production of glucose, decrease glucose absorption from the small intestine, and/or increase peripheral glucose uptake at the cellular level. It does not increase the number of insulin-producing cells, nor does it replace receptor sites or insulin.

41. b. Nonsulfonylureas include biguanides and alpha-glucosidase inhibitors that decrease glucose production by the liver. They can cause hypoglycemic reactions. Biguanides decrease, not increase, the absorption of glucose from the small intestine. Nonsulfonylureas are oral antidiabetic drugs that decrease serum glucose level, not increase it.

42. b. Ginseng and garlic can lower blood glucose level; garlic may increase insulin level. Concomitant use of these complementary and alternative drugs may necessitate a change in the insulin or oral antidiabetic drug dose.

43. b, c, d, e. Aspirin, oral anticoagulants, and cimetidine can increase the action of sulfonylureas, especially with the first-generations, by binding to plasma proteins and displacing sulfonylureas. The action of sulfonylureas may be decreased by taking several different types of medications, including anticonvulsants such as phenytoin.

Case Study

1. Although there are a variety of causes for these symptoms, when a diabetic client presents with a headache, confusion, slurred speech, and a glucometer reading of "low," a hypoglycemic reaction should be suspected. Readings may vary depending on brand of glucometer, therefore, a reading of "low" may be in the 20 mg/dL range. This is an emergency and must be treated quickly.

2. As long as the client is conscious, hard candy, sugar-sweetened fluids, or glucose paste may be given. Other options include fruit juice or peanut butter crackers.

3. Once the client becomes unconscious, other options must be explored. The client may receive glucagon to stimulate glycogenolysis. A benefit of giving glucagon is that it may be administered IM,

IV, or subcut. The blood glucose level begins to increase within 10 minutes after administration.

CHAPTER 48: URINARY DISORDERS

1. b
2. e
3. d
4. f
5. e
6. d
7. c
8. a
9. e
10.

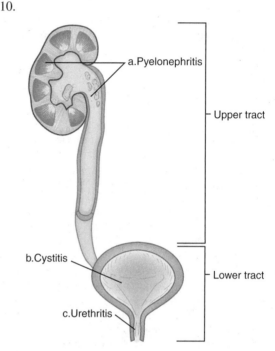

11. c. When methenamine is given with sulfonamide, crystals in the urine can form. Methenamine can cause hematuria, even when used alone. Chest pain and intestinal distention are not known to occur when given with sulfonamide.

12. b. Cranberry juice can help lower the pH and make the urine more acidic. Whole milk may make urine more alkaline and increase the pH. Although increased fluid intake is important when a client has a urinary tract infection (UTI), simply increasing the amount of water alone will not decrease the urine pH. Prune juice will make the urine acidic, not alkalotic.

13. b. Flavoxate is an antispasmodic that has a direct action on the smooth muscles and is contraindicated in clients with glaucoma. Antispasmodic has the same effects as anticholinergics.

14. c, d, e. Ertapenem, an antiseptic, has side effects that include diarrhea, headache, and nausea. Other side effects include drowsiness, confusion, agitation, and elevated hepatic enzymes.

15. a, c, d. Urinary antiseptics can inhibit and/or prevent bacterial growth in the kidneys and bladder but are not effective for systemic infections. Antacids decrease absorption of other oral drugs when taken together.

16. d. Tingling or numbness of extremities could be a sign of neuropathy, which can be irreversible and needs to be evaluated immediately. Brown- or rust-colored urine and diarrhea can be side effects of nitrofurantoin, but they do not need to be immediately reported to the provider. Frequency in urination is common with UTIs.

17. a, b, e. Urinary analgesics, such as phenazopyridine, are used to relieve symptoms associated with cystitis (pain, burning, frequency, and urgency).

18. c. Phenazopyridine is a urinary analgesic. Bethanechol is a urinary stimulant, flavoxate is an antispasmodic, and trimethoprim is an antiinfective.

19. d. Bright reddish-orange urine is to be expected when taking phenazopyridine. This can be very startling to the client if not told in advance to anticipate the change. Undergarments can also be stained orange while taking this drug.

20. b. Oxybutynin is an antispasmodic that is prescribed for urinary tract spasms. Phenazopyridine is a urinary analgesic, not an antispasmodic, Bethanechol is a urinary stimulant. Trimethoprim is an antiinfective.

21. a, c, d, e. Bethanechol is a urinary stimulant and would not benefit this client who has overactive bladder. Nitrofurantoin is an antiinfective and, unless this client has a UTI, there is no need for it. Oxybutynin and tolterodine tartrate, although beneficial to clients with overactive bladder, are contraindicated in clients with glaucoma. Dimethyl sulfoxide (DMSO) is a urinary analgesic that is used to treat urinary frequency and urgency.

22. b. Bethanechol chloride is a urinary stimulant that increases bladder tone. It is prescribed when bladder function is lost because of spinal cord injuries, such as with paralysis.

Case Study

1. Oxybutynin chloride is a urinary antispasmodic that has direct action on the smooth muscles of the urinary tract. By relaxing these muscles, the spasms are decreased.

2. Clients who have urinary or GI obstruction as well as those with narrow-angle glaucoma should not take oxybutynin. Oxybutynin blocks acetylcholine receptors that mediate parasympathetic function. Should the client experience severe abdominal pain, constipation, or urinary retention, the health care provider should be contacted immediately.

3. Common side effects include dry mouth, drowsiness, blurred vision, headache, insomnia, tachycardia, GI distress, and constipation. The client should be encouraged not to participate in any activities where dizziness could be an issue (climbing, skateboarding, etc.). The client should be warned not to drive or operate heavy machinery until he knows how the drug will affect him. If any of these symptoms are severe, his health care provider should be contacted.

4. No, the dosage range is 5 mg bid/qid, with a maximum of 20 mg/day.

CHAPTER 49: PREGNANCY AND PRETERM LABOR

1. g
2. f
3. j
4. i
5. a
6. b
7. d
8. e
9. h
10. c

11. c, d, e. Maternal physiologic changes seen during pregnancy affecting drug actions include increased maternal circulating volume, resulting in dilution of drugs; increased glomerular filtration rate and rapid elimination of drugs; and increased liver metabolism. Other changes are reduced GI motility and increased gastric pH, making the environment more alkaline; and the clearance of drugs is altered during late pregnancy, resulting in decreased serum concentration.

12. a. Drugs crossing the placenta is analogous to drugs infiltrating breast tissue. Lactation causes increased blood flow to the breast and drugs accumulate in the adipose tissue through simple diffusion.

13. a, b, d. Timing, dose, and duration of drug exposure are crucial in determining the drug's teratogenicity. The teratogenic period begins 2 weeks after conception and exposure to teratogens can result in birth defects and/or death of the fetus.

14. b. Corticosteroids, such as betamethasone, accelerate lung maturity and surfactant development in the fetus in utero, thereby decreasing the incidence and severity of respiratory distress.

15. b, d, e. Gestational hypertension can have devastating maternal and fetal effects. Gestational hypertension can progress to preeclampsia and/or eclampsia, increasing the risk of HELLP syndrome and seizures. The goals for clients who develop gestational hypertension include prevention of HELLP syndrome, delivery of an uncompromised fetus, reduction of vasospasms, and prevention of seizures.

16. a, c, d. GI complaints, such as heartburn, nausea, and vomiting, are the most common during pregnancy, possibly resulting from elevated levels of progesterone, which causes decreased gut motility and relaxation of the cardiac sphincter.

17. c. In maternal iron deficiency anemia, iron supplements will show a modest reticulocyte count increase in 5 to 10 days; a rise in the hemoglobin level will be seen in 2-4 weeks.

18. a, c, d, e. Nausea and vomiting or "morning sickness" are frequent complaints during early pregnancy. To decrease nausea and vomiting, clients should avoid fatty or spicy foods; eat high-protein snack. Also, eating crackers, dry toast, or other carbohydrates before rising can also decrease frequency and severity of nausea. Fluids taken between meals rather than during meal can also help. Fluids should not necessarily be avoided before arising. Sometimes small sips of flat soda or apple juice may be beneficial.

19. b, c, e. Iron supplements should be taken 2 hours before or 4 hours after antacids so the medication can be absorbed. Although best taken on an empty stomach, iron can be taken with food if necessary. Jaundice should be reported immediately to the health care provider. Vitamin C found in orange juice can enhance iron absorption.

20. a. Foods that are rich in iron include broccoli, red meat, nuts, spinach, and iron-fortified cereal.

21. b. The recommended dosage of folic acid is 400 mcg-800 mcg. If planning pregnancy, folic acid should be started one month before and for the first 2-3 months after conception. The American Congress of Obstetricians and Gynecologists recommend that all women of childbearing age take 400 mcg of folic acid and 600 mcg during pregnancy.

22. a. Acetaminophen is the most commonly OTC drug for pain relief during pregnancy. It is safe to use during all trimesters of pregnancy. Aspirin and ibuprofen use during pregnancy is contraindicated. Diphenhydramine is an antihistamine.

23. a. Beta-sympathomimetic drugs, such as terbutaline, stimulates beta-2 receptors on uterine smooth muscle to decrease the frequency and severity of uterine contractions. Terbutaline has significant adverse effects. Pulmonary edema and cardiac arrhythmias can occur. Breath sounds should be auscultated at least every 4 hours and assessed for the presence of wheezes, crackles, or coughing.

24. b, d, e. The loading dose of magnesium sulfate 4-6 g is given over 20–30 minutes as an IVPB. It is administered via a pump. Too-rapid administration of magnesium sulfate can lead to cardiac arrest. Clients receiving magnesium sulfate are on bed rest while receiving therapy and should be monitored continuously. Calcium gluconate is the antidote for magnesium sulfate toxicity and should be at the bedside for emergency. Decreased or loss of DTRs is an adverse reaction to magnesium sulfate.

25. a, b, c. NSAIDs, such as aspirin and ibuprofen, can cause maternal anemia and greater blood loss at delivery, and the overall homeostasis of the fetus can be compromised. Additionally, ibuprofen, when taken late in pregnancy, can prematurely close the ductus arteriosus.

26. a, b, d. Side effects and adverse reactions are generally dose related and include flushing, nausea, and slurred speech. Other side effects include feelings of increased warmth, perspiration, nasal congestion, lethargy, decreased gut motility, tachycardia, and hypotension.

Case Study

1. Some priority questions to ask include if K.R. has been receiving regular prenatal care and the date of her last visit. The nurse should inquire if there are any known complications with this pregnancy such as gestational diabetes, gestational hypertension, or hyperemesis gravidarum. K.R. should also be questioned regarding membrane rupture and for any bleeding or changes in fetal movement. Other questions should include substance use, including herbals, caffeine, and tobacco use.

2. K.R. is at high risk because of her age, history of miscarriage, and previous PTL.

3. Nonpharmacologic measures that the nurse can suggest while K.R. is waiting to hear back from the health care provider include lying down on her left side, or if that is not possible, at recline and put her feet up. Dehydration may lead to PTL, so K.R. should maintain hydration. Having an empty bladder may also help, so the client should be advised to void. If nonpharmacologic measures are not effective, the client may require tocolytics. There are no FDA-approved drugs for PTL. But, beta sympathomimetics (terbutaline), magnesium sulfate, or prostaglandin inhibitors are used "off label" to halt or delay labor. One of the major goals in tocolytic therapy is to interrupt or inhibit uterine contractions to create additional time for fetal maturation in utero.

4. Although the survival rate of a fetus at 33 weeks is fairly high, the baby is preterm and will require close observation. The mother may be given corticosteroids, such as betamethasone or dexamethasone, to accelerate fetal lung maturity and development of surfactant to decrease the incidence of respiratory distress syndrome in preterm infants.

CHAPTER 50: LABOR, DELIVERY, AND POSTPARTUM

1. a. spinal block; b. epidural block
2. b
3. d
4. e
5. a
6. c
7. b
8. d
9. a

10. c
11. latent; active; transition
12. neonatal
13. mu; kappa
14. should not
15. saddle block
16. oxytocin; also ergot alkaloids, prostaglandins
17. decreases
18. $Rh_0(D)$ immune globulin
19. d. Postdural headaches are caused by leakage of cerebrospinal fluid through a puncture site. The decrease in pressure exerted by the CSF causes the headache.
20. a, b, c, d. Postdural headaches can occur with regional anesthesia, such as epidural or spinal anesthesia. Client should be advised that bed rest, oral analgesics, and/or caffeine can help relieve the headache. At times, an autologous blood patch may be needed.
21. d. Opioids can cause maternal or neonate respiratory depression. A reversal agent, naloxone, is given.
22. a. Before administering general anesthesia, antacids or other drugs that decrease gastric secretions are given to decrease gastric acidity. They may also prevent nausea and vomiting, but these are not the primary reasons for their administration just before general anesthesia.
23. d. Clients with hypotension are positioned on their left side to facilitate placental perfusion. Isotonic fluids will need to be rapidly infused, and ephedrine or phenylephrine may need to be administered. Oxygen may be needed but it is not the first thing the nurse would do.
24. c. Bishop score is an objective measurement to determine the readiness for labor induction. The elements assessed by the Bishop score are dilation, effacement, station, cervical consistency, and cervical position. Scores of 8 or greater are associated with a successful labor induction.
25. d. Ergot alkaloids should not be used during labor. Instead, it is used after delivery to sustain uterine contrations to prevent or control postpartum hemorrhage and to promote uterine involution. The fourth stage of labor is the "early postpartum" that consists of the first 4 hours after the delivery of the placenta.
26. a. Clients with hypertension should not receive methylergonovine. When this drug is given IV, dramatic increases in blood pressure can occur.
27. a, c. During assistance in all types of regional/local anesthesia, the nurse would continuously monitor the client. If the anesthetic is injected into a vessel, the client may experience dizziness and metallic taste in the mouth. Other indications of vascular access is ringing in the ears or numbness. Hypotension, not hypertension, can occur with local anesthesia. If hypotension, the client should be placed on her left side to increase placental blood flow.

28. b, c, d, e. Deep tendon reflexes are usually assessed on a client receiving magnesium sulfate, not oxytocin. A type and crossmatch should be obtained in the event that the client will need an emergent cesarean section. The fetus may become hypoxic, and there is an increased risk for uterine rupture. If uterine rupture is suspected, assess for FHR deceleration, sudden increased pain, loss of uterine contractions, and hemorrhage.
29. c, d. Somatic pain occurs during the transition phase and the second stage of labor. Pain is caused by the stretching of the perineum and vagina.
30. b, c, e. Anesthesia for cesarean delivery may be general, spinal, or epidural. General anesthesia allows for rapid anesthesia induction and control of the airway.
31. a, d. Topical agents used for pain relief for perineal wounds include benzocaine and witch hazel.
32. b. Use of heat lamp after applying benzocaine topical spray to relief perineal pain is not recommended. Heat lamp can cause tissue burn.
33. b. $Rh_0(D)$ immune globulin is given when there is a maternal/fetal blood mixing of incompatible blood. The Ig should be given at 28 weeks gestation and within 72 hours of giving birth. It is not given at 38 weeks gestation or before amniocentesis. It can be given after amniocentesis.

Case Study

1. Inductions are based on several factors, including intrauterine growth retardation. At 38 weeks' gestation, K.E. is considered full-term. There are several options to induce labor. Before delivery, the cervix must efface, or thin, and dilate. A mechanical device such as a urinary catheter can be placed through the cervical os, and then 30 mL of sterile saline instilled into the balloon. This will act similarly to manual stripping of the membranes to start labor. Another method is to place prostaglandin E_2 (PGE_2) either intracervically or intravaginally. It is usually left in place for approximately 12 hours and then synthetic oxytocin is started intravenously to augment labor. Once the cervix has dilated to approximately 5 cm, an amniotomy ("breaking the bag") may be performed under sterile conditions. Labor will tend to get into an established pattern within a few hours of the amniotic sac being broken.
2. Priority teaching for this client includes advising her to communicate her needs and desires to the health care team regarding analgesia and delivery. Ideally a "birth plan" will have been developed by the client and her partner in advance. This plan is usually submitted to the health care provider and is brought with the client to the hospital. As much as is possible and safe, the client should be able to control her delivery.
3. Analgesia may be provided by intravenous narcotic agonists, mixed agonist-antagonists, and regional anesthesia (epidurals, blocks). The client should also have the option of refraining from the use of analgesics if she desires ("natural childbirth").

CHAPTER 51: NEONATAL AND NEWBORN

1. Respiratory distress syndrome; surfactant
2. endotracheal
3. Hyperoxia; hypocarbia
4. newborn
5. ophthalmia neonatorum
6. d. Surfactant replacement, such as beractant, is given to premature newborns with immature lung development.
7. c. Exogenous surfactant must be warmed before administration by warming it in the hands for 8 minutes or at room temperature for 20 minutes. The vial should not be shaken.
8. b, d, e. Exogenous surfactants are administered to newborn with premature lung development and treatment of respiratory distress syndrome. Drugs of this class include beractant, poractant alfa, and calfactant.
9. a, b, d. Complications during and following administration of surfactant can cause bradycardia and hyperoxia. Desaturation can also occur because transient esophageal reflux can obstruct the ET tube. Cyanosis, not pallor, is another complication.
10. b. Generally, complications such as cyanosis and hypoxia after surfactant administration do not lead to severe complications when properly managed. The nurse should assist in repositioning the neonate to disperse the drug throughout the lung. Suctioning is appropriate if an obvious sign of airway obstruction is noted.
11. d. HBIG should be given to the newborn if the mother is hepatitis B positive. The first of three series doses of recombinant hepatitis B should be given as a separate injection at a separate site. The HBIG provides passive protection while the newborn's body develops acquired immunity to the recombinant hepatitis B vaccine.
12. b. Erythromycin is an antiinfective administered to a newborn's eyes within the first hours of birth to prevent blindness. Blindness in newborns can occur because of vaginal infections, such as chlamydia and gonorrhea.

Case Study

1. Hepatitis B virus transmission occurs vertically at the time of delivery when the neonate is exposed to the mother's blood and body fluids.
2. The nurse should acknowledge J.G.'s concerns and inform her that her baby will receive medications to decrease the risk of developing hepatitis B.
3. The nurse would anticipate administering hepatitis B immune globulin (HBIG) and the first dose of recombinant hepatitis B. HBIG should be administered within 12 hours of birth. HBIG provides immediate passive protection against liver damage. Recombinant hepatitis B stimulates the body to produce antibodies against hepatitis B viruses.

4. Recombinant hepatitis B vaccine is given in three series. The first one is given within 12 hours after birth. Subsequent doses are given at 1 month and again at 6 months of age.

CHAPTER 52: WOMEN'S REPRODUCTIVE HEALTH

1. b
2. e
3. d
4. c
5. a
6. menarche; menopause
7. estrogen
8. spironolactone; diuretic
9. 48
10. anovulation; amenorrhea
11. hypoestrogenic
12. b
13. d
14. c
15. a
16. e
17. c. A woman with breast cancer should not take oral contraceptives because the hormones could accelerate tumor growth. Other contraindications include history of endometrial cancer, history of thromboembolic disorders, liver disease, coronary artery disease, undiagnosed vaginal bleeding, and endometriosis. A person who is not sexually active may not need oral contraceptives, however, it is not contraindicated.
18. a, b, c. There are no contraindications for using combined hormone contraceptives (CHCs) in epilepsy, but other medications that the client takes must be evaluated. There is no contraindication for a client with depression taking CHCs. The 45-year-old client is, in all likelihood, perimenopausal, so there may not be a need for CHCs, but they are not absolutely contraindicated. A person who smokes or has diabetes requires extra caution because of the risk for thromboembolism.
19. c. If only one dose has been missed, the client should take the dose as soon as possible and then resume the regular schedule with the next dose.
20. a, b, c, d, e. Common side effects with conjugated estrogen include acne, breast tenderness, leg cramps, fluid retention, and nausea. Other common side effects are vomiting, breakthrough bleeding, and chloasma.
21. a, d, e. Aspirin toxicity can occur, increasing the anticoagulant effects. Barbiturates such as phenobarbital and topiramate, which can be used either for seizures or for migraines, are contraindicated in clients taking oral contraceptives. All women of child-bearing age should take supplemental folic acid.
22. c. Potassium levels should be monitored closely. Drospirenone causes the body to retain potassium.

Hyperkalemia is possible, especially in clients with undiagnosed kidney disease.

23. c. Ethinyl estradiol and etonogestrel transvaginal ring is inserted vaginally and left in place continuously for 3 consecutive weeks, then removed and wait 1 week before inserting a new one. If the ring has been out less than 3 hours, it can be rinsed with lukewarm water and reinserted. If the ring has been out for more than 3 hours, it should be reinserted and use an alternative form of contraception until the ring has been in place for 7 days.

24. b. As part of the ACHES mnemonic [*A*bdominal pain (severe), *C*hest pain or shortness of breath, *H*eadache (severe), *E*ye disorders, *S*evere leg pain], severe headaches could be indicative of cardiovascular side effects and should be reported to the health care provider immediately.

25. c. Progestin hormone therapy decreases the risk of ovarian and cervical cancers but

Case Study

1. With these presenting symptoms and at her age, the client is likely menopausal. Dyspareunia, frequency, urgency, thinning vaginal epithelium, and decreased elasticity on speculum exam are due to estrogen deficit. Frequency and urgency can also be associated with a urinary tract infection (UTI), so a urinalysis should be obtained; however, a UTI would not account for the findings on speculum exam. By definition, a lack of menstruation for 1 year is defined as menopause. Other symptoms associated with menopause may include hot flashes and night sweats.

2. Treatment may be symptomatic and include taking cool baths, using a fan, and sleeping in light clothing. Another option is hormone therapy (HT). HT should be administered at the lowest doses and for the shortest amount of time possible. HT improves vasomotor symptoms such as hot flashes, and it also improves vaginal dryness and irritation. It does, however, come with increased risks of cardiovascular events such as DVT, stroke, and MI, and certain cancers (breast, ovarian, and lung). The health care provider should discuss the risk-to-benefit ratio with the client to help her decide the best option.

3. HT also decreases the risk of osteoporosis. C.W. is thin and Caucasian, which are two risk factors for osteoporosis. Using HT, increasing vitamin D and calcium intake, and exercising (such as walking) may help prevent bone loss. The use of medications for osteoporosis includes bisphosphonates and SERMs. These medications help prevent the breakdown of bone.

CHAPTER 53: MEN'S REPRODUCTIVE HEALTH

1. g
2. h
3. j
4. f

5. e
6. i
7. b
8. c
9. a
10. d
11. d. Sildenafil is indicated for erectile dysfunction. Its action is enhancing blood flow to the penis to facilitate an erection. Sildenafil is contraindicated in clients with significant cardiac disease or persons with anatomic deformities or conditions that predispose them to priapism. Sildenafil is also contraindicated in persons who are on nitrates. Age is not a contraindication.

12. d. Androgens (i.e., testosterone) are male sex hormones to control the development and maintenance of sexual processes, accessory sexual organs (i.e., hypogonadism), cellular metabolism, and bone/muscle growth.

13. c. The use of hormones to "bulk up" or improve performance occurs at all levels of sports competition. Side/adverse effects from the use of excessive intake of anabolic steroids include increased low-density lipoprotein cholesterol, decreased high-density lipoprotein cholesterol, acne, high blood pressure, liver damage, and dangerous changes in the left ventricle of the heart. Adverse effects may not be recognized until years later.

14. a. Blood glucose levels may be decreased in clients with diabetes when taking androgens. The client should be instructed to carefully monitor blood glucose levels for changes so the insulin dose can be adjusted.

15. a, c. Androgens can be used to treat advanced breast cancer and endometriosis in women. Other uses include management of severe menopausal symptoms in women, refractory anemia in both genders, and tissue wasting associated with severe illness.

16. a, b, d. Males on androgens can experience frequent, and often time painful, continuous erection called priapism. They can also experience gynecomastia and sperm counts can decrease or even stop. Other side and/or adverse effects include abdominal pain, nausea, insomnia, diarrhea, or constipation. Androgens can cause hypercalcemia which can cause frequent urination.

17. a, c, e. Androgen antagonist blocks the synthesis or action of androgens and are indicated for benign prostatic hypertrophy (BPH), advanced prostate cancer, and endometriosis. Androgen antagonists are also used to treat male-pattern baldness, acne, hirsutism, virilization syndrome in women, and precocious puberty in boys.

Case Study

1. Erectile dysfunction can occur in men at any stage of life. It occurs due to lack of sufficient blood flow to the penis. It may be seen in men with diabetes. Some of the drugs used to treat hypertension, such

as diuretics and beta blockers, may also cause erectile dysfunction.
2. One class of drugs that the client may be referring to is the phosphodiesterase (PDE-5) inhibitors, which includes sildenafil, tadalafil, and vardenafil. They work by increasing blood flow to the penis so the client can maintain an erection.
3. Side effects may include upset stomach, blurred vision, flushing, and headache. The most serious side effect is a sustained erection (priapism) that lasts longer than 4 hours. Priapism is an emergency because a thrombosis may form in the corpora cavernosa, which can lead to permanent loss of function.
4. The nurse should teach the client not to use any herbal preparations without discussing their side effects with his health care provider. The client should also be advised to not use any nitroglycerin or nitrate-containing drugs while taking PDE-5 inhibitors because the combination can cause marked hypotension. PDE-5 inhibitors should also not be taken with grapefruit or grapefruit juice because it increases the amount of PDE-5 available. Side effects, such as headache and vision changes should be taught to the client.

CHAPTER 54: SEXUALLY TRANSMITTED INFECTIONS

1. c
2. e
3. b
4. f
5. a
6. d
7. b
8. d
9. f
10. c
11. a
12. d or e
13. True
14. False. Washing bed linens of a client diagnosed with scabies *is* necessary. All bedding and clothing should be decontaminated and anyone in close contact with an infected person should also be examined and treated if necessary.
15. False. Nitroimidazoles and alcohol *are* contraindicated. Like metronidazole, drinking alcohol concomitantly can cause a disulfiram-like reaction.
16. False. Pediculosis pubis is treated with topical *permethrin 1% cream rinse.* Alternatively, malathion lotion can be applied. Both will need to be rinsed off after certain period of time has lapsed. An oral drug, ivermectin can be taken to treat pediculosis pubis.
17. c. Clients with gonorrhea should also be tested for HIV, *Chlamydia*, and syphilis.

18. a. Abstaining from sexual activity is the safest practice to prevent any further transmission; however, if that is not an option, all partners should wear a condom during sex. Partners do not need to take antibiotics; however, all partners should be tested.
19. d. If the client wants to participate in sexual activity, using a condom is the safest, even if gonorrhea was treated. However, if abstaining or using a condom is not possible, then the client should wait at least 7 days after treatment to resume in sexual activities.
20. a. Gonorrhea and syphilis are two different types of sexually transmitted infections. If a client is diagnosed with one sexually transmitted infection, then the client should be tested for the other, including HIV and *Chlamydia.*
21. a, b, c, d. HIV is a virus that is spread through sexual contact and blood and body fluids. Blood and body fluids include breast milk, blood, vaginal secretions. There are no indications that HIV is transmitted through mosquitoes.

Case Study

1. The presumptive diagnosis is gonorrhea involving both her genitourinary and oral mucous membranes caused by *Neisseria gonorrhea.* Oral infections caused by *N. gonorrhea* cause pharyngitis and dysphagia. She may also have a fever, and if left untreated her infection can cause tubal scarring.
2. Dual drug therapy is recommended with ceftriaxone 250 mg IM *plus* azithromycin 1 g PO, both as a single dose. Dual therapy improves treatment efficacy and decreases the development of drug resistance.
3. K.E. should be informed that she is at risk for other infections, such as chlamydia, HPV, and HIV, and that she should be further tested. She should abstain from sexual activities until therapy is completed and her partners should be treated. If she cannot abstain from intercourse, then instruct her to use condoms. Review with the client how STIs are transmitted and how they could be avoided.

CHAPTER 55: ADULT AND PEDIATRIC EMERGENCY DRUGS

1. h
2. g
3. k
4. e
5. i
6. a
7. f
8. b
9. d
10. c

11. j
12. f
13. d
14. a
15. d
16. b
17. c
18. e
19. g
20. a. Nitroglycerin is a vasodilator and can cause a rapid drop in blood pressure, especially in first-time users. Tachycardia or bradycardia can also occur, but it is not as common as hypotension.
21. a. Morphine can cause respiratory depression so the client's respiratory status must be monitored closely. Naloxone can be used to reverse respiratory depression if needed.
22. d. Myocardial ischemia can occur when a client is receiving dobutamine. The nurse must monitor carefully for signs of myocardial ischemia, including chest pain and dysrhythmias. Dobutamine can cause tachycardia, not bradycardia.
23. b. Procainamide is an antiarrhythmic for ventricular dysrhythmias that are unresponsive to adenosine. Procainamide is discontinued if hypotension develops. Other end points to procainamide include ECG changes (i.e., widening of the QRS complex by 50% or more), when the maximum dose has been given (17 mg/kg), or when the dysrhythmia is successfully treated.
24. b, e. Amiodarone is appropriate to treat ventricular tachyarrhythmia, such as ventricular fibrillation and atrial fibrillation that is not controlled by other measures. The dose to administer is dependent on the presence or absence of a pulse. Amiodarone is not given in clients with bradycardia or atrioventricular blocks, such as second-degree block.
25. a. Sodium bicarbonate is indicated to treat severe metabolic acidosis as well as hyperkalemia related to specific drug overdose situations. It is not a first-line drug to treat cardiac arrest.
26. c. Intracranial pressure can increase following head trauma or malignancy. Mannitol is an osmotic diuretic used to treat increased intracranial pressure by causing fluid to shift from the brain tissue back into the vasculature. Strict fluid intake and output must closely be monitored due to possible significant fluid loss.
27. c. This client is exhibiting signs of an allergic reaction. Besides receiving epinephrine, the client will receive diphenhydramine. Diphenhydramine reduces histamine-induced swelling and itching that occur in allergic reactions.
28. c. Naloxone is an opiate antagonist and naloxone 0.4 mg IVP is within the dose range to be administered. If this is an opioid overdose, the drug should reverse fairly rapidly, and the client will become responsive. If this is not an opioid overdose, there will be no response. Benzodiazepines, such as di-

azepam, are also used for back spasms, but they do not produce pinpoint pupils. Flumazenil is the reversal agent for benzodiazepines.
29. a, d, e. Dopamine is a vasopressor and may be used to treat hypotension in cardiogenic, neurogenic, and septic shock after adequate fluid and/or blood product resuscitation. However norepinephrine may be preferred in neurogenic shock. Hypovolemic shock should be treated with fluids, either crystalloids or blood. *Insulin shock* is actually misnamed and refers to a hypoglycemic reaction. It should be treated with glucose, not vasopressors.
30. a. Dobutamine is a sympathomimetic drug with beta-adrenergic activities. It is used in shock states. Blood pressure is elevated only through the increase in cardiac output.
31. b. Norepinephrine is a catecholamine that acts on the alpha-adrenergic receptors and has potent vasoconstrictor actions, and as with other adrenergic agonists, abrupt discontinuation can cause a profound drop in the blood pressure.
32. d. D_{50} is used to treat severe hypoglycemia, most commonly attributable to insulin shock. Increased urine output and hyperglycemia can occur because of D_{50}. D_{50} is highly irritating to the vein and should be administered through a large peripheral or central vein.
33. c. Adenosine is a first-line drug for supraventricular tachycardia. It has a very short half-life of less than 5 seconds. Adenosine 6 mg is given IV push over 1-3 seconds followed by 20 mL of saline. If a second dose is needed, a 12-mg bolus is given 1 to 2 minutes after the initial dose.
34. a. Once the dysrhythmia has been suppressed, if a total of 3 mg/kg has not been exceeded, a maintenance drip of lidocaine at a rate of 1–4 mg/min is started.
35. b. The correct solution to utilize for IM injection is 1:1000 solution.
36. a. The standard concentration of 1:10,000 epinephrine is used in cardiac arrest.
37. a. Usual dosage for atropine in adults is 0.5 mg and may be repeated q3-5 min. Anything less than 0.5 mg can produce a paradoxical bradycardia.
38. b. Diazepam is a benzodiazepine. Flumazenil is a reversal drug for benzodiazepines. Naloxone is a reversal drug for opioids.
39. c, d, e. Magnesium sulfate is an essential element needed by the body for multiple functions. The primary indications for emergent magnesium include refractory ventricular fibrillation, cardiac arrest associated with hypomagnesemia, and torsades de pointes. It is not indicated for atrial dysrhythmias or for hypokalemia.
40. d. Furosemide is a loop diuretic that inhibits reabsorption and promotes renal excretion of water, sodium, potassium, magnesium, calcium, and hydrogen. It also promotes vasodilation and diuresis, which can lower blood pressure.

41. b, d, e. Nitroprusside sodium is a drug used to reduce arterial blood pressure in hypertensive emergencies. Blue or brown color indicates the solution has degraded and should not be used. The bottle should be protected from light. Because this drug is a potent antihypertensive, the client will need to be monitored continuously in the critical care unit. As nitroprusside breaks down, the byproducts include thiocyanate or cyanide; therefore, levels must be monitored closely, and the drug should be used for the shortest amount of time necessary. Nitroprusside should be tapered, not discontinued abruptly.

42. a, c, d. Atropine is an anticholinergic and can cause dry mouth, mydriasis (not miosis), and urinary retention. It can also cause myocardial ischemia, restlessness, anxiety, and thirst.

Case Study

1. M.E. self-administered three nitroglycerin (NTG) tablets before calling EMS. NTG dilates the coronary arteries to improve blood flow and oxygenation to the ischemic myocardium. IV NTG infusion is reserved for chest pain related to unstable angina or acute myocardial infarction. BP and HR must be continuously monitored because hypotension is a common adverse effect.

2. An aspirin is given to clients having chest pain to decrease platelet aggregation in acute coronary syndrome and for acute myocardial infarction. Oxygen is given to provide adequate supply to the myocardium. It can be administered either by nasal cannula, nonrebreather mask, simple mask, or endotracheal intubation to maintain the oxygen saturation at >94%. This client does not, at this point, require endotracheal intubation. Morphine is used to relieve pain, dilate venous vessels, and reduce the workload of the heart. IV nitroglycerin is reserved for clients with unstable angina or an AMI. A nitroglycerin drip is usually initiated at a rate of 5 mcg/min and increased by 5 mcg/min every 3–5 minutes, based on chest pain and blood pressure response.

3. The nurse would prepare to administer epinephrine 1 mg IV q3-5 minutes while continuing CPR and shocking any shockable rhythm. If the client continues in ventricular tachycardia, then amiodarone 300 mg IV can be given and may be repeated once at a dose of 150 mg. The client should be evaluated periodically for a pulse and/or change in rhythm.